T0186310

A NEW BEGINNING IN SIGHT

A NEW BEGINNING IN SIGHT

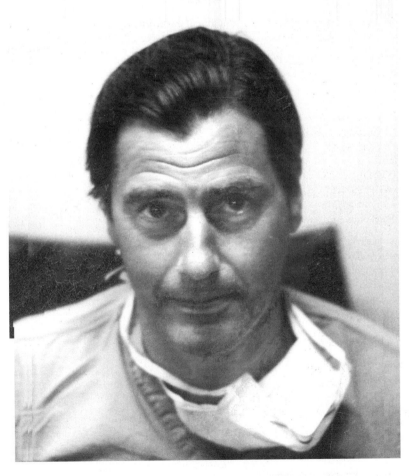

Eric J Arnott

Published by the Royal Society of Medicine Press Ltd
1 Wimpole Street, London W1G 0AE, UK
Tel: +44 (0)20 7290 2921
Fax: +44 (0)20 7290 2929
E-mail: publishing@rsm.ac.uk
Website: www.rsmpress.co.uk

British Library Cataloguing in Publication Data
A catalogue record for this book is available from the British Library

ISBN 1-85315-730-9

Distribution in Europe and Rest of World:
Marston Book Services Ltd
PO Box 269
Abingdon
Oxon OX14 4YN, UK
Tel: +44 (0)1235 465500
Fax: +44 (0)1235 465555
Email: direct.order@marston.co.uk

Distribution in the USA and Canada:
Royal Society of Medicine Press Ltd
c/o BookMasters, Inc.
30 Amberwood Parkway
Ashland, Ohio 44805, USA
Tel: +1 800 247 6553/ +1 800 266 5564
Fax: +1 419 281 6883
Email: order@bookmasters.com

Distribution in Australia and New Zealand:
Elsevier Australia
30-52 Smidmore Street
Marrikville NSW 2204, Australia
Tel: +61 2 9349 5811
Fax: +61 2 9349 5911
Email: service@elsevier.com.au

Typeset by SR Nova Pvt. Ltd., India

Printed and bound by Replika Press Pvt. Ltd., India

This book is dedicated to my wife Veronica.

CONTENTS

ACKNOWLEDGEMENTS

This book is dedicated to my darling wife Veronica, with whom I shared so many happy years raising our family and practising ophthalmology. Her memory has been a constant source of inspiration to me. She was my soulmate and my life. She accompanied me on every step of my journey, becoming a forceful generator of ideas and organizer of events in the ophthalmic world. I would not have been able to achieve anything I did or survive in today's world of hospital bureaucracy without her.

The greatest thanks go to my son Stephen, who helped me write this book and without whose constant help, support and advice this project would never have been completed. My thanks also go to my other children, Tania and Robert, who were always available to listen and make suggestions.

I am most grateful to Sir Ranulph Fiennes for kindly agreeing to write the foreword. I am most grateful also to Herve Byron, Howard Fine, Tom Stuttaford, Patrick Condon and Bob Sinskey for the trouble they took in reading the book and relating their comments.

Throughout the writing of *A new beginning in sight*, I sought the help of many others – to all of whom I am most grateful. These include: Joy Andrews, my private practice manager, who tactfully helped in the description of the many patients mentioned in the script; Professor Charles Kelman, with his wife Ann and his manageress Diane Spiro, who advised me on parts of the book dealing with the US; Bradley Geist, our American attorney, who edited the section on the American trial; Nils Burwitz, a celebrated artist, who conceived the idea for the book cover; Michael Gallagher and Julie Rampton of the Cromwell Hospital and David Karcher and Manus Kraff of the American Society of Cataract and Refractive Surgery, all of whom have supported me in promoting this book as a tribute to the leaders and pioneers of modern ophthalmic surgery; David King of the Carlin Company, who has been so instrumental in helping to record the activities of the innovators in our profession. Many thanks also to Yvonne Light, who stepped in to do a masterful edit, and to the Royal Society of Medicine Press for their sponsorship.

I'm grateful to many friends and colleagues who read each section as it was completed. These include Veronica's relatives Hester and Susan Cattley and Natalie Dipple. My own cousin, Guy Arnott, living in far off Australia, was able to give a very impartial criticism of my work. My ophthalmic colleagues Richard Packard, Paddy Condon, John Grindle, Mike Sanders and Professor Upadhyay regularly reviewed the script. Also called upon were the services of our friends Marcella, Lady Dashwood, Anthony Spooner and Peter and Nicola Davies.

Finally, I would like to pay particular tribute to all the friends, relations, medical colleagues and patients who form the basis of these memoirs and together embody all our endeavours.

FOREWORD

It gives me great pleasure to write an introduction to this exciting book. While the author and I forged very different lives and careers, we have, over the decades, shared many situations.

The book starts with his early upbringing and medical studies. During his time at Trinity College, Dublin, he stayed in the same remarkable house as my mother Audrey and sister Celia, who was a fellow medical student. When learning ophthalmology at Moorfields Eye Hospital, London, he spent many weekends with my family in Lodsworth, where he witnessed my first calls to explore the unknown.

We were both blessed in having adoring wives who settled into our lifestyles and did much to enhance their qualities. My wife Ginny supported me on my polar trips and was responsible for organizing the Transglobe Expedition. In a very different clime, Veronica was with Eric and joined him on his travels, which focused on India and America but encompassed all five continents. As described in the book, her experiences imbued in her a need to spend many hours each day raising money for ophthalmic charities. She managed (among many other causes) their son's bicycle ride around the world, the Great London Treasure Hunt and, finally, the Mobile Eye Surgery Unit – built for the eye camps of India.

Eric's memoirs contain anecdotes about many patients, from all walks of life, who were treated in his practice. He describes one of my own visits to his rooms shortly after my return from the Antarctic with Michael Stroud, still sporting the polar beard and cross-eyed from having walked for weeks in the featureless land of the Antarctic. To make my appearance even more bizarre, I was suffering from severe frostbite and both my feet were covered in sacking.

Just as I have attempted to follow in the footsteps of my peers – Scott, Shackleton and Amundsen – so did Eric. He was associated with and knew well Svyatoslav Fyodorov of Moscow, who developed refractive surgery, Harold Ridley of London, who invented the plastic lens implant, and Charlie Kelman of New York, who developed small-incision cataract surgery. All of these innovators are fully described, as are the handful of pioneers who, with the author, followed their lead and helped to develop these procedures.

My ultimate link with Eric was witnessing the result of the transforming surgery he performed on my mother, who was suffering from a cataract.

Sir Ranulph Fiennes Bt., MBE

PREFACE

My adult life started the day my mother died, on 19 January 1948. She had been diagnosed with terminal cancer 14 months earlier, as a result of which my call up for RAF officer training at Cranwell College was deferred on compassionate grounds. During the ensuing period, at the tender age of 17, I nursed my mother, looked after my frail father and ran our home in Swanage. No doubt my nursing abilities were inadequate and my cooking diabolical. Nevertheless we managed.

One night in January, I went into mother's bedroom. The scene was very peaceful: the rays of a full moon were shining into the room and mother, lying in her bed untouched, seemed to be merely sleeping. I had spent the previous months living in the shadow of a progressively relentless disease, feeling a mixture of hopelessness, frustration, sorrow, compassion and love. In the serene tranquillity of the surroundings, I made a dedication to practise medicine and attempt to live my life through Christianity.

On 3 July 2001, my existence turned a full circle with the departure of my adored wife, Veronica, with an illness not dissimilar to my mother's. It is said: 'One must look back with gratitude, forward with hope and upwards with faith' ... but it's not always that easy!

Between 1960 and 2001, I shared with Veronica 41 years of idyllic married bliss. We led an exceptional life in ophthalmology, devoting much of it to working together on advances in ophthalmic surgery with a handful of colleagues from around the world. Over this time, the cataract operation was developed from a crude procedure to a technique that today has the ability to instantly restore normal vision with no convalescence.

After my retirement in 1999, Veronica and I found a small house on the south-westerly tip of Cornwall, at Porthleven in Mounts Bay, which has panoramic views over the Atlantic Ocean. It had been our intention to write our memoirs in this Haven of Peace. We had wanted to relate how, working with these pioneers, ophthalmic innovations had been developed that have so markedly improved the quality of life for many millions of patients. This I have tried to do, with the help of Veronica's spiritual presence.

The brain, the heart and the eye are arguably the three most important organs of the body. The brain is the centre for the spirit, the soul, learning and the body's intellect. The heart is responsible for the circulation of our blood and epitomizes life's very function. Yet the eye must surely be the most beautiful and intricate part of our whole system. An organ that receives sight, it plays other roles beyond relaying vision to the brain. Enveloped as they are by the lids, the eyes can express sensuality, love and understanding. They reflect an individual's feelings and emotions.

The eye may be compared in its structure to a camera. A camera is essentially a box with a glass window through which light enters. A biconvex lens focuses these rays of light onto a film and a diaphragmatic shutter opens and closes to take the picture. The eye is very similar. The anterior surface consists of a clear cornea, comparable to the glass face of a watch. Some 3.5 mm behind the cornea is the coloured iris, the most delicate structure in the whole body. In the middle of the iris lies the pupil, essentially a black empty hole that dilates in the dark and constricts with stimulation by light. Immediately behind the pupil is the lens, which, with the cornea, focuses the object onto the retina. From the retina, the visual image is sent up to the brain for interpretation.

Although any part of the eye may become diseased, more than 75% of ocular surgery is related to the lens. The cornea and the lens are the only two translucent parts of the body, and this translucence needs to be maintained by active metabolism. Any breakdown of this metabolism in the lens will lead to its opacification. There are many causes for this, the most common being the ageing process. The only treatment for this condition, known as a cataract, is the removal of the lens from the visual pathway.

The best way to remove the cataractous lens has wracked the brains of the most eminent ophthalmic surgeons for thousands of years. The very first recorded reference to cataract surgery appears in a Sanskrit manuscript dating from the second century BC. This depicts, in picture form, a Hindu surgeon named Susruta, the father of Indian surgery, performing a cataract operation, watched by his pupils. Susruta simply passed a sharp probe into the eye and couched the lens into the inert cavity of the posterior compartment of the eye. The obstacle preventing the passage of light to the retina was thus removed. Although this created a marked improvement for the previously blind patient, the patient would only have been able to appreciate the vague form of surrounding objects, as the eye had lost the focusing mechanism of the lens.

It is possible that the 'miracles' in the Bible, which relate to Christ's healing of the blind, are associated with the dislocation of the cataractous lens into the posterior cavity. This is illustrated by the tale of the blind man in Bethsaida, in the Gospel of St Mark.

They came to Bethsaida, and some people brought a blind man and begged Jesus to touch him. He took the blind man by the hand and led him outside the village. When he had spat on the man's eyes and put his hands on him, Jesus asked, 'Do you see anything?' He looked up and said, 'I see people; they look like trees walking around.' Once more Jesus put his hands on the man's eyes. Then his eyes were opened, his sight was restored, and he saw everything clearly.

Again, in St Mark, it is quoted:

As Jesus and his disciple were leaving Jericho, a blind man, Bartimaeus was sitting by the roadside begging. When he heard that it was Jesus of Nazareth, he began to shout: 'Jesus, Son of David, have mercy on me!'

'What do you want me to do for you?' asked Jesus. The blind man said, 'Rabbi, I want to receive my sight.'

'Go,' said Jesus, 'Your faith has made you whole.' Immediately he had his sight restored.

It is possible that the blind cured by Christ's miracles were suffering from cataracts. The 'laying on of hands' could have dislocated the opaque lens, giving the same result as that achieved by couching. Of some interest is the fact that couching or dislocating the lens deprives the eye of more than 50% of its focusing power, as the lens is no longer in place and functioning. With Christ's healing in Bethsaida, the formerly blind man initially said: 'I see people; they look like trees walking around.' When Jesus again touched his eyes, his vision was totally returned. Had Jesus miraculously restored his lens? Of note also is the fact that the man must have been born with vision, as he knew what trees looked like.

For thousands of years, the only treatment for dealing with the cataract was couching or dislocation of the lens. Some ophthalmic surgeons made their fortunes from this technique, most notably Chevalier Taylor. With a retinue of more than 30 'assistants,' he travelled extensively throughout Europe, and after each operation his retinue would yell 'another miracle!' He and his team would then leave before their patients had the time to develop postoperative infections. Despite these poor results, Chevalier Taylor had a vast following and operated on popes, princes and many distinguished people of the day, including JS Bach, Fredrich Handel and Gibbon, the author of *The decline and fall of the Roman empire*.

In 1748, Jacques Davial, a French ophthalmic surgeon, was the first to manually remove the lens from the eye. During an operation, while trying to push the opaque lens into the back of the eye, it started to break up. Davial made a much larger opening into the eye and removed the fragments of the disintegrating lens. Thus, after many thousands of years, the operation known as 'extracapsular cataract extraction' had been introduced. This was more sophisticated than the couching procedure, entailing the need for many more instruments, and took longer to perform. It must have caused terrible pain to the poor patient, as even cocaine anaesthesia was not available at the time. Patients were merely sedated, with the liberal use of brandy or whisky, and then held down.

The operation, while an improvement on couching, was relatively crude and could be used only on patients with an advanced or mature cataract. As stitches had yet to be developed, patients were required to keep the operated eye closed for many days until the wound had fully healed. For his great contribution to surgery, Davial was recognized by being depicted on a French postage stamp.

Von Graeffe, an eminent German surgeon in the nineteenth century, considered that a simpler form of cataract surgery would be to remove the lens in one piece instead of breaking it up before its removal. As in Davial's operation, a large incision was made into the eye. It was through this incision that forceps were introduced, so that, like a terrier shaking a rat in its teeth, the intact lens was gripped and dislocated from its retaining zonule, before being wrestled through the pupil and out of the eye. The 'intracapsular cataract extraction' joined the 'extracapsular cataract extraction' as a recognized procedure for the removal of cataracts in the mid 1880s.

Until the mid 1950s, these three forms of cataract extraction were all that was available. Although general anaesthesia was now obtainable to relieve the pain of the procedure, postoperative convalescence remained traumatic. Patients had both eyes double-padded and closed for 24 hours, during which time they had to stay totally still. Some surgeons even requested that the patient's hands be tied to the frame of the bed to prevent rubbing of the eye. Patients remained bedridden for some 10 days. Six months of convalescence was required before the patient could return to normal activities. Having suffered this quite harrowing ordeal, only limited vision was restored, and the patient had to wear thick 'pebble lenses' or contact lenses to regain any semblance of precise vision. The 'aphakic spectacles' created a Galilean telescopic effect and caused enormous distortion to the patients' perception of depth and peripheral vision. For example, when going through a doorway, the sides of the door would seem to close in. Nonetheless, this form of limited vision was preferable to the alternative state of blindness.

Part One. Creatures of Circumstance

CHAPTER 1
Origins

My great grandfather John Arnott left his native Scotland to seek a new career in the 'Emerald Isle' in the early nineteenth century. By all accounts he was a remarkable man who possessed the Midas touch. He amassed a huge business empire that included a chain of Arnotts department stores throughout Ireland and Scotland, steamship companies, railways, breweries, the Cork Park Racecourse and two newspapers – the *Irish Times* and the *Northern Gazette*.

Throughout his long life, his principal endeavour was to help the poor in his adopted country. During the Great Hunger of the mid 1800s, he became the Westminster Member of Parliament for Kinsale, County Cork. He was instrumental in championing 'The Irish Poor Law Relief Bill,' which helped to reduce the rate of child mortality. Under this reform, orphans from the Union Homes in cities such as Cork, Limerick and Galway were sent onto farms around the country to replace the young farmers who had died in the typhus epidemic or had emigrated to America. Vast depopulated areas of the country were restored by this influx of young city children, who, in many cases, were welcomed as a part of the family.

In an effort to reduce the cost of a loaf of bread, he built mills in Limerick, Cork and Dublin to demonstrate that it was possible to produce a poor man's loaf for a quarter of the normal price. These bakeries supplied a considerable part of Southern Ireland and were later given to those who had helped to build and run them.

In 1859, he was made Lord Mayor of Cork and was later knighted by the Lord Lieutenant, the Earl of Carlisle, on the occasion of the laying of the foundation stone of St Patrick's Bridge. This bridge joined the two sides of the city, which were divided by the River Lee. Sir John was created a baronet in 1897, an honour he enjoyed for only a few months, as he died in March 1898. The Bishop of Cork was at the funeral service, and an old friend, the Reverend CB Harley, gave the address:

'A merchant prince has fallen, one who was loved of the poor as a helper of all who were in need. He was a philanthropist from first to last. What strange decision marked his life, what wondrous evidence of will, what promptness of action? After a fire had destroyed his store, Arnotts in Dublin, he stood by the smouldering ruin and said: "We must see that the men suffer not; employment must be provided immediately for them."

'For years he allowed me to lift the veil and see the principles which had actuated his life, principles which he never spoke of in any public way. These were based on his love of the Bible and Jesus Christ. He told me that far back, he had learned to love that wonderful epistle of St James, because it showed him the duty of faith with good works. He loved best of all to visit the fatherless and the widows in their affliction. He did good even to those he thought had wronged him. At one time I saw him distribute a sum of £1000 to the poor and it was then that I recognized in him a thoughtful benefactor, an intellectual giant, a noble faithful and true-hearted man.

'In his attempt to establish a home for the consumptives in Youghal, he showed the same compassion. So much of his charitable commitment was done without any publicity and remained unknown to the general public. There was hardly a clergyman in Cork, no matter what denomination, who had not from time to time sought help from him for some troubled member of his flock. Help was always forthcoming.

'I was sitting by his bedside in the company of all his family at his death when he said: 'Take care of the orphans and widows, whatever you do.' I, his poor servant, was favoured by administering the Sacrament of the Lord's Last Supper. With psalm, hymn, peacefulness and surrounded by his loving family, he passed into everlasting life.'

The second Sir John Arnott, my grandfather, shared his father's concern for the poor and was particularly worried about how the inhabitants of the slums could thrive, either morally or physically, amid squalid surroundings and on a starvation diet. He set up dining halls in Dublin and Cork, where the working classes could have well-cooked meals at a nominal price. He enjoyed the unstinting support of his wife, who was extremely active in several charities, most particularly as Secretary of the Soldier's and Sailor's Help Society. Here, disabled servicemen were taught new trades such as making baskets, toys, tables and mats. During the First World War, she was made a Dame of the British Empire for her unstinting work for the Red Cross. For many years, the second Sir John was chairman of the *Irish Times*. Under his control, the paper flourished and became the most influential paper in the country without being provocative about religious and political differences. He was a military man who rose to become Honorary Lieutenant-Colonel of the 4th Battalion Cheshire Regiment, and those who served under him were always willing to acknowledge his commanding abilities. After the Boer War, he organized the *Irish Times* Widows and Orphans War Fund, by which he relieved 265 widows and 410 orphans out of the raised sum of £1500.

At the turn of the century, the Cork Park Racecourse was sold to the Ford Motor Company, as it was considered that an assembly plant in Cork would generate employment for thousands of workers. To make up for this loss, my grandfather, together with Major E Loder and two others, established the Phoenix Park Racecourse in Dublin, modelled on three British racecourses: Sandown, Hurst Park and Kempton Park.

King Edward VII and Queen Alexandria attended the opening meeting in August 1902. This was one of the last times a British monarch visited

Southern Ireland before the Easter Risings of 1916 that eventually led to Irish Independence.

Grandfather had seven children, three daughters and four sons. One daughter, Vickey, married the Lord De Freyne – hence our association with Frenchpark, home for most of our young lives. Mary married Count Van Cutsen, one of the Pope's standard bearers. Grandfather's eldest son, Johnny, had a noble but short life. After Eton, he joined the 15th King's Hussars and spent most of the next four years in the trenches of France. In 1918, he was killed in action and for his heroism was awarded the Military Cross. Unbeknown to the rest of the family, he had an Irish actress girlfriend who he had been unable to marry because of the problems of those war years but who bore him a son, John, in 1912. Grandmother, Caroline Arnott, educated him at Downside and he became Head of School and was an outstanding athlete. Trapped in Italy at the start of the Second World War, his only avenue of escape was to Hungary, where he spent the next few years under first German and then Russian occupation. He married a Hungarian lady, and their one son, Patrick, after many decades is now reunited with his family in England.

The youngest of Grandfather's children, Tommy, had the identical up-bringing as his eldest brother but, being younger, was able to enjoy, with his wife Lettice, the years between the world wars in the regiment, enjoying the pleasures of peacetime. He had a passion for horses and became an expert polo player, who on the field was known as the 'galloping major'. In 1939, the 15th King's Hussars were mechanized with armoured cars and lost their horses. Uncle Tom, keen to continue his army career working with horses, transferred to the 'Mules', a poor substitute for the horses of the Household Cavalry Regiment. Tommy served with distinction during the war, using the mules, in the allied advance up Italy, to carry supplies along mountainous terrain unsuitable for vehicles. On one occasion, he rescued his sergeant, who had been blown up in a minefield. Major Arnott carefully picked his way through the minefield to the wounded soldier and carried him out of danger on his shoulder. For this act of gallantry, he was awarded the American Silver Star. The army was very much in the blood of Tommy Arnott's family. Both his sons, Peter and Guy, joined the regiment. Guy, after serving in Malaya, went to Australia, where he built up a successful chain of stores.

After my grandfather's death in 1942, the second son, Lauriston, became head of the family. He had joined the army after leaving Wellington College and was twice severely wounded in the trenches during the Great World War. Like his father, he spent many years as chairman of both the *Irish Times* and the Phoenix Park Racecourse. He was also was very active in the Soldier's and Sailor's Help Society, which by this time had been renamed 'The Lord Robert's Work Shop.' He lived on the Hill of Howth in Shearwater. This was a part-wooden house with an uninterrupted panoramic view of heathland sweeping down to Dublin Bay and the Dublin Mountains in the distance. He remained a lifelong bachelor, and the love of his life was his dog Jester.

Grandfather's third son, my father Robert, born in 1896, was educated at Eton, which he did not enjoy. Like so many of his generation, he became embroiled in the horrors of the Great War. He served in the Dardanelles and witnessed action in Gallipoli. He was not injured but suffered from 'black jaundice' and returned to England on a hospital ship. While still semi-conscious, he overheard a doctor say: 'That young officer will not be with us for much longer.' These few words galvanized him into making a recovery. On leaving the army, he went to Cambridge University, where he studied agriculture. While at Cambridge, Father owned a racehorse, and our family still retains his racing colours, which have a plain purple jockey shirt and cap. After Cambridge, he was given a job in the London office of the *Irish Times*. In 1926, while staying in a hotel in Sevenoaks, he fell in love with Cynthia, the 22-year-old daughter of the hotel manager, Mr James. They had two sons – my brother John and me.

CHAPTER 2
A dedication

As my father had a passion for golf, it was only natural that our family should live by the side of a golf course. Our house was in Sunningdale, and it was here that I spent my early years, along with my brother John. It was inevitable, with father being 'married' to golf and our very beautiful mother living a life of solitude, that our parents would drift apart. Father went to live with his sister Vickey in Frenchpark, County Roscommon, and we moved to Bournemouth.

One of my earliest recollections as a child of four is sitting on my mother's brother's shoulders in the middle of the night, as we made our way to our small house perched on the side of a hill in the outskirts of Bournemouth. Despite the separation, our home was warmed by the absolute love and dedication of our mother, who had refused a divorce so as to protect our interests.

As there was little for us to do in the holidays in Bournemouth, we spent the majority of them at Frenchpark, with the De Freyne family. Looking back, I realise the incredible debt of gratitude we owe my cousin Francis and Aunt Vickey for their enormous understanding and hospitality over so many years.

The trip to Frenchpark, in a remote part of Ireland, was an adventure in itself. We would leave London Euston on a large London Midland & Scottish red steam train with brightly coloured sleeping carriages. Walking up to the engine, we watched the sweating fireman shovelling enormous quantities of coal into the roaring red-hot furnace, while copious amounts of steam billowed out of its funnel. The journey from Holyhead to Kingstown, Ireland, was completed on the overnight ferry. With no stabilizers on the ship, the crossing could be very rough. Then there was a drive of 100 miles from Dublin to Frenchpark. The first 50 miles of the drive to Mullingar was through English Home County countryside. This was the area of Ireland that was 'in the pale', where the landlords had protection from the British in the 1800s. After Mullingar, we were in land previously considered to be 'beyond the pale.'

Here the whole nature of the landscape changed. Instead of woods and fields, there were bogs as far as the eye could see. It was through this mystical countryside that we drove to Frenchpark. The road undulated and passed over the Shannon River and into the hinterland of central Ireland, where donkeys and carts were more often seen than cars. The village had a cluster of houses and shops, many with thatched roofs, and in the winter all gave out smoke from the turf fires burning within. Beyond the village was a high stone wall, in which were large wrought-iron double gates framed by colonnades topped with a statue of an eagle on a golden ball.

To the left of the curving drive was the old deer park, and on the right was the wonderful Palladian red-brick house, dating from 1667, which had curved wings containing the old kitchen and laundry, the chapel and billiard room. In one of the garages there was still a hansom cab and other horse-driven carriages – relics from the previous century.

The interior was as impressive as the exterior. The large hallway had an ornate Waterford glass chandelier, and the curving staircase swept up to the drawing room, which extended the whole length of the building and had a fireplace at either end – always lit in winter. The Frenches had lived here for 300 years. In the 1800s, the family was elevated to the peerage. Father's sister, Vickey, married Frankie De Freyne in 1914 and after having four daughters, Patricia, Johnnie, Patience and Faith, produced their son and heir Francis in 1927. Frankie died when Francis was only six, and Aunt Vickey ran the estate until he became of age.

On our first visit to Frenchpark, electricity had not yet been installed, and dozens of paraffin lamps lit the house at night. Similarly, there was no mains water supply. Water was drawn from a deep well by a pump driven by a very aged Perkins engine. This was used twice a day and was worked by an equally aged retainer, Mike O'Brien, who by this time was well into his 80s and had lived on the estate forever. The sterility of the water was questionable. On being told of a dead rat in the well water, Aunt Vickey retorted: 'Well no one during the last 300 years has died from drinking this water.'

In those pre-war days of the 1930s, John and I spent many happy and memorable holidays with our cousin Francis. We were a 'terrible trio', and every day we'd explore the hidden wonders of the countryside. We hunted rabbits and went ferreting with the gamekeeper. We would bicycle daily to the village to buy chocolate bars from our friend Mr Tulley, the grocer, and visit Mr McManus, the butcher, who still did his own slaughtering. The relationship between the house and the village was one of mutual respect, and the villagers often came to seek advice from Aunt Vickey.

One of the neighbours was the First President of the Republic of Ireland, Douglas Hyde – an outstanding scholar who was fluent in the Irish language. As children, we would often see him at parties, and I remember once playing with the revolver of one of his security guards. Another neighbour was Aunt Vickey's brother-in-law William French. He and his very beautiful wife Louise lived at Croghan and had three daughters: Timmy, Candy and Mariebelle. I remember bursting into tears at one particularly dreadful children's party. Mariebelle came to my rescue and led me by the hand over a bridge, across a stream, into the garden. Gazing up at this beautiful girl, my tears evaporated, to be replaced by smiles. Like other members of the French family, they have been not only relatives but also lifelong friends.

John and I were at Frenchpark on 3 September 1939, the day war was declared. We were crouched under the table in the library when Neville Chamberlain came on the air and gave his historic address. This news would change the world forever, but as young ignorant boys, we just felt relief that our schooling would be interrupted.

Indeed it was. For the next few months we had private tuition in the billiard room given by Ian Thompson, a Cambridge graduate who was enjoying his gap year. He lived with us all at Frenchpark, before returning to England to join the armed forces. In the spring of 1940 we returned to England.

At about the time I started at Harrow in 1942, Father had decided to return to the family roost! So we left Bournemouth and moved into Whitecliffe Manor in the Isle of Purbeck, north of Swanage.

Harrow School was not evacuated during the war. Both at school and at home, the war seemed ever present. During my first two years at Harrow, many sleepless nights were spent in the basement. The Germans were concentrating on night raids, and London was their main target. Night after night, after a little sleep, the sirens would sound and we were herded to the basement. Despite the bombs blasting off all over London, there was never any sense of alarm or imminent danger. It was a normal part of our existence and all we could think about were our comfortable beds upstairs.

By 1944, the menace to London had changed from the bomber to the V1 "doodlebug". This amazing invention was a jet-propelled, unpiloted, mono-plane bomb. Launched from pads in France, it flew over Kent, London and the Home Counties. When it ran out of fuel, the jet engine cut out and the plane would plummet to the ground. Thousands of these doodlebugs were launched during the summer of 1944.

A state of emergency was declared in London. All students were sent home, except the few due to sit exams. The following weeks were rather exceptional, with only a skeleton staff of masters and a few dozen boys living on an otherwise almost totally abandoned Harrow Hill. During every exam session, several doodlebugs would fly towards our school. We were instructed to carry on working during the approach of these flying bombs but were warned that we must dive under our desks the moment their engines stopped. This plane had a very unique undulating rasping drone. There would suddenly be a menacing silence when we would duck for cover, waiting for the inevitable explosion. With the departure of imminent danger, we could recommence our exam. Extra time was allowed for the time spent under our desks! I passed, but surely the examiners would not have had the heart to fail anyone who had had to endure this trial by bomb.

Prime Minister Sir Winston Churchill used to make an annual visit to the 'Speecher', Harrow's distinctive semicircular speech room, and one time he passed within two feet of me. He would sit in the middle of the stage facing the boys, who were seated in the semi-circular tiers of seats. By tradition, the most junior treble in the school would stand, looking up at Churchill and singing a solo Harrow School song, 'Five hundred faces and all so strange'. It was an incredible sight to see our war leader with tears streaming down his cheeks.

John and I would return to Whitecliffe Manor for the holidays. Being wartime, cars were only used for essential services. Our mother Cynthia solved our transport problems by buying two New Forest ponies named Twinkle and Winkle and an open four-wheeler, four-seater trap. These two magnificent ponies, galloping side by side and pulling the buggy on which mother sat wielding a very large riding crop, became a much-loved sight in Swanage, at a time when there was very little diversity from the war. The fact that our mother had no previous experience with ponies and trap did not deter her in any way. Shopping could not have been easier. She would pull up in the middle of the high street, and the shopkeepers would come out to take her orders and carry out the provisions. Once General Montgomery, driving past in his staff car, saluted her.

The children of Swanage were always clamouring for a ride in this unique form of transport, and accordingly a day of charity was arranged, called 'The mile of pennies'. For one penny, a child could have a ride up and down the beach in the trap. Every penny was placed in a line on the path and by the end of the day extended almost the length of the seafront. Hundreds of children had enjoyed an experience of a lifetime and much money was raised for the British Red Cross, but one mother and two ponies returned home totally exhausted.

Swanage often suffered 'hit and run' raids from Me109s or Focke-Wolf 190 fighter planes, which carried a single bomb. One Monday morning we were all going to have our photographs taken, but my brother was stricken with severe diarrhoea and our appointment was cancelled. Instead I took our dogs for a walk up Barrow Downs. At precisely midday, a Focke-Wolf 190 shattered my peace, passing overhead with all guns blazing. It passed so close that I could see the pilot's head. The bomb hit the middle of the High Street, killing the ironmonger Mr Bruton and destroying Musprat's photographic studio. But for my brother's gippy tummy, our buggy would have sustained a direct hit in the high street.

That night, Lord Haw-Haw, the ignoble William Joyce, who was later executed as a traitor to England, stated on the German evening news that a successful raid had been made in Swanage against the scientists who were on their way to the radar installations in Worth Matravers. Haw-Haw had not realized that these installations were now safely located in Malvern and that the death of one civilian ironmonger was all that had been accomplished.

The Isle of Purbeck was used for the dress rehearsal of the Normandy Invasion, for the training of fighter pilots and as a practice area for the American Super Fortress 'Tedder carpet' pattern bombing. One evening in the spring of 1944, a large army contingent was billeted in the farm in front of our house. At dawn, John and I climbed to the top of the hill and watched from under a gorse bush – just 200 yards from General Eisenhower and Field Marshal Montgomery as they made preparations for D-Day.

In July 1946, I left Harrow School after a rather undistinguished sporting career but academically with slightly more distinction. I immediately volunteered for the Royal Air Force (RAF), with the intention of going to Cranwell to gain a commission and earn my wings as a pilot. That summer I went to the wedding of Desmond Murphy to my first cousin May Van Cutsem. As John was serving in the army in Palestine, I escorted Mother to London, where we stayed at the Basil Street Hotel. I was so proud of her, looking so beautiful at this first meeting of the clans after so many war years.

After a holiday of adolescent fun at Wighill Park in Yorkshire with my Uncle Tom, Aunt Lettice and their children Peter, Guy, Marigold and Caroline, I returned home to Swanage to find that all had changed.

Mother had not been feeling well for some little time and had consulted a surgeon in Bournemouth, who had diagnosed cancer of the ovaries, with extensive pelvic secondaries. I well remember our kindly GP, Dr Pearce, talking to my father with a gloomy countenance behind closed doors. Father was so sad as he told me that Mother's prognosis was deemed hopeless and survival was only a matter of time. He also suggested that I defer my call up to the RAF.

As she became progressively weaker, my temporary job of cook and housekeeper also included nursing. Despite being only 17 and very inexperienced, I really enjoyed that year. I used to drive around the countryside on John's battered pre-war BSA (Birmingham Small Arms Company) motorbike. Every Saturday night I'd go to the theatre in Bournemouth with Mother's friends. One bitterly cold night, I made the 25-mile return journey by the light of the moon, as the bike lights had failed. Luckily there were fewer police in those days!

I was very close to Mother and I hated witnessing her pain and suffering, which seemed to be more and more progressive. Yet, even at this time, the thought that she might die did not, quite honestly, enter into my head.

With my national service call up imminent, Dr Pearce would issue a certificate every two or three months stating that my presence at home was essential. Towards the end of 1947, I was summoned to attend the Deferment Board in Admiralty Arch, Whitehall. Duly armed with a sealed envelope containing Dr Pearce's report I was confronted by the senior dignitaries of His Majesty's Services. They all looked extremely old, rather solemn and extremely sceptical. I presented them with the envelope. Immediately their countenances changed to one of extreme condolence. Without further interrogation they wished me well and I was given another four months' leave. I returned home to Swanage amazed at the simplicity and success of my mission.

In January 1948, I realized why they had been so sympathetic. Mother's condition took a rapid turn for the worse and John was called back from Palestine. On 19 January, her condition became extremely serious and in the evening Dr Pearce was summoned. I remember sitting with Father and John in the morning room, reading Somerset Maugham's *Creatures of circumstance,* when Dr Pearce came down to say that Mother had died. She was only 44.

That evening, Father asked John and me to join him in his bedroom to discuss our future. Despite his grief, it filled me with gratitude and affection that his main concern was for our welfare. There was now no point in staying any longer at Whitecliffe. John said that he would like to resign his commission in the Royal Irish Fusiliers and start a career in the *Irish Times*. Without hesitation, I said that I wanted to study medicine at Trinity College, Dublin. Later that night, I returned to Mother's room to make my solemn obligation for life.

Before leaving Swanage, we scattered my mother's ashes over the field where the ponies had grazed in front of the house and, in her memory, donated an eagle lectern to the Church of St Mary the Virgin, New Swanage.

Part Two. Into The Unknown

CHAPTER 3
The Dublin years

Within days of my mother's death, we went to stay with Aunt Vickey at Frenchpark. Later I started as a premedical student at Trinity. John and I found a place to stay at Woodville with the Hamiltons of Hanwood. These wonderful four ladies, all well into their mid-70s, seemed to have eternal youth on their side. Like so many Irish families, they had very little money and lived off their own talents and rent from paying guests.

Connie, the youngest, was a landscape gardener, and two were artists. Letitia, known as May, was a member of the Royal Hibernian Society and specialized in oil paintings, usually composed with a pallet brush. The merit of her work was only truly appreciated after her death, and today her paintings are very valuable. In later years, May gave us, as a wedding present, an oil painting of the Parade Ring at the Phoenix Park Racecourse. May's elder sister Eva was also a very accomplished painter, but her work has never received quite so much acclaim. One of my most treasured possessions is a painting of my dog Flossy lying in the sunlight on the front steps of Woodville, which was painted by Eva in 1950. The other sister Amy was in charge of the housekeeping.

The Hamiltons were the most loving people. In this large rambling house, warm with friendship (although not by central heating), the paying guests were treated as members of the family. Life with the Hamilton sisters and their guests was one of perpetual fun and gaiety, which deflected me from my serious and often sad studies. There was an element of eccentricity about the whole place. The dining room was separated from the kitchen by a bookcase, through which the parlour maid, Bridget, would appear with the dinner – to the astonishment of any new guest. The quality of the food was questionable. It was repetitious and on many occasions inadequate for the number of guests. The comfort of the bedrooms could, at times, leave much to be desired. One guest, too frightened to complain, came down to breakfast and said that her bed had not only lacked sheets and blankets but also a mattress. She had slept fully clothed on the springs!

During one lunch, Georgie Payne, the gardener, who had been with the family for more than 40 years, came in unannounced and said, quite rightly, that the house appeared to be on fire. He returned to the garden and the family finished lunch before calling the fire brigade, who fortunately arrived in time to put out the fire before too much damage had been done. The sisters shared all their parties with us, and we were privileged to meet many of the mainstream writers and artists of Ireland at that time. Most notable was Evie Hone, who followed John Piper in producing the last four windows in the Eton Chapel, Windsor.

Another of the paying guests was Commander Arthur Rickards RNVR who had spent the war in motor torpedo boats and was now working for a pharmaceutical company. He certainly brought with him a new dimension of humour. At this time, my cousin Patience was making frequent visits to Woodville. It took some time for me to realize that Arthur and Patience were having an affair. When they became engaged, Arthur came to Frenchpark to receive Aunt Vickey's permission for her daughter's hand in marriage. The visit took place on a cold winter's night. Lady De Freyne prepared herself by a blazing fire at one end of the drawing room. The front door bell rang and the parlour maid brought the guest into the drawing room. Aunt Vickey rose and offered him a drink. She made polite conservation for a few minutes before realizing that she was entertaining the local corn merchant, who had come to see Francis on business matters. A few minutes later, Arthur arrived and proceeded to mistake the corn merchant for Francis!

In 1952, John was made London Editor of the *Irish Times* and went to live in London. John's journalistic abilities were quite considerable. Every day he would write a column about current events and gossip in London. His biggest scoop was breaking the news, in 1956, that Sir Anthony Eden was planning to invade Egypt to save British interests in the Suez a full 24 hours before any other news agency. The Suez Canal invasion was, as is well documented, a fiasco and lead to the Prime Minister's resignation.

Trinity, Dublin, unlike most other universities, had a premed year of physics, chemistry and biology. One therefore entered the university in limbo, as a student trying to obtain a place in the medical school. My chances of success seemed rather gloomy. Of an initial intake of 120, only 80 would pass into the first medical year. Chemistry was relatively easy, but soon I decided that physics was boring and almost impossible to comprehend. In November, the morass of difficulties I had lifted, like morning mist on a lake, when Professor Walton gave his first lecture. It was like hearing Sir Malcolm Sargent conducting the Proms at the Albert Hall. From his opening words he brought wit, comprehension and depth of meaning to the subject. I sat mesmerized by the way he could turn this subject, previously so meaningless to me, into one of such profound interest. After my initial surprise, I put pen to paper and recorded every word he uttered throughout the whole year. I revised and rewrote the whole lecture – most time consuming but well worth the trouble. Absorbing knowledge from good lecturers is far more beneficial than learning from textbooks.

This great lecturer turned out to be the Professor of Physics who had been working with Professor Cockcroft, during the 1930s at Cambridge University, on the splitting of the atom for nuclear energy. Professor Cockcroft was subsequently awarded the Nobel Prize for Science and the premise 'that matter can neither be created nor destroyed' was shattered. When Professor Walton realized where these studies were leading and the possible destruction that could be unleashed on the world, he resigned from Cambridge and obtained his post at Trinity College, Dublin. I sat the exams in July with much trepidation, knowing that failure would result in the end of my dream of joining the Medical School. I was fortunate enough to pass.

On an autumnal Monday in October 1949, I entered Trinity College, Dublin, as a first-year medical student. As a late teenager who may have suffered tribulations in life, in my case the recent loss of my mother, I was still unprepared for the assault on the system that occurs the moment you enter the precincts of the Medical School. The training starts with the study of anatomy and the many failures that can occur in the body. It becomes immediately evident that spirit and soul are entrapped in a frail body that is forever changing and can so easily disintegrate. The manifestations of the body are given – not self-made. A beautiful model, with inherited looks and beauty, has done nothing personally to acquire them.

The anatomy school caused me some disquiet. It was bright and airy, with large overhead glass windows under each of which was the naked body of an intact corpse, where we medical students congregated with scalpels and textbooks. The sight of an extremely attractive 19-year-old girl dissecting the leg of one of these corpses amazed me. How could such a pretty innocent-looking girl be taking part in such a macabre scene? It was only a few days before I did the same thing.

I was so proud to be sitting with the next generation of doctors in that anatomy hall. Our Professor of Anatomy, Dr Erskine, a distinguished gentleman with a totally bald and very shiny scalp, reminded us that we were on hallowed ground and that no parts of the bodies were to be removed from this consecrated area. Over the years, many patients from the various hospitals in Dublin had willed their bodies to the school, ensuring that their demise would benefit others. One of my distinguished patients of later years, David Niven, then a young unemployed actor in Hollywood, reputedly bequeathed his body for $50.

I now joined my fellow students and began dissecting. As first-year medical students, we studied anatomy, physiology, histology and biochemistry. This is a time that the dreams of childhood and the fantasies of living become the realities of life and death. Over the years I have since realized that there are basically two types of doctor: those who have deep abiding faith in a particular creed or those who become obsessed with the scientific rather than religious beliefs in life. I have always felt that doctors who lead and run their professional lives under the edicts of religious belief give a better and more sympathetic service to their patients.

Anatomy is relatively straightforward but requires endless hours of dissection. Many of our great painters and sculptors, such as Michelangelo, have learned this discipline. During the year, I spent much of my time studying in my little Wolseley 8 car, parked in the front drive of Woodville and scaring away potential paying guests, who were terrified to see the skull on my lap!

In the second year, I studied the more tranquil subjects of pathology, bacteriology and biochemistry. The study of pathology and disease further confirmed my awareness of the body's frailty. Professor Fearon, a world authority who had written the standard textbook on biochemistry, once said to us: 'If over the years you forget all that I have taught you, remember one thing. The most important substances in biochemistry are the B vitamins, which help to support the metabolism and general wellbeing of the body.' I took these vitamins throughout my training.

For the summer, I joined John in London. Night after night we would dine at a little restaurant in the haunt of journalists in Fleet Street called Ninos. It was in July at the annual Eton v Harrow cricket match at Lords that, through one of my girlfriends, Victoria de Rutsen, I met the 10-year-old Veronica Mary Langué, who would later become my wife, soulmate and the real love of my life.

The next year studying surgery, obstetrics and gynaecology, I had my first contact with patients and the hospital. Spring had arrived after a long winter.

The working day would begin with a clinic – a demonstration given by a surgeon or physician, usually alongside a patient's bed. One of my favourite teachers was Dr Brian Mayne, consultant to the Meath Hospital. His years as a Japanese prisoner of war had not been wasted. He fortunately had with him a copy of Saville's *Medicine* and had learned the text by heart. Attending these morning clinics was one of the highlights of my learning years. Not once did a patient ever object to this form of examination: most seemed to enjoy the experience, particularly when students displayed their abysmal ignorance.

At this time, a cousin was getting married at a large social occasion in Dublin. As an usher, I had planned to take most of the day off but felt that it would be a good idea to nip into the Adelaide Hospital for the morning clinical round, so I dressed in my morning suit and top hat to save time. To my dismay, the clinical round that day was a post-mortem. I sat in the autopsy room in my finery looking like an undertaker. It was a poignant insight into life and death.

I spent most of the summer of 1953 trying unsuccessfully to court Victoria de Rutsen and together we visited Frenchpark for the last time. Shortly after, the contents of the house and farm were auctioned, and the roof was removed to avoid payment of taxes.

It was in the climate of my failed love affair with Victoria and the loss of Frenchpark, with all its memories, that I reluctantly returned to Trinity to finish my studies. I was so wrong to be sceptical, as the next few weeks demonstrated the real benefits that medicine can bring, while at the same time enhancing the experience and awareness of the givers.

I became resident at the famous maternity hospital, the Rotunda. It served the greater part of Dublin on the north side of the River Liffey, including the area around Mountjoy Square – once the most fashionable part of Dublin – which contained many gracious Georgian squares and terraces. Yet in the confines of these buildings, whole families lived together in poverty and abject misery.

After only a few days in the Labour Ward of the Rotunda mastering the intricacies of childbirth, we were considered to be capable obstetricians and thrust into the district in groups of three or four. Mothers who were having their first baby or had anticipated complications were admitted to the hospital. All the other patients had their delivery in the district, with the assistance of a midwife or medical students. Almost without exception, when we arrived at the patient's house, the mother's face would light up with pleasure and she would exclaim: 'Thank God we've got the young doctors and not those awful midwives.' Little did they know!

Our group of four – including David Hall, Mike Norman and Austin Darragh, whose father wrote *The riddle of the sands* – had a set routine for each delivery. One was assigned to look after the mother, another the newborn baby and the third would do the cleaning, sterilizing and preparation of the instruments. The final member of the group was in reserve, in case of an emergency such as untoward bleeding. In that event, they would immediately summon the wagon from the hospital. We were credited for each case we attended, even if the patient had to be admitted. As can be imagined, more were admitted to the Rotunda than was absolutely essential!

On one occasion, a patient told us, when taking her history, 'Doctors, I had a severe bleed last night.' We panicked and rushed her into the Rotunda as an emergency. When we visited, an elderly battleaxe of a sister met us in the doorway of the ward and marched us over to the woman, now lying comfortably in a bed with clean linen sheets. The sister pulled back the bedclothes and, without any ceremony, separated the woman's legs, snarling: 'I can see very little bleeding.' The woman said: 'Don't be so stupid, I wasn't bleeding from there – I had a bad nose bleed.' We failed to get credit for that case.

It was accepted practice that, when summoned, we were expected to stay with the patient until after delivery. This could take two or three days, after which we wretched young doctors would return bedraggled, dirty and unshaven. Having attended several very protracted deliveries, we had a stroke of luck. While waiting for events to take their course, we were surprised by the entrance of a woman into our improvised labour ward. She strode over to the mother-to-be and, peering between her legs, declared: 'You'll never get anywhere sitting around doing nothing.' She then seized a pair of Spencer-Wells forceps, opened the woman's legs even wider, inserted the forceps and ruptured the amniotic membrane. There was an immediate outpouring of amniotic fluid and within an hour the baby was delivered. We looked in wonder at the woman, who it transpired was the theatre sister of the rival Holles Street Hospital.

The patient was her sister. We carefully noted this novel procedure, and it became the first manoeuvre we performed on every subsequent patient. Our colleagues were perplexed at how our group, on each call, was always finished in two or three hours. Induction, as it is now called, is a standard procedure today.

One of our patients, a pretty Romany girl, lived in a small thatched cottage alongside the main Navan Road, which had only a single window. During delivery, the baby showed signs of fetal distress, and it became obvious that the umbilical cord was wrapped around the neck. We became desperately concerned that we would lose the baby but there was no time to get to the hospital. This was a major emergency. Once the baby's head had presented, one of us supported it while the other cut the umbilical cord, and we then expedited the delivery. After resuscitation, thankfully both mother and baby did well. Thrilled at our success and feeling terribly proud of ourselves, we let out our pent-up energies by carousing around the town, waking up all our fellow residents in the early hours of the morning. For this misdemeanour, we lost our credit for this case. Such are the vagaries of life.

So we started our final year in earnest. We worked harder than ever to complete our studies in medicine, surgery and gynaecology. The final surgical exam moulded my future career, as 10% of the marks were for ophthalmology. In my naivety, I thought this an easy subject and bought a small textbook on the subject that I learned by heart. The consultant examiner was Beecher Somerville-Large, an eminent eye surgeon. My little textbook held me in good stead, and I scored 80% in ophthalmology, despite having little knowledge of the subject.

I passed my exam in Medicine, Surgery and Gynaecology, and Aunt Vickey proudly escorted me at the passing-out ceremony, as recorded in the *Irish Times*.

Many of my friends went on to eminent careers: Peter Payne became a consultant obstetrician and gynaecologist, as did William Crawford and Ian Dalrymple. Adrian Henry became an orthopaedic surgeon and pioneered keyhole arthroscopy of the knee. Most of my colleagues, such as Nancy (Kevany) Butler, Mike Norman, Des Bell, David Hall and Lettice Bowen, become general practitioners.

CHAPTER 4
The wonders of life and death

I had considered training as a neurosurgeon, a specialty still in its infancy, but this all changed after I was invited to dinner with Beecher Somerville-Large and his wife Sammy at their home Brooklawn. I subsequently found out that Somerville-Large had been given a brief to study the incidence of retrolental fibroplasia, a severe ocular condition that affects premature babies. By a cruel twist of fate, his daughter Faith was one of the few babies with this condition in Ireland.

Beecher Somerville-Large had the unusual distinction of being Elected President for two years of the Ophthalmologic Society of the UK, now renamed The Royal College of Ophthalmology. Although slightly deaf, he always claimed that this disability helped him through his presidency. Chairing the committee meetings, he would occasionally turn off his hearing aid and, after a while, switch it back on, saying: 'We have discussed this subject for long enough, let's turn to the next item on the agenda.' He had an abiding love of ophthalmology, which he instilled into all his students. Beecher's hobbies were gardening and archaeology. He spent part of every summer holiday in West Cork studying archaeological relics along the coastline and presented many lectures on the subject. During dinner, he told me that, in a few years, there'd be a vacancy for a consultant ophthalmic surgeon in Dublin and asked if I'd consider a career in ophthalmology. After little persuasion, I agreed, and for the next few years he acted as my guardian, mentor and friend. I left, pondering that it would take me another 10 years studying to achieve this goal.

Before specializing I had to spend a year as a junior house officer doing six months of surgery and six months of medicine. I was fortunate to be given a position in the Adelaide Hospital and privileged, in 1954, to get a surgical appointment with Nigel Kinnear. Nigel had a perfect bedside manner, showing courtesy and compassion at all times to his patients, but in the operating theatre his demeanour could change and he'd become a tyrant.

He was a dapper man, sporting a finely cut moustache. He expected his house surgeon to be equally immaculately dressed. Out of youthful stubbornness, I bought myself a pair of yellow suede shoes, which I wore on my first surgical ward round. On noticing my gaudy shoes, he raised an eyebrow but said nothing and thereafter accepted my bizarre outfit. I wore these ghastly shoes on every ward round over the next few months.

There is always a unique atmosphere in the operating theatre: a mix of drama and excitement. It starts with the meticulous scrubbing up of hands and forearms, followed by the ceremony of being cloaked in a sterile gown, hat, mask and gloves. The surgeons then enter with sterile gloved hands raised as if in prayer and supplication, which on occasion are badly needed. The theatre sister, nurses and technicians silently pad around like altar boys before a priest at mass. Meanwhile, the patient, having been swathed in drapes, lies anaesthetized on the operating table, with a mask over the mouth, from which protrude tubes leading to the anaesthetic machine. At the patient's side, the anaesthetist hovers over his machine like an ice-cream man with his barrow.

Having cleansed the skin, the surgeon makes the incision with a deft stroke of the scalpel. Blood immediately pours into the incised area. With pressure packs and forceps, the ruptured vessels are clamped before the incision is extended to the deeper layers of tissues. Apart from his inherent expertise, a surgeon's skill lies in his knowledge of anatomy and comprehension of the patient's condition. When dealing with the abdomen, surgery is made very much easier if the patient is not too overweight.

Although the majority of operations involved the abdomen, the surgeon was always trespassing into other areas of the body, which are now regarded as subspecialties. One surgical list might include removal of the stomach, gall bladder, part of the colon and a kidney, an appendectomy and, to finish the day, an exploratory operation on the vessels to the leg. In most cases, surgery involved removal of the offending organ. Mercifully, many of the organs, such as the gall bladder and appendix, are not essential for the patient's wellbeing and some are duplicated, so the loss of one is not too serious. The worst scenario was to open up the diseased area only to find a cancer that had spread well beyond the limits of its own organ, making surgery was impossible. The responsibilities of the surgeon are enormous, and decisions have to be taken that will markedly influence the future lifestyle of the patient. Throughout my career, I always entered the operating theatre with some degree of apprehension, as you never know what you might be confronted by.

I had the feeling that Nigel thought I was a rather clumsy surgeon, as he affectionately nicknamed me 'Butch', calling me this even in front of the patients. Nigel was one of the original pioneers of vascular surgery, a very difficult and delicate area. During one week we operated on six patients, each of whom failed to make the end of the operation. After the final list, while having tea in the surgeon's room, Nigel turned to me and sadly commented: 'Butch, it hasn't been our best week, has it?'

Despite these losses, Nigel had great success with his general surgery. He had a beautiful pair of hands, and it was a true delight assisting him at surgery. At times he would reverse the roles and would act as my assistant. I can so well remember doing my first appendectomy and the thrill I felt when the offending organ was localized, ligatured and removed.

On one Saturday afternoon, before going racing at Phoenix Park Racecourse, I did a final round of my patients. The last patient I visited was one of our ward sisters, who had been admitted with a clot in the main artery of one of her legs. As young interns, this elderly sister had mercilessly bullied us but, despite her strict discipline, she was loved and respected by all. On examining her, I was appalled to find that the blood clot had progressed up to her left groin. Horse racing was now of little importance, and I immediately summoned Nigel Kinnear. Together we did an emergency exploratory operation to establish where the obstruction of the artery commenced. Every time we enlarged the initial incision, hoping to get above the blockage and seal the artery, the progressive blood clot preceded us. After many hours of surgery, we knew we were beaten and felt extremely sad at the loss of an old colleague and friend.

The house surgeons took it in turns to be on emergency night duty. On these nights, we would dread to hear the residency door opened and slammed shut by the night sister, followed by the sound of her footsteps marching down the corridor. Huddled in our beds, we would wait for the tap on the shoulder, knowing that the rest of the night would be spent dealing with an emergency – the complexity of which could possibly be way beyond our expertise.

All junior doctors, nurses, and interns were expected to be on duty for the whole of the Christmas period. The hospital took on a new look, with a Christmas tree in every ward, gaily decorated with bunting and crackers. Everyone worked hard to ensure that the patients had as happy a Christmas as they would have had in their own homes. Indeed, for many of the Dublin poor, they probably had a Christmas such as never before.

But on Christmas Eve, there was nothing I could do for a terminally ill patient except sit beside her in the darkened room as she clutched a crucifix to her breast. I watched the candlelight procession of the hospital nurses and medical staff singing *Ave Maria* as my patient's life ebbed away.

During my second six months as an intern, I was house physician to Dr Mitchell, who kindly allowed me to spend part of the week studying ophthalmology at the Royal Victoria Eye and Ear Hospital. I was also able to attend Beecher Somerville-Large's outpatients' clinic at the Adelaide Hospital.

I found being a physician far less fulfilling and missed the excitement of the operating theatre. In the 1950s, we had few treatments for patients with leukaemia or other malignant diseases. Chemotherapy was in its infancy and radiotherapy was rather basic. Cortisone had just become available and seemed to be the panacea for almost every condition.

One of my patients was a young beautiful girl with radiant long red hair. She had Hodgkin's disease, which at that time was untreatable. We managed to stabilize her condition with empirical therapy – therapy that is useless but keeps the mental condition of the patient buoyant. She looked outwardly well and was in no pain. The hospital chaplain visited her one afternoon and asked her whether or not she was prepared for her impending death. Having, I think, quite rightly not been made aware of the seriousness of her condition, the chaplain's comment came as quite a shock. From that moment on she rapidly deteriorated, became totally hysterical and had to be kept heavily sedated until her demise some days later.

One of the most difficult tasks for a young intern, who has much closer contact with the patient than the consultant, is to determine how much information should be divulged to the patient. Although many patients wish to know all about their illness and its prognosis, others require a discreet veil to be placed over their condition. I've always found that a patient is most helped by an element of optimism. The chaplain who had been so tactless with my patient had, however, helped many others in the hospital, but he felt that his calling as 'saviour of the soul' was more important than our efforts of trying to save the body. He considered us to be totally ignorant about the facts of spiritual life and once asked us over tea: 'What is faith?' I had recently been to St Patrick's Cathedral and heard an uplifting sermon on the subject, so I was able to quickly reply: 'Faith is the substance of things hoped for, the evidence of things not seen.' He looked at me in amazement and never again challenged my religious beliefs.

CHAPTER 5
Over the hurdles

After my year in the Adelaide Hospital as an intern, I left in July 1955 as a fully qualified doctor. Now I had to concentrate on studying to be an ophthalmic surgeon. It is not easy to continue studying well into manhood without the sheltered financial support of a family. At 25, I needed to spend a further year obtaining a Diploma in Ophthalmology with no income and no way of getting a grant. To my rescue came a very old friend Sir Richard Musgrave, who lent me £500 without interest. But for his generosity it would not have been possible, and I remain eternally grateful.

Another friend, Hubert Morris, kindly allowed me to share his bedroom in his Mayfair flat for a nominal rent. We shared with John Duckworth Bradshaw, Peter Herbert and Charles Stewart-Menteith, all of whom worked for Poland's insurance brokers at Lloyds of London. A smell of burning woke me one day at 4 am and Peter burst into the room enveloped in smoke. The flat was on fire! We raced down the stairs but the lower corridor was a raging inferno and almost impassable. We called the fire brigade, alerted the other tenants and then waited in the street. When they finally arrived, one of the firemen turned to Peter Herbert and asked: 'Are you going for a swim, sir?' None of us had realized that Peter was standing in the middle of this Mayfair street stark naked!

So I started my studies at Moorfields Eye Hospital and the Institute of Ophthalmology with a mixture of clinics and lectures. I was now studying in London and living with friends who, while working hard during the day, were busy socializing in the evenings. All my time was spent studying for the next exam.

Between lectures I could attend outpatient sessions in the London teaching hospitals, such as Bart's, St Thomas' or Charing Cross. It took only a short time to realize who the 'greats' were in this discipline.

My favourite surgeon was Sir Alan Goldsmith, who was knighted for being the queen's oculist. It was obvious that Alan did not enjoy teaching. His clinic took place every Tuesday at 1.30 pm, but he would invariably say: 'Please excuse me if I don't teach you today. I have a bad migraine.' All the students would then leave but, knowing the form, I would arrive back at his clinic at 2 pm. He never had the face to turn away one student and I effectively had six months' private tuition from this brilliant teacher. From him I learned a considerable amount of my basic ophthalmic medicine. His shyness was probably why he didn't enjoy teaching large numbers.

Even in these early days I befriended Sir Harold Ridley, the inventor of the lens implant. He offered me a residency at St Thomas' Hospital, which I reluctantly had to decline, as I had promised Beecher Somerville-Large that I would return to Dublin. If I had accepted that post I might have met Dr David Owen, who was Harold's intern before he turned to politics. Edgar King was another outstanding teacher whose practice in Harley Street I later inherited.

At the time, Keith Lyle was considered one of the most eminent ophthalmic surgeons for squints – a condition whereby the eyes are non-aligned. Keith worked from his private rooms in Mayfair. At a cocktail party, a debutante making polite conservation to him asked whether or not he had rooms in Harley Street. On being told no, she retorted: 'What bad luck, but not everyone can be successful.' He wrote the standard textbook on squints with Worth, who practised in Bournemouth, and was equally well known for his manual on sailing. Such are the diverse interests of surgeons.

On occasional weekends I would go to stay at Smugglers, in West Sussex, with the Twisleton-Wykeham-Fiennes family. Celia Fiennes had studied medicine at Trinity and had also lodged at Woodville. On my first visit to Smugglers, I passed a shirtless boy riding a pony bareback down the lane to her house. This was how I met Sir Ranulph Fiennes, who was later to become the world's greatest living explorer, an accomplished novelist and a tireless charitable fundraiser. His father Ranulph was killed in 1943 before Ran was born. Weekends with Celia, Ran, his sisters Gillian and Susan and mother Audrey were always amusing. Ran was still a schoolboy at Eton, but even then his adventurous streak was becoming apparent. The family remained lifelong friends. Celia married a missionary doctor and practised medicine in Africa. Many years later, I operated on Lady Fiennes for cataract and would regularly administer to Ran between his various expeditions. On one occasion, he had double vision, as weeks travelling over the Antarctic snowy terrain with no horizon, where the endless expanse of snow merges into the overcast sky, had made his eyes focus at a distance of one metre in front. It took some weeks for this convergence of the visual axises to relax. He had come into my waiting room the day after his return with both feet heavily bandaged, still sporting his Polar beard, as my other patients gazed at him in awe. He looked like the Yeti.

The Diploma in Ophthalmology course ended just before Christmas, which I spent in Ireland before accepting an appointment as house surgeon at the Royal Victoria Eye and Ear Hospital in Dublin. This was stimulating and rewarding, but I still had to pass my exam for the Diploma in Ophthalmology. Thus in the middle of my internship, I returned to London and rejoined my friends in Hertford Street.

The final part of this exam was a practical, during which we examined selected patients under the watchful eye of the examiner, Sir Stephen Miller, ophthalmic adviser to the queen. Initially, all went well. The first patient had an old retinal detachment; no problem. The second patient had a long-standing inflammation of the eye and opacification of the lens, again no problem. The third, however, presented some difficulties. This patient had a squint, which in my opinion was caused by adhesions and not muscle paralysis. Sir Steve started to question me about paralytic muscles of the eye and, in my youthful arrogance, I replied: 'This questioning is not relevant to this patient's condition.' A heated argument developed. I temporarily forgot that he was the examiner and we became locked in a debate about the patient's condition, while the poor patient observed us with some bemusement. Our altercations came to the notice of our senior examiner, Mr Lister, who asked what was going on. We both stated our cases. After deliberating for some little time he said that he agreed with me, the humble student, and then he personally conducted the rest of my clinical examination. That evening I learned that I had passed.

Six years later, I met Sir Steve in the consultants' canteen at Moorfields Eye Hospital. He asked me if we had ever met. When I reminded him of the incident, he at once launched back into the same argument. We never did come to an agreement. Later Steve became a great friend, and towards the end of his career I operated on most of his patients.

Having passed my Diploma in Ophthalmology, I returned to Dublin for the second six months of residency. I was now permitted to perform some surgery. My first operation was on a patient with a severe injury to one eye. I may not have had the experience of my senior consultants, but no patient could have had more care taken over the surgery. Over the next few months I performed many other eye operations, but not as yet the cataract procedure, which is considered the ultimate operation.

I attended all Beecher's ward rounds and surgical sessions and from him learned how to relate to patients and gained an immense knowledge of ophthalmology and an appreciation of the delicacy and precision required. In my year at the Royal Victoria Eye and Ear Hospital, I also discovered the importance of conducting a thorough examination of the patient before surgery. Beecher was a perfectionist who showed enormous compassion for his patients and in return received great respect.

On New Year's Eve 1956, I said farewell to all my friends and colleagues at the Royal Victoria. I now had to return to London to study for the Fellow of the Royal College of Surgeons' (FRCS) degree. That evening I joined Uncle Laurie for midnight mass in Howth Church.

In February 1957, I started at Nuffield College, an annex to the Royal College of Surgeons in Lincoln's Inn Fields. By miraculous luck, on my first trip to the canteen I met Professor Frank Stansfield, the foremost teacher of anatomy in the country. By the end of tea he had accepted me onto his anatomy cramming course for the Primary Fellowship of the FRCS degree. His classes had been fully subscribed for many months, and I was lucky to have so unexpectedly been given a place.

Passing the primary exam involved general anatomy, physiology and other basic sciences, which now seemed almost irrelevant. Sir Stewart Duke-Elder, the most eminent British eye surgeon of his time, explained why this anomaly had occurred. He told us that he had been actively involved in formulating the special FRCS degree and considered that, as eye surgeons, we must have the same skills and education as surgeons in the other specialties. He considered it imperative that we should share the initial part of the FRCS with all the other specialities, such as general surgery, neurosurgery, vascular surgery or cardiac surgery, while the second part of the FRCS dealt exclusively with ophthalmology. The world changes – not always for the better. Ophthalmology has now departed from the Royal College of Surgeons and has its own royal charter and set of exams. I am grateful that I was able to obtain the highly respected FRCS; we were all awarded an honorary FRCOphth, when the examining system changed in 1988.

Professor Sloames, our physiology professor, was the consummate professional and did much to help us in our quest to pass. But the anatomy lectures with Professor Stansfield were quite inspirational. Frank Stansfield was a master at teaching the three-dimensional study of anatomy – on a two-dimensional blackboard. Starting with one single red line, he would develop before our eyes the most incredible illustrations. He would often linger in front of one of his pupils and rest his enormous paunch on the student's desk. His teaching was simple, explicit and pure perfection. Once again I wrote down his every utterance and, with my friends Johnny Cockril and Mike Norman, refurbished and edited his brilliant work every night. So complete was his teaching that I did not once look at an anatomy textbook.

He was a tremendously warm-hearted person and always made sure his overseas students enjoyed the cultural attractions of London. Such were his skills as a teacher that his students were sent to take their exams in Glasgow, Edinburgh or Dublin so that other students did not have to compete with too many pupils who had been on his course. I was naturally sent to Dublin for my primary examination. Mr TG Wilson, the President of the Royal College of Surgeons of Ireland, and the father of one of my colleagues, telephoned me at Shearwater a few days later to tell me that I had passed. Johnny Cockril and Mike Norman failed the exam, gave up any idea of becoming surgeons and subsequently became excellent general practitioners. So much do our peers influence us throughout our training!

CHAPTER 6
Battle of Britain pilots

Having passed the first part of the FRCS exam, I rejoined Hubert Morris in Hertford Street, London, with my brother John and Gerard Dent. For the first time, at the age of 28, I was able to earn a little money in my chosen career.

The consultant surgeons at both branches of Moorfields, City Road and High Holborn, held regular outpatient clinics supported by a staff of senior and junior assistant ophthalmologists. Moorfields was considered to be the jewel in the crown and everyone wanted some association with it. Locum appointments would occur when any of the permanent surgical staff took annual leave. This was ideal for a half-trained ophthalmic surgeon, such as me.

Beecher Somerville-Large had already written letters of introduction to his ophthalmic friends in the hospital, which were of great help to me. His colleagues included Henry Stallard, Cyril Dee-Shapland, Edgar King, Arthur George Leigh and Harold Ridley, who in later years became my teachers and friends.

One of my regular sessions was a refraction clinic, where I had to prescribe glasses and try to improve the corrected vision of patients who had had complicated ophthalmic surgery. I shared this clinic with an optician, Mr Hudson, and at lunchtimes we would often walk through the bomb-devastated city, seeing few intact buildings, until reaching St Paul's Cathedral some two miles distant. It was said that: 'God preserved St Paul's Cathedral for the services of his people, and Whitbread's Brewery for the worker's beer.'

After a few months at Moorfields, I was invited to do a short-term locum internship by Cecil Thornhill, one of the residents at the hospital. Each resident was expected to do weekend duty every fourth week, being on standby from Saturday morning until Monday evening, sometimes dealing with more than 100 emergencies. Weekend duty was done in pairs, with one resident responsible for accidents and emergencies, the other for the wellbeing of all inpatients, including those being admitted for surgery on the Monday. During my month as a locum resident, I accepted being on casualty for the first weekend and the second, but I objected to being asked to cover for the third weekend in a row. This was Cecil's only lapse of consideration, and at all other times he gave me great assistance and remained a good friend.

The following spring I returned to Dublin to attend the annual meeting of the Ophthalmological Society of the UK, of which Beecher Somerville-Large was the president, with Susan Gaisford St Lawrence acting as his secretary. Beecher was extremely popular and highly regarded by his ophthalmic colleagues and this meeting attracted the ophthalmic hierarchy from around the world. As Beecher's protégé I was invited to all the academic and social functions of the week.

Dublin is at all times a romantic city, with its turbulent history and magnificent architectural heritage, and Beecher produced a meeting that showed it to its full. The official functions were held in the College of Physicians in Kildare Street. Beecher hosted a reception at Brooklawn. Most of the ophthalmic surgeons attending the congress were invited to this cocktail reception, among them Sir Benjamin Rycroft, whose son, Peter, would later be one of my colleagues at Moorfields. At this time Sir Benjamin was only the second London ophthalmic surgeon to have received a knighthood. During the Second World War, he was ophthalmic surgeon at the Queen Victoria Hospital, East Grinstead – the foremost unit for the treatment of burns and reconstructive surgery. All of the Battle of Britain pilots who suffered burns when bailing out of their blazing Hurricane or Spitfire fighter planes ended up in this hospital under the care of Sir Archibald McIndoe. Many of these young men had indescribable burns to their body and faces. Benjamin Rycroft had to deal with the eyes of these patients, many of whom had lost their lids as a result of severe burns. These exposed eyes needed very special treatment to ensure that they did not become dry and infected. Sir Benjamin ably supported the plastic surgeon, Sir Archibald, who had to deal not only with burns to the face but to the whole body.

Through pioneering plastic surgery techniques, Sir Archibald, with Sir Benjamin's help, was able to repair much of the damage done to the body. Inevitably there would be some distortion to the facial features, which still disturbed those who saw them. To address this situation Sir Archibald formed the Guinea Pig Club to provide psychological support. He gave these men the strength to go out and face the world beyond the safe confines of the hospital. He was a truly remarkable man, whose ability to inspire is movingly described in Richard Hillary's book *The last enemy*.

The final day of the Dublin conference coincided with the spring meeting at the Phoenix Park Racecourse. I invited many of my peers, and our family grandstand and bar were made open to them all. I was just a non-entity, yet I played host to the most senior in my profession.

After the races I returned to Shearwater House on the Hill of Howth, with Uncle Laurie, to join my Aunt Vickey and father for a quiet dinner. It was to be the last time I would ever see Uncle Laurie. On 2 July 1958, he died after an anaesthetic blunder during a minor operative procedure.

At around this time in 1958, we moved into a Victorian flat in Kensington High Street. It was vast, with a kitchen that could have come straight out of a country mansion. The hall was so long that we could play miniature bowls along it, and many of our parties ended up there. We had only been in this flat a few days when Gerard Dent proposed the addition of a Sudanese manservant. The Suez Crisis of 1956 had compelled many expatriates to return to the UK, some of whom had brought their staff back with them. Gerard's parents had friends who had done so and could no longer afford to keep their servant. Bogy duly arrived at Old Court Mansions. A most impressive figure, short and stout, coal black in complexion, he had frizzy greying hair and sported a perpetual grin. He spoke perfect English with an eastern accent.

Every morning he'd prepare a full English breakfast for us. He did all the shopping and kept the apartment immaculately tidy. He would buy the morning groceries from Barker's food store but would announce to the other shoppers: 'I will not join you peoples in the queue – my gentlemens are hungry and I have to look after thems.' And nobody dared gainsay him.

Uncle Laurie's estate sent me a trunk of silver sporting trophies – a treasure trove of polo cups, candlesticks, golf trophies and artefacts won by two generations of our family. Bogy polished them and placed them around the flat. It really was a very smart bachelor pad. We held impressive dinner parties in the vast dining room, illuminated by our recently acquired silver candlesticks. One female guest commented: 'This flat is like an Indian Palace, I expect at any minute a coloured servant to enter this room with our dinner.' At that precise moment Bogy came in with our steaming food, served up on one of my uncle's silver salvers!

Part Three. The Dancing Years of Spring

CHAPTER 7
Veronica and her family

In August 1958 I holidayed at Shearwater, where my father was now living. I greatly missed Uncle Laurie and was not at all ready for the parties and dances that were part and parcel of the Dublin Horse Show week.

John and I were now in control of the Phoenix Park Racecourse, under the management of the Director Mrs Peart and the Club Secretary Teddy Tighe. On the Saturday after the horse show we had our most important race of the year – the 1500 Stakes. We hosted a party in the private stand. Alcohol had by now replaced afternoon tea. Uncle Laurie had tried to limit drinks to one per guest, but when John and I inherited the stand all discipline went by the board. We were unable to control the crowd of friends and hangers on and I felt depressed that in memory of my uncle, so recently departed, we had to give a party such as this. But life had to go on and we entertained the winners of the various races, in particular Lester Piggott.

The following Thursday, 14 August, my life changed forever. I went to Howth Castle to collect Susan St Lawrence and her house guests, Veronica Langué and Sarah Fletcher. I drove them back to Shearwater for tea with my elderly great aunt, Emmy Bloomfield. Even at that time I must have had some strange inkling about our future, as I felt sad at being unable to introduce Veronica to Uncle Laurie. I so well remember saying to Veronica that she had missed him by only a few weeks.

Two days later the girls and I walked through the grounds of Howth Castle. We climbed between the massive rhododendron bushes and around the Druid Stone to the top of the hill, where we sat and gazed at the panoramic view. To one side were Dublin Bay and the city, with the backdrop of the Dublin mountains, and on the other side the harbour of Howth and Lambay Island. I had to put up with their girlish banal conversations about how they were missing their boyfriends. I really cannot remember who Veronica discussed on that occasion, but it was not a boyfriend of great import. That Sunday I took Susan and Veronica to West Pier, where we joined Desmond Bradley and friends in his Dublin Bay Class 24-foot sailing boat, Arandora. We took up our stations for the impending race. It was perfect racing conditions – a cloudless sky with a stiff breeze. Leaving Howth Harbour, we rounded Lambay Island and had a beat up to the Kish Lighthouse. Veronica and I were in charge of the port sheet of the jib. This was the first of hundreds of occasions we would be boating together. Our boat was laden with too many people, but Desmond Bradley was a masterful skipper and Arandora had an easy run home with the wind to our backs. We raced towards Lambay and passed the finishing line third overall and first in our class of ten.

I hadn't yet realized that I had met my partner for life.

A few weeks later I saw Veronica again: I returned from a dance in Yorkshire late Sunday night. She was sitting demurely in the drawing room with Hubert Morris, his fiancée Joyce, John, and Susan St Lawrence. She was breathtakingly beautiful. She had blonde hair and the most incredible pair of deep sapphire blue eyes; her 17-year-old body was finely slim with long shapely legs. Yet she seemed totally unaware of her beauty.

I was still taking out other girlfriends and living a bachelor's life, but over the next few months I fell progressively under her spell, even though she was some 12 years younger than me.

On my return from Ireland, Harold Ridley told me that I would get the next house appointment at Moorfields in four months' time. He seemed to have total responsibility for making the appointments of the resident surgeons and was not a man who said idle words, so I took it for granted that the job was mine, even though there were at least 44 applicants.

Although I might go for days without seeing Veronica, our relationship continued to develop. We enjoyed the simple things that young people do, like the zoo in Regent's Park and boating on the Serpentine. My relationship with Veronica was different to that with any other girl. From the time we first met there was no pretence or attempt to show off to each other. We dined out at inexpensive restaurants, and she would sit with me knitting or reading for hours while I studied.

Veronica had been educated at The Arts Educational School, Tring, specializing in dance, although at this time she was studying health and beauty at Atkinson's in Bond Street. She introduced me to ballet and we had wonderful nights watching Margot Fonteyn in Swan Lake or at the Royal Opera House, Covent Garden, or the Russian Georgian Ballet at the Albert Hall.

Veronica gradually became absorbed into our circle of friends. Our mutual relationship with Susan St Lawrence continued and we would go away for weekends together to Veronica's parents at West Green or to Lodsworth to see the Fletchers and Fiennes's. Susan, after a few months, married Robert Constable-Maxwell, and to this day they are living happily in Bosworth Hall, Lincolnshire.

One Saturday in late September, Veronica, Susan and I drove to Windsor Great Park. We had a picnic lunch on the side of the road, sitting under one of the park's large oak trees, which have since been cut down. We made an odd trio: me with my long-term platonic 'sister' of a girlfriend and the young ballerina with whom I was quietly falling in love. After lunch we all drove to Veronica's home, West Green Cottage, Hartley Wintney, Hampshire. This romantic cottage lay at the end of a narrow country lane, with farmland on one side and a common on the other, and had its own apple orchard. The drawing room led out through French windows to a patio, on which I would later spend many evenings having cocktails with the family. The house was beautifully furnished with antique furniture that Joy Langué had inherited from her parents. I received a very warm welcome.

Arvid Langué was then aged 61. He walked with a limp – a result of his war wounds – and spoke with a slight Russian accent. He was upright and very well preserved, with aristocratic features, round spectacles and thick grey hair. His wife Joy, some 16 years younger, shared Veronica's good looks. This was my first meeting with the family who would soon be part of my own. Our relationship started as it continued for the next 40 or so years. Never a cross word was exchanged between Arvid, Joy or myself. At that first lunch, Veronica's 10-year-old brother Charles tried to embarrass me by placing a whoopee cushion under my seat. The spontaneous peals of laughter from the family epitomized the easy atmosphere of the house.

Both sides of Veronica's family had an interesting history. Veronica's father was proud of his full name: Arvid Langué Querfeld von der Seedeck. The last part had been given to a Prussian general during the prolonged Franco-Prussian wars of the eighteenth century. Despite this Prussian ancestry, Arvid was very much a Russian and had an abiding love for his homeland and its people.

Arvid's father, Carlo, had had business interests in both Pskov and Riga. In 1905, he bought a leather factory and house in Pskov, which, among other items, produced the soft leather riding boots used by the Russian Imperial Cavalry. The factory employed more than 80 skilled workers, and although its profits were meagre it was a major contributor towards the prosperity of the city.

Their main residence was in Riga, then part of the Russian Empire and, until the outbreak of war in 1914, Carlo Langué was the Baltic States Consular General to Brazil. The property was requisitioned by the Germans and then given to the people in 1920 by the Bolsheviks, who controlled the Baltic States for a short time after the war. It later became the Russian Embassy in Riga.

During the calm before the storm that was to shatter Europe, the Langués lived a peaceful life and had four sons, Oscar, Werner, Arvid and Didio, and one daughter, Marguerite, whose lives so reflected the adversities of that generation.

Arvid was born in 1896 in Riga. At 16 he joined the military academy at Pskov and then the senior military academy in St Petersburg before joining the Imperial Russian Grenadier Guards. In the winter of 1914 he was sent to the Eastern Front, where his regiment was fighting the Germans, near the border between Warsaw and Minsk.

He was awarded the Order of St Stanislaus for bravery in 1915 and the Order of St George IV Class (the highest military order) for extreme bravery in 1916, and he was promoted to captain. Once again, the Grand Duke Nicholas presented the order in the Tsar's absence. The citation for the award read: 'For saving the battalion from encirclement; for penetrating the

German lines; destroying machine gun lines; taking prisoners and for starting a major retreat of the German army and so relieving Warsaw from the German advance.' In later years, these actions caused him untold grief.

After a two-month rest in Finland to replenish their losses, his battalion returned to the front near Minsk at the end of 1916. In March 1917, Tsar Nicholas II abdicated and a provisional government headed by Kerensky was formed. Despite the onset of the revolution, the regular army remained loyal and continued to fight the Germans. In July 1917, the Russian Army mounted one final initiative, known as the Kerensky Offensive. Little progress was made and after the Germans rushed reinforcements from the Western Front, the Russians retreated, the army revolted and the way was paved for the Bolshevik Revolution.

During this offensive, Arvid was injured with severe machine-gun wounds to his legs and a shrapnel injury to his right temple. In recognition of his bravery for 'personally leading his troops in rout of a superior enemy force', he was awarded the silver Cross of St George by the Duma. The medal was sent to him at the Old Imperial Hospital, Minsk, where he was being treated for his injuries. After the Russian surgeons had operated on his legs, although still gravely ill, he was allowed to return to the family home in Pskov.

When the success of the revolution became apparent, his parents and sister escaped to Riga but, as Arvid was too weak to move, he stayed alone in the house to await his fate. When the Germans finally reached Pskov, Arvid was captured and sent to a German military hospital at Bad Elster in Saxony. Pretending to be an injured German officer, he escaped from the hospital on crutches, carrying a large bottle of morphia. His desire to escape was fuelled by the knowledge that the terms of the Brest-Litovsk Peace Treaty between Germany and Bolshevik Russia included the repatriation of all White Russian prisoners of war, who would surely be shot on their return.

By some incredible means and despite his excruciating pain, Arvid managed to get to Denmark and then, at the invitation of the Imperial Russian Embassy in London, made his way to England. He was admitted to the Queen Alexandra Hospital for Officers, where he was intermittently an inpatient until the end of 1921. Between numerous operations, Arvid worked in the Imperial Russian Embassy in Chesham Place and became very involved with the Russian Red Cross. The embassy was closed and the Russian Red Cross disbanded after the British government's recognition of the Bolshevik Regime in 1921.

When Arvid first arrived in the UK, he contacted the Chance family and it was through their introductions that he was able to establish himself. The Chances owned Christie's Auctioneers and, mixing in their circle of friends, Arvid developed a new interest in antique furniture and old houses. He had a natural artistic ability and made a living refurbishing old houses. Arvid spent the winter months in the South of France, supplementing his income playing cards and roulette with other dispossessed White Russians.

General Chance's son Peter was at Eton College with Eric Cattley, who was invited for the weekend to the Chance's home, and took Arvid Langué with him. Peter had been invited to become better acquainted with Joy, Eric's beautiful 17-year-old sister. But as soon as Joy saw this exceptionally good-looking Russian war hero, she showed little interest in Peter. Thus started a relationship that would come to fruition only after several more years. The home had belonged to Reginald and his wife Marguerite before he passed away. This couple had lived for some years in the house. Although Reginald had lost two brothers and two nephews, his wife Marguerite was more fortunate in having one sister Edith Owen and one brother Sackville Owen. When they died, the house was left to their two children, Eric and his younger sister Joy. Eric was not yet 18, yet these two young people were allowed to enjoy the privileges of the house with its servants. It was to this house that Peter came with Arvid.

Despite his impeccable Russian background, Arvid, as the impecunious White Russian émigré, was considered unsuitable for Joy. The Cattley family trustees tried to prevent the continuance of this blossoming romance and sent Joy on a trip around the world, with a companion, to forget about Arvid. Joy then lived with her brother Eric and his new wife Hester in Grosvenor Square, London.

Love always finds a way to fire Cupid's arrow: Arvid and Joy met again, by chance, at a cocktail party. From then on, the passions of their love could not be extinguished and, despite continued reservations from the family and trustees, they finally married in 1934. Peter Chance was the best man and Joy's brother Eric gave her away.

They initially lived in a large country house, Mendom Abbey, in Norfolk, with their two large Alsatian dogs. This was not ideal, as they had no friends in that part of the country and were miles from London. So they returned to the Home Counties, where Arvid designed their new home in Dogmersfield, Hampshire, besides the Basingstoke Canal. Despite their happiness in Barley Mow House, they suffered many tribulations. Joy had numerous miscarriages and gave birth to a stillborn boy. Then the Second World War started and Arvid was called up into MI6 and sent to Evesham, Worcestershire. He was assigned to the decoding department on account of his knowledge of Russian, German and French. He sat alongside a great friend, Bruce Keith, who worked in the Japanese section. Here they monitored signals between Japan and Germany. One intercepted message contained information about the proposed Japanese attack on Pearl Harbour. The British Government was immediately contacted and the information was transmitted to the American government. As the world knows, the Americans took no action and the American Pacific Fleet was almost obliterated.

Arvid and Joy's happiness was fulfilled when their daughter Veronica was born on 12 March 1941. For their safety, shortly afterwards, Joy and Veronica were sent to Tenby, South Wales, to stay with an elderly aunt, Edith Owen. One day, during their stay in Wales, when the young Veronica should have been having her late-morning rest in her bed, a Polish RAF pilot, coming in at zero height over the sea, clipped a tree and crashed his crippled Spitfire into the aunt's house. Joy, watching from the High Street in Tenby, came rushing home, sure that her baby daughter had been killed. Thanks to the forgetfulness of the nanny, she was still playing in the garden, but the pilot lay dead on the bed and lying under him was Veronica's golliwog totally intact. After the war, in 1947, the Langués had a son, Charles, and they moved to West Green Cottage, Hartley Wintney.

CHAPTER 8
Moorfields – just the way it was

In 1958, John and I briefly spent Christmas with my father, now Sir Robert Arnott, and my Aunt Vickey. My father's fortunes had dramatically changed with the death of his brother Lauriston. He had sold Shearwater House and had bought Ounavarra, which overlooked the River Liffey in Lucan. It had a mile of river frontage along the Liffey and was opposite Lucan House, which was occupied by the Italian Embassy.

As Harold Ridley had promised, I became Resident Intern of Moorfields. This was in fact a misnomer, as I was only in residence two nights a week on casualty duty, seeing patients off the streets, or house duty, looking after the inpatients. Despite spending only two nights and every third weekend on duty, the weekdays from 8 am until 10 pm were exacting and busy.

The internship was for a period of two years spread into intervals of four months. The first four months were spent understudying the senior resident officer – a New Zealander, Lindsey Poole – who was responsible for the general medical running of the hospital. After four months, I graduated to casualty officer, which was an extremely strenuous role.

12 March 1959 was very special; I went to Veronica's 18th birthday party, given by her parents in Peter and Paddy Chance's house in Chelsea. The following weekend Veronica and I went to a point-to-point in Berkshire. As so often happened throughout my career, I was delayed in the hospital and we did not arrive until the last race. We later went for dinner at West Wycombe Park, the home of Sir Francis Dashwood, an old prep-school friend. Francis was now married to Veronica's cousin, my ex-girlfriend Victoria de Rutsen.

In April, I spent the first of a few wonderful weekends at Bodees, a small eighteenth-century cottage in East Sussex, on the opposite side of the estuary to Bosham, with my friends Gerard Dent, Charles Orme and 'Doc' Desmond Keogh. Bodees looked exactly like the cottage in *Snow White and the Seven Dwarfs*. It was perched on the edge of the mudflats in Bosham estuary and surrounded by a small orchard. To the right of the front door was a plaque with the inscription;

Kind hearts are the roots
Kind thoughts are the seeds
Kind words are the fruits
Kind acts are the deeds

This was meant as a sailing retreat, so a boat now had to be found. Fortunately the United Hospital Club was replacing its wooden racers with sleeker fibreglass boats, and we were able to buy an ancient clinker-built 17-foot sailing boat that was Bermuda-rigged, with a forward sail and mainsail spreading from the single mast. Instead of a conventional keel, it had a retractable centre plate made of heavy steel.

Siobhan, our ramshackle old tub, gave us all many hours of immense pleasure pottering around Chichester Harbour and the Solent. She looked a total wreck but had all that we needed. Charles and Doc, the more experienced sailors, took on the maiden sail in the estuary. As they lowered the rusty centreboard, it immediately dropped through the hull to rest in the mud at the bottom of Bosham Harbour. The boat, now totally uncontrollable, went spinning onto a mud bank.

After a new centreboard had been fitted, we sorted out the rigging and fittings. At high tide, we tied Siobhan alongside the Bosham jetty and proceeded to strip the boat down. No doubt we were a scruffy bunch. The harbour master, in his yachting cap, blue blazer and white trousers, immediately ordered us to remove our 'junk from the jetty' and move off. We complied, and Siobhan rested on the flats opposite our cottage, where at low tide she resembled a complete wreck.

Later that evening I had an inspiration. I remembered a connection between Aunt Vickey and the Earl of Iveagh, who owned most of the moorings in the Bosham estuary. The following weekend, I made a point of seeing the fierce Harbour Master, Commander Lannoway. I copied his dress, wearing a blue blazer and white trousers, and hoped that he did not recognize me. Luck was on my side. I introduced myself and asked if the earl had communicated with him about the possibility of a mooring. 'Indeed he has,' the Commander replied: 'His Lordship's boat is moored in the channel just off this jetty. There is another deep mooring nearby that you can have. How long is your boat – 10 or 20 metres in length?' I nodded and pointed across the estuary to our semi-derelict old boat, which at this time was looking its worst with the tide fully out. The commander groaned, but he could not go back on his word. We enjoyed the mooring for the season, but next year's mooring was not so close to the jetty.

When not sailing we would go for long walks along the bank of the estuary. The shoreline was studded with wrecks, including a Second World War midget submarine. Chichester harbour is renowned for its bird life, and we saw many rare species of birds. In the evening we often drank in the Anchor Bleu pub in Bosham. Here Rex Whistler did his last sketch, before being killed in the Normandy invasion in 1944. It depicted a gnome sitting astride a triple-star wooden casket of brandy.

My time in Bosham was limited, as my duties of casualty officer in Moorfields Eye Hospital were becoming more demanding. When Lindsey Poole, the senior resident officer, left in June 1959, I also became house officer for two consultants, Terry Perkins and Barry Jones. I had to admit, examine and discharge all the patients under their care, as well as attend each consultant's clinical session and two surgical sessions per week. Thus I learned from their ward rounds and their expertise in the operating theatre.

Mr Kapoor, the senior resident officer who preceded Lindsey Poole, was an Indian, and he decided to give Lindsey's leaving party in the residency at Moorfields and personally cooked a meal of culinary delicacies from the Indian continent. The dinner was an outstanding success. Retribution came in the morning, when every guest was confined to bed with acute abdominal colic. For the first time in the history of Moorfields Eye Hospital, the senior consultants of the hospital had to service both the casualty and inpatient sectors.

Each of the consultant surgeons had a very different personality and set of skills. Mr Perkins, who later became the first professor of research at Moorfields, loved gadgets. He constructed an instrument for measuring intraocular pressure that is still in use today. It was while working with Mr Perkins that I did my first cataract operation. After 10 years in medicine, I at last performed the operation that is the hallmark of our ophthalmic profession. All young ophthalmic surgeons record their surgical accomplishments by the number of cataract operations they have performed, although it is only one of many ophthalmic surgical procedures.

In the UK, it is, quite rightly, illegal to practise surgery on animals, and surgical skills have to be learned from operating on our patients. So consultants have the responsibility of not only treating their patients, but of teaching their residents how to operate on these very patients.

It is rather like learning to fly, with the flying instructor showing the pupil how to take off, fly and land the plane. After a period of time, the instructor will hand over to the student, but if a problem occurs he can regain command of the aircraft, as it is fitted with dual controls. But with surgery, there are no dual controls. Only one surgeon can operate and once the consultant has handed over, he can only give advice and can't actively interfere with the procedure. It is therefore a huge decision as to when an intern is considered safe to perform their first operation. I was always very grateful for the help given to me by my senior colleagues at this most important time in my life.

It is a strange feeling operating on a patient, knowing that his or her future sight is dependent on my actions over the next few minutes. The outcome of an operation must never be taken for granted, and total care and concentration must be applied throughout the whole procedure. Many surgeons are often as hyped up as athletes before a race, but in surgery the stakes are so much higher!

My other teacher at this time was Barry Jones, from New Zealand. He was clinical instructor to the interns, but later became professor of clinical studies at Moorfields.

That August I took my quarterly leave and travelled to Ireland to stay at Ounavarra with my father, Aunt Vickey and my cousin Johnnie French. Veronica had arranged things so she could stay with her cousin Sheila Dunsany at Dunsany Castle, County Westmeath. After the usual week at the Dublin

Horse Show, my holiday took a turn for the better. I had organized a tennis party at Ounavarra to which I had invited Veronica. This was the first time that she had seen the house, and together we walked through the newly cut hay in the fields below the house and along the River Liffey. The bees were buzzing among the wild flowers of the riverbank, and the occasional fish disturbed the surface of the water. It was a magical afternoon that was over too quickly.

The next day I started my duties in the fourth 'firm' at Moorfields. The three surgeons I now assisted were John Ayoub, Alex Cross and Arthur Leigh. John Ayoub had a great big beak of a nose and massive hands. His hobby was sailing and he seemed to be forever cleaning and painting his boat. After every weekend his fingernails were ingrained with black oil, which refused to shift even after the 10-minute surgical scrub. Many years later, I was impressed when he arrived at an ophthalmic meeting in Amsterdam, having crossed the North Sea in his own Norwegian-built boat. He became a great friend of mine and, when I finally became a consultant, was responsible for putting me on the staff of the Royal Masonic Hospital in Ravenscourt Park, London – one of the most prestigious appointments in London.

Alex Cross was the world's expert on tuberculotic conditions of the eye. He was a gentle unassuming man, who more resembled a priest than a surgeon, and was always generous with the amount of surgery he allowed his assistants to do under his guidance. On one occasion he allowed me to operate on a patient who had been blind with cataract and inflammation of the eyes for 20 years. The case was considered hopeless. I dissected through the scarred tissues and reached the cataractous lens, which, before it could be gripped with forceps, spontaneously floated towards the back of the eye. I rapidly picked up a scoop from the theatre trolley and passed it into the depths of the eye to retrieve the lens before it hit 'rock bottom' in the back of the eye, which it would have destroyed. I finalized the operation by putting in sutures to close the wound. That evening, I realized that this patient was developing an acute intestinal obstruction and arranged to have him immediately transferred to St Bartholomew's Hospital, where he underwent his second operation of the day – this time on his abdomen.

He recovered from both of these operations and, with sight restored, would sit by the window all day and gasp whenever a red London bus passed by. The press heard about this patient, and my name was in print for the first time in my professional life. Apparently, when he first saw his wife after the operation, he tactlessly said: 'Lord, love, how you've aged.'

The third surgeon I joined was Arthur 'George' Leigh, a small rotund man with an infectious laugh. He was a beautiful surgeon to watch: he specialized in corneal transplantation and cataract surgery. He taught me a great deal, and under his direction I performed my third cataract operation. When visiting the patient the next day, he took off the eye pad and examined the eye. Turning to his staff and visitors he said: 'This is the first cataract operation my intern surgeon has done with me and look at the magnificent result!' The patient's face was a mixture of relief and alarm at realizing the inexperience of the surgeon who had performed it!

At this time my ophthalmic surgical skills increased enormously. I also performed my first squint, glaucoma, corneal transplant and retinal-detachment operations. I felt such pride at doing them but was very aware that the consultant could probably have done them better. I was gradually starting to do more and more surgery without the supervision of my seniors. There was a great element of trust, and each intern was careful not to abuse the freedom or go beyond the barrier of their capabilities. In this way, NHS patients got the best treatment without an excessive wait for their operation, and everyone benefited. The consultants and their entrusted medical staff made all decisions about patient care. How much better this was than the present shambolic system, where patients have to wait on average over six months for a cataract operation and overseas doctors are being drafted in to reduce the waiting lists. Regrettably, consultants are no longer in control of their clinical lists. Instead these are monitored, doctored and fudged by administrators who do not understand the real needs of the patients.

Apart from my growing relationship with Veronica and my time-consuming duties at Moorfields, two other events occurred in late 1959: the purchase of a new car and the Christmas concert in Winchfield Village Hall.

My ancient Triumph Mayflower needed to be replaced. It was some 10 years old and my Great Uncle Loftus Arnott had just left John and myself a magnificent inheritance of £500 each, which enabled me to consider buying a new car. Veronica and I went to the Motor Show at Earl's Court, where quite the most beautiful car in our fairly meagre price range was the convertible Hillman Minx. I sold my Triumph Mayflower for £200 to my old school friend, Johnny Staniland, who had a car agency in Cirencester. He later told me that this had been a bad deal, as the car stayed in his showrooms for months. How much would this classic car be worth today?

On a cold clear Friday 10 days before Christmas, Veronica and I had one of the most memorable days of our life. In the morning I did a surgical list at Moorfields, but joy of joy, I was able to leave at 11 am. Picking up Veronica, we drove west in my ancient car. We stopped for lunch in Lechlade, where we sat oblivious to all those who were lunching around us. When we finally reached Johnny Staniland's garage, our new moonstone white Hillman, with red-leather upholstery and black roof was waiting for us. The car had elegance and beauty, which was in such contrast (with a few exceptions) to the blancmange moulds of today. With my little Scottie Dog mascot screwed onto the bonnet, we made our way back to the Langué's house, so Veronica could attend her last rehearsal for the Winchfield Christmas concert. I can still recall every detail of this drive.

We sat snugly in our new car, with the hood up, singing to the radio. We would have had no more pleasure in a brand new Rolls Royce.

The following Saturday was typical of the slightly dichotomous life most of us lead before settling into marriage. In the morning I operated at Moorfields and then went to a wedding at Sandhurst. After the reception I hot-footed it to the Langués, where I met up with Gerard Dent and his friend David Lord. Gerard known affectionately as 'G' had been one of my closest friends and a flatmate for many years. He was a Bertie Wooster character. We all pitched up at Winchfield Hall for the long-awaited Christmas show. Many of the Langué's family friends were there, including Miranda Marling, Veronica's best friend. Gerard and David gave their interpretation of 'There's a green eyed goddess to the west of Kathmandu,' with G's upper-class accent nearly bringing the house down. Following other sketches, Veronica performed 'The dance of the swans' from Tchaikovsky's Swan Lake. She looked so wonderfully beautiful, gliding over the small village hall stage as if her feet didn't touch the ground. Her performance was equal to that of any prima ballerina and was received with rapturous applause.

Towards the end of January 1960, I went to see my father in Ounavarra. On the overnight ferry crossing to Rosslare, I had a quick supper and realized as soon as I had done so that I had eaten a contaminated tomato with my grill, but I thought no more about it. On reaching Ireland, I drove north to Ounavarra. I had a pleasant few days doing little but talking to Father and going for walks with his adored dog Noely.

Noely was the daughter of Flossie and had been born in my bedroom at Frenchpark on Christmas Eve some few years previously. He looked as if he might have been half fox, which he probably was. As nobody wanted him, he was shipped off to Dulwich to live with Patricia Johnson, my cousin. Since Mother's premature death in 1948, Father's constant companion had been a dog called Lucky, who was the father of my dog Flossie. When Lucky died in 1958, Patricia kindly agreed to hand over Noely to father. Noely had a long journey from London to Ireland. He was put on the wrong plane at Heathrow, ended up in France and had to go into quarantine for six months. British Airways paid his quarantine expenses and gave a cheque for £50 to compensate for the lack of companionship. When Noely at last arrived at Ounavarra he became inseparable from Father. Noely lived to a ripe old age, and when he finally succumbed, Father survived him by only a few weeks. It is quite incredible the relationship that can grow between a lonely person and his dog.

On returning to London, I joined the third 'firm' at Moorfields. This time my surgeons were Jimmy Doggart, Henry Stallard and Pat Trevor-Roper.

Jimmy Doggart must be one of the most charismatic ophthalmic surgeons of all time, as well as a respected Latin and Greek scholar. He was a member of the Garrick Club and is portrayed in a painting of club members going to the 1954 Epsom Derby. As was his wont, he is shown in the forefront of the painting, wearing his straw hat and pontificating to other members of the club. Some years later I inherited his practice without any advance knowledge: he had suddenly sent me an Indian tea chest crammed full of his patient notes and an accompanying letter explaining that he had retired and wished me to continue to look after his patients.

He was a fine physician but not particularly interested in the surgical aspects of ophthalmology. In fact, he almost never attended the operating theatre. To my knowledge, the last time he actually set foot inside the theatre was when Bill Thornhill, as a rather too anxious resident at the end of the first day's ward round, turned to Jimmy and said: 'Well sir, I will now go and do the list.'

'You will indeed not,' replied Jimmy Doggart, who stormed into the operating theatre and proceeded with the list. Remembering this incident, after finishing my first ward round with him, I dutifully waited until he invited me to do his operating list. With his permission I entered the operating theatre to do my first full surgical list without the supervision of a consultant.

Henry Stallard, in his day, was arguably the best cataract surgeon in the world, as well as being the author of *Eye Surgery*, considered to be the world-wide standard textbook on ophthalmic surgery. Despite his surgical brilliance, he is probably best known for having been a member of the triumphant English athletics squad in the 1924 Paris Olympics and was one of the four runners in the film *Chariots of Fire*. Henry was rather pleased that his Olympic record for the 220-yard sprint was never challenged as this length was never run again.

His surgery was also a joy to watch, although he was of the 'old school' and insisted on complete silence with the theatre door locked. He operated with a slow, methodical, brilliance. When operating on the posterior confines of the eye, although still demonstrating expertise, his surgery became even more prolonged. During retinal operations the theatre lights had to be turned off, so the back of the eye could be examined with the retinoscope. On one occasion, when the lights were turned back on, the anaesthetist was found to be fast asleep.

Sadly one of his specialties at Moorfields cost him his life. He was in charge of putting cobalt plaques onto the surface of the eyes in children suffering from ocular cancer. He achieved remarkable success with this treatment, but unfortunately the radiation from these plaques gave Henry bone cancer. Henry Stallard was a great teacher and from him I learned much of my expertise in anterior-chamber ophthalmic surgery. It was wonderful to watch his surgery and then try to reproduce his results.

My third consultant teacher at this time was Pat Trevor-Roper, brother of Professor Hugh Trevor-Roper, the historical scholar who infamously authenticated Hitler's diaries before they were later found to be a hoax. Pat was also a keen historian who wrote several excellent textbooks on ophthalmology and its history. Some years after I was his surgical intern, he gave a prize lecture at a symposium, in which he likened my small-incision cataract surgery to 'the shooting of pheasants with guided missiles'. Such was the dogma and abysmal ignorance I encountered from so many of my peers when championing modern forms of cataract surgery. Despite our professional differences, we were good friends.

One week at around this time, having worked solidly for two weeks, I operated on a child of five who had received a severe perforating injury to his eye. This was a particularly complicated operation and I felt drained, so Veronica and I decided to leave London for the weekend. We drove, with the hood down, to Bodees Cottage, Bosham, where the Ormes and Doc Keogh greeted us. Our arrival made quite an impact. Veronica was blue from the cold, and I was yellow. I had developed jaundice – from the infected tomato I had eaten six weeks earlier on the crossing to Ireland. We immediately turned around and, feeling very despondent, drove back to London.

Being ill in a bachelor flat in central London would not have aided my recovery, so it was agreed that I should return to Ireland to convalesce. By the time I was tucked up in bed at Ounavarra, I began to feel really ill. I spent the next few weeks alone with Father. In the evening, while I clutched my aching liver and he smoked endless Players Navy Cut cigarettes, we chatted together as father and son. He reminisced about his horrors of the First World War and his own jaundice. We talked about his time at Cambridge University studying agriculture, his short venture into racing, which started so well and ended so disastrously, his latter years of misery and the companionship he had had since with his dogs. I realized with thanks to God that I had been given these few weeks to get to know my father, who had previously seemed so remote.

Before meeting Veronica, I had been very fond of one of my first girlfriends, Barbara Lloyd, who called herself 'Bar'. Veronica's nickname as a child was 'Barr', as it was one of her first baby words because of a bib she wore with a picture of a sheep on it. In my delirious jaundiced state, I spent some time on the phone in Ireland talking to the wrong Barr.

Every week Dr Dillon would come to examine me and say that I needed a further week's convalescence. Early in April, Veronica came to visit me and gave me a brown cable woollen jersey that she had knitted. From the moment she arrived my illness dramatically improved. In a few days I was well enough to drive for lunch at the Kildare Street Club. By the Saturday of that week my stamina had almost totally returned. Veronica and I spent a romantic day driving out to Powerscourt, County Wicklow, in John's new MGA car, to sit by the famous waterfall. I spent several more days convalescing in Veronica's company, before she had to leave me to visit the other love of her life, Patrick Hodson. Despite the fact that Patrick proposed to her at this time, I felt no jealousy towards him. I had known and respected him as a friend for many years.

Fact is stranger than fiction. After leaving the Hodsons, Veronica returned to Ounavarra and brought with her another of her boyfriends, Peter Dawney, who I also knew. I was sure he was no real threat, as he had the unfortunate habit of being sick every time he took Veronica out to dinner. We all drove to Howth Castle for the wedding of Robert Constable-Maxwell to Susan St Lawrence in my father's old Ford Consul, which broke down on the way to the wedding. I got my guests to the service, but missed it myself, waiting for the car to be repaired. I did make it to the reception, which seemed to be attended by all of Ireland.

By the end of April, our spring solstice was almost coming to an end. Yet we had one more memorable day in Ireland. We went to the Punchestown Races, one of the best cross-country race courses in the world, with its unique setting, some 30 miles from Dublin, and in the evening attended a large dinner party at the Shelbourne Hotel. The owner, Peter Jury, was hosting the party and, as a joke, had been told that one of the guests was a world-famous prima ballerina. He hailed her as the guest of honour and placed her next to him at dinner. Poor Peter was slightly surprised to see that Veronica, the prima ballerina, was obviously still in her teens.

Two days later, my jaundice and a wonderful few weeks behind me, I returned to Moorfields, where I had been barely missed. Gordon Krolman had to reluctantly relinquish his elevated status on my return. Gordon was a Canadian from Winnipeg, already married to a beautiful woman, Maureen. I had first met him when he was a fellow student studying for the Primary FRCS in Lincoln's Inn Fields. Gordon and his wife became my closest friends. He arrived from Winnipeg speaking in a broad Canadian accent, but after a few weeks attained a very distinctive BBC accent, which would disappear whenever he returned home.

Gordon was an Anglophile at heart and had the largest Jaguar car then available on the UK market. After he had completed his residency at Moorfields he returned to Winnipeg, just as a new professor was to be appointed in the chair of the ophthalmic hospital. As so often happens, the private sector could not agree with the public about the choice of applicant until Gordon returned home. Impartial to either side, he was immediately offered the chair. With his impeccable Moorfields training, he was a very successful professor and brought many innovations into Winnipeg.

Friday 6 May 1960 was the day when Princess Margaret married Tony Armstrong-Jones. That morning I did an operating list with Henry Stallard and returned home to find Veronica and my flatmate, Tony Tisdell, huddled closely together on the sofa watching the royal wedding on TV. Nothing was amiss, yet I felt it was time for us to frankly review our relationship. Veronica and I walked into Kensington Gardens and sat on a bench overlooking the Round Pond. We said virtually nothing to each other, but I think we both realized that a mutual bond was being tied.

During the following week I managed to see Veronica on my two evenings off duty and on the next Saturday we planned a weekend away. Veronica packed my weekend bag – the first time a girl had ever done this for me. We drove to Virginia Water and walked through the woods to the Indian

Pogo Sticks, eventually arriving at West Green Cottage rather later than we had planned. After a quick change, we went to dinner with Sir John and Lady Marling, whose daughter Miranda was one of Veronica's closest friends. Veronica, in a stunning, full-length, blue-silk cocktail dress, with great pride took the driving seat. Despite our not being officially engaged, there seemed to be a festive atmosphere in the air and we all became rather merry! Later, Arvid drove us home in his ancient Austin car. He was still enjoying the evening enormously and took us on a merry-go-round tour of the local petrol stations on the way home.

On Sunday, Veronica and I drove her brother Charles back to his boarding school near Amersham. We stayed for the morning service, and I was mesmerized by the bright sun streaming in through the windows directly onto Veronica in a blue and white polka-dot dress, which caused amazing flickering shadows on the aisle and pews – the dancing lights of spring. After the service, we gave the headmaster and his Alsatian dog a lift back to the school. We had a wonderful picnic on the grass, while Charles played in the wood, and then hired a rowing boat at Pangbourne. Charles was not an accomplished oarsman and we made very little progress. Every few yards we would bump into the bank, which caused us much amusement. On returning Charles to his school, we were driving across Pangbourne Bridge, over the River Thames, when I turned to Veronica and said: 'Isn't it about time we got married?'

Despite this unromantic proposal being made with Veronica's younger brother listening to every word, she accepted.

The next day I rushed to Lambert and Harman in Bond Street, just before they closed for the night. I collected the family sapphire ring, which had been given to our family by the Williams, of Carhays, 100 years earlier. This had a large blue sapphire stone, guarded on either side by a diamond, and was so cleverly constructed that it was difficult to see how the stones had been set into the ring. It had been my grandmother's engagement ring and also my mother's.

I gave Veronica the ring, and we immediately had an impromptu party with John, Gerard Dent, John and Ger Powell and Hubert and Joyce Morris, who, on hearing the news, had all rushed over to join us. At one o'clock in the morning, John and I went to the Jacaranda Club to collect more 'fizz'. At two I drove Veronica back to her flat before spending the rest of the night in Moorfields.

The following morning I was scheduled to assist Pat Trevor-Roper in the operating theatre. He kindly invited me to perform the surgery, while he assisted. This was the only time in my whole career that I declined to operate, as I was suffering from a bad hangover. Pat was very sympathetic.

It was almost a week before we could have our first evening alone, when we dined in the Candle Light Room at the Mayfair Hotel, Piccadilly. We danced to a Caribbean steel drum band and watched a South Seas-style cabaret. There are a few times when you are young and in love when you can escape the restrictions of this world and find a different level, where love and trust take on a new dimension. This was one of those times, and we realized that our feelings towards each other were as much spiritual as sexual. We left the Mayfair Hotel at midnight and drove slowly home along the river embankment to Old Court Mansions, where we talked until 3 am. Veronica slept in John's bedroom, as he was away for the night.

Our brief courtship came to a temporary halt the following day, when Veronica had to honour a contract with the Swedish Ballet Company in Stockholm. She had given me a premature birthday present of an Asprey's alarm clock, which to this day is on my bedside table. Together we had lunch in our favourite restaurant, Nan's Pantry, and I was left miserable, watching her train leave for the ferry to Stockholm. With nothing better to do, I drove down to Bodees, our cottage in Bosham, for the night. On the drive down to the coast, I used the time to compose a letter in my mind to Barbara Lloyd. It was a very difficult letter to write, as she was one of the few other girls with whom I had enjoyed a great friendship and I was anxious not to hurt her, particularly as her father was recovering from a heart attack. Later I wrote the first of many letters to Veronica.

During these few weeks I was kept very busy at Moorfields, along with my fellow interns Neil Dallas, Peter Rycroft, Gordon Krolman, Anthea Connel, John Cairnes and Peter Watson. I frequently visited Veronica's parents at West Green and they would come to dinner in London. Taking out girlfriends was now a thing of the past.

Meanwhile, Veronica had very little to do during the day in Stockholm. Her colleagues wasted no time in meeting Swedish men and three of her company had received marriage proposals in as many weeks. The work, although enjoyable, was exacting, with performances every night of the week. During one show everything went wrong and all the girls ended up in the middle of the stage, doubled up in laughter. The audience loved it, and fortunately the management turned a blind eye.

Veronica was asked to become the lead dancer, but she had already made up her mind to return home as soon as she could. She wrote to me saying she would not stay away from me, even if she was offered the part of the 'principal dancer in the Bolshoi'.

Eight weeks later she came home, and we celebrated with her parents by going to see Lionel Bart's musical *Oliver!* followed by dinner at the 400 nightclub.

Thus started for us what must be one of the most wonderful periods in the life of any couple – the limbo period between the engagement and the wedding. So much had changed in six months. Veronica was now my constant companion and no longer the girl whose attention I was vying for against other equally amorous suitors. On a trip to Ireland we spent some of our time at Ounavarra and the remainder driving around the west of Ireland. On our first night we drove towards the Wicklow Mountains to have dinner with Denny and Hillary Wardell at their house Tullygobbin. With typical Irish hospitality, they had organized a surprise party of all our greatest Irish friends. The next day we went to the races at Phoenix Park Racecourse, which drew a record attendance. The president of Ireland, Shaun T O'Kelly, the Lord Mayor of Dublin and the British ambassador were all introduced to Veronica.

I wanted to show Veronica Frenchpark. The once-magnificent Palladian house was now a scene of devastation. There was no roof or floors. The basement, however, remained intact, and we were able to walk along the lower corridor throughout the whole length of the house. We walked past the derelict stone kitchen and scullery and climbed up the stairs, down which John, Francis and I had once rather cruelly launched Mrs Despard, the elderly cook, on a tray. Standing in the hall and looking up, we could see only the sky, where previously the large crystal chandelier had hung from the carved ceiling.

We then went on to Galway, getting very lost on the way. We joined Dennis and Hillary Wardell with our hosts, her parents the Palmers. The weather was ideal for Veronica's tour: showers interspersed with sunshine. The four of us drove from Glenlow Abbey to Galway and then to the Bloss-Lynches house in Ballinrobe. One of the Bloss-Lynche's ancestors was Judge Lynch, who was famous for committing his own son to be hanged. This macabre event gave rise to the term 'lynching', when a furious mob from Galway hung the judge on his own petard. After lunch, we took the coast road past CroaghPatrick Mountain, from where legend has it St Patrick banished all snakes from Ireland.

That evening we went with the Wardells and Palmers to the Twelve Pins Inn for dinner, which was thick with the smells of pipe smoke and Guinness. During the course of the evening everyone became more and more 'merry' and the conversation ever bawdier. Veronica was still only 19 and totally unprepared for the excesses of an Irish night out. We left the party early with a rather distressed Veronica wondering whether or not she would ever be able to cope with my Irish life.

By the following morning all was forgiven but never forgotten. This was the only time during our engagement that we had any dissent.

That morning I took Veronica to experience a mass in Galway. Being Protestants, we couldn't understand a word of the Latin service, but it was very uplifting. Then I showed Veronica Connemara, which at all times of the year is a verdant green. We held hands to walk up a small mountain and laid two stones on the pile already there, marking the success of previous climbers. We sat for an hour on the peak, admiring the panoramic view of one of the most beautiful scenes in the world.

We stopped to have lunch at Dunsany, where Charles was staying, and our last two days were spent with my father, during which time we had dinner at Brooklawn with Beecher and Sammy Somerville-Large.

CHAPTER 9
Sir Harold Ridley and fellow inventors

As the second resident surgical officer at Moorfields, I was assistant to Arthur Lister, Cyril Dee-Shapland and Harold Ridley.

Arthur Lister had been my saviour some few years earlier, when I had had my altercation with Sir Stephen Miller during the Diploma of Ophthalmology exam. He was the grandson of Professor Joseph Lister, who had introduced the concept of antiseptics in the 1870s. His recognition of the need for hygiene and sterility in the operating theatre was instrumental in reducing the incidence of postoperative infections that accounted for the death of more than 45% of all patients recovering from amputations. He was one of the greatest pioneers in medicine of all time. Arthur Lister upheld his family tradition. He was a perfectionist, with an almost obsessive need to perform perfect surgery on his patients. He drove an ancient open-top Lagonda V6, and he often would stop halfway on his journey home and return to once again inspect the patients on whom he had operated only minutes before.

Cyril Dee-Shapland was already 60 years old and close to retirement. He came from a military family and his brother was a famous general. Cyril believed in strict discipline, as a result of which his interns found him very demanding. I always considered him a surgeon who required only to be pandered to, and I much enjoyed working with him.

He always wore a frock coat, liberally splattered with remnants of food, and grey pinstriped trousers – the garb of a previous generation. Cyril was very keen on salmon fishing. Each summer he would take a rod on a river accompanied by two elderly friends, Colonel Sanders and an ophthalmic colleague Mr Moffat. On one occasion, Cyril parked his ancient Lagonda in a farmyard and the three friends walked down a valley to the river. At the end of the day's fishing they climbed back up the hill and came upon a bull in a field. Cyril and the colonel took a circuitous route around the field to avoid it. But Moffat, showing no fear, strode through the field and was chased the whole way up the hill by this charging bull. He eventually reached the safety of the farmyard and sank exhausted onto the front seat of the car. Cyril, after relieving himself against the wall of a farmyard building, turned around to find that his friend had died from a heart attack. In some respects, this may be the best way to pass on from this world, painlessly, having spent the day enjoying one's favourite pastime.

Following the lead set by Professor Gonin in the 1920s, when he became the first surgeon to successfully treat a retinal detachment, Cyril was responsible for making important improvements to the procedure. The retina is the light-sensitive concave inner layer of the eye. When holes develop in this fine membrane, the fluid in the centre of the eye will pass through them and lift the retina away from the choroid, the overlying layer of tissue to which it is bound. It is analogous to stripping wallpaper. When this happens, as the retina detaches, the patient experiences progressive loss of the visual field, like the tide of the sea coming in and covering the sand.

Professor Gonin realized that these holes could be sealed by heat thermocoagulation, and in some cases his treatment was successful. Cyril Dee-Shapland thought that a contributory factor in retinal detachments could be that the stretching of the overlying coat of the eye caused these holes to appear in the retina. He perfected an operation in which an elliptical strip of the outer coat of the eye was removed, thereby releasing the tension on the retina. This scleral resection was performed over the area of the reti-nal hole. In the bed of this elliptical area, he placed the thermocoagulation that had been the basis of Gonin's operation. I assisted Cyril at dozens of these operations, and his success rate was very high. This combination of Gonin and Shapland's operation brought real relief and restoration of sight to thousands.

Cyril Dee-Shapland would do several retinal-detachment operations, each taking up to two hours, on every one of his operating lists. These extended surgical sessions overlapped his clinics and, during the four months that I worked with him, he never once entered the outpatients department. His presence in his clinics was not really required, as he had an outstanding senior clinical assistant, Dr Johnny Mallet, who was not interested in performing surgery but very ably managed Cyril's outpatient sessions.

Johnny Mallet had been a resident surgeon at Moorfields during the Second World War and was on duty the night a bomb hit the hospital. He helped to rescue patients from the blitzed portion of the building. Every Tuesday he shadowed Cyril from Moorfields Hospital to the Brompton, being not only medical assistant but also unofficial chauffeur. He had to wait for hours while Cyril completed his operating session and finally, in desperation, he hatched a scheme designed to break this habit. On a cold winter's day with ice and snow on the roads, he drove Cyril between hospitals in his open-top Lagonda. When they arrived Cyril stepped out of the car and said: 'Dear Boy, what fun. Let's do that again.'

I was doing a ward round with Cyril Dee-Shapland when he was called away to an administrative meeting. He was gone for only a few minutes. When he rejoined me, he was in tears. The chairman of the medical board had advised him that if he did not pay more attention to his outpatient clinic, he would be asked to resign. This shabby treatment was typical of the way our country rewards those who have done the most for it.

The third surgeon I worked with was Harold Ridley, inventor of the artificial intraocular lens, whom history will judge to have been the most influential British ophthalmic surgeon of the twentieth century, second only to Sir Stewart Duke-Elder.

When I joined him in August 1960, he was a senior consultant at both St Thomas' and Moorfields but as yet had not found world fame. Rather to the contrary, many senior consultants in both hospitals were openly critical of his work.

Nicholas Harold Lloyd Ridley can remember sitting on Florence Nightingale's lap shortly before she died at the age of 90 in 1910. Harold's most famous ancestor was Nicholas Ridley, Bishop of Rochester, who was burnt at the stake for heresy in 1555 during the reign of Queen 'Bloody' Mary.

At the age of 31, in 1938, Harold was made the youngest ever consultant at Moorfields. He immediately became a 'terrier', yapping at the heels of his senior colleagues. Harold had a mission to ensure that the Moorfields' staff was of the highest calibre – both in ability and integrity. This would account for his future influence on the appointment of the resident surgical officers, including my own many years later.

When Harold joined the staff, consultants held an honorary appointment and were not paid for their services. If a consultant did not feel like going to the hospital on a particular day, the surgical resident officer would deal with the outpatient and operating sessions. Some of the consultants rarely, if ever, went to the hospital to see their outpatients, and others did virtually no surgery. Harold Ridley lost no time making it clear to his colleagues and the board of governors that consultants who did not fulfil their commitments should be encouraged to leave. The young Harold was taking on the establishment and made some very powerful enemies. Among these was Sir Stewart Duke-Elder, the doyen of world ophthalmology, who had been a consultant since 1929. Harold's changes in the working practices were very instrumental in his resignation from the hospital in 1938.

When the Second World War started in September 1939, most surgeons remained in their civilian appointments until called up, which, in many instances, could be deferred for months or even years. Harold Ridley carried on as a consultant at Moorfields until 1941. He was there during the Battle of Britain, where he was in charge of the emergency services that dealt with the eye problems of the military and civilian casualties. Although Harold treated several pilots who had suffered eye injuries, the actions of only one pilot, who inadvertently formulated the history of lens implantation, are fully documented.

15 August 1940 was the day that the Battle of Britain began to be won by the RAF, with the Luftwaffe suffering massive losses. Flight officer 'Mouse' Cleaver was one of the 'few' who helped Britain to this eventual victory. In his late twenties, Mouse was considered rather elderly to be a fighter pilot. Having been brought up with planes on an estate in Ireland, it was only natural that he

would join the elite '601' City of London Squadron. This squadron contained a number of well-known society names of that time, including Max Aitkin and Prince Macintosh. They were equipped with Hawker Hurricane fighter planes, as at this stage in the conflict there were only a few Spitfires.

On that day in August, '601' squadron took off from their base and rallied over Goodwood Park, West Sussex, to be as close as possible to the South Coast, thus minimizing the time required to intercept the enemy. There was a scramble for action in the early afternoon, but it was a false alarm. The pilots landed again and went into the officers' mess for tea, before being almost immediately alerted for another take-off.

Mouse ran to his plane and, jumping into the cockpit, instinctively pulled out the choke before firing the engine. In his rush for a quick take-off, he had forgotten that the choke floods a warm engine and there was no way the engine would fire. He was hurriedly given a brand new Hurricane that had been delivered only the day before. As he climbed into the unmarked Hurricane, he realized that he had left his flying goggles in his other plane. He carried on, without goggles, thinking that it would be just another routine patrol. It was not. The squadron found a dozen Junkers JU-88 bombers coming in over Selsey, and the clash developed into a frantic chase towards Salisbury Plain.

Cleaver's plane was hit by cannon shell from the bombers' escort, which he had not seen. The canopy of his plane was shattered, and fragments of it entered both eyes. Now totally blind, he had the incredible sensation of being in a fully functional fighter plane and being unable to control it.

He had no option but to bail out, but how? He had to turn the plane upside down in order to fall out of the cockpit. Misjudging the angle, he hit his left shoulder on the plane's rudder, but thankfully his parachute opened and he landed on a farm near Twyford. His troubles were not yet over. Blinded and in appalling pain, he was confronted by angry farmers who prodded him with their pitchforks. It took a little time for Mouse to convince them that he was a British not German pilot. Official war records state that Cleaver landed his own plane, which was actually true, as it was the new unmarked Hurricane that crashed.

He later came under the care of Harold Ridley, as his eyes were riddled with plastic fragments. Over the next year Harold performed 17 operations on his eyes. The right eye never saw again, but Harold's brilliant expertise saved the sight of his left eye, and Mouse Cleaver was able to return to a normal civilian life. His one seeing eye had a small scar on the cornea and a hole in the iris through which a small piece of plastic had passed before entering the lens. Some 50 years later a cataract developed in this eye, and I performed a cataract operation, replacing one piece of plastic with another!

The relationship between Mouse Cleaver and Harold Ridley changed ophthalmology forever. Before Mouse's severe injuries, it was considered that any retained material in the eye, would over time destroy the eye due to the immune process of the body. Harold Ridley learnt that these fragments of plastic remained harmless, unless they had a sharp edge which could cause mechanical damage. Thus, eight years later, he developed one of the outstanding innovations in medicine – the intraocular lens to replace that lost at cataract extraction.

Shortly before going overseas with the forces, Harold married Elisabeth Wetherill, a voluntary nurse, which started a most perfect marriage that would last for the next 60 years. Sir Stewart Duke-Elder was put in charge of deciding who went where and, maybe still holding a grudge about his resignation from Moorfields, he dispatched Harold to Ghana in West Africa – the remotest outpost of the war.

There, with little to do, Harold put his fertile mind towards solving another of mankind's great problems – onchocerciasis, or 'river blindness,' which caused millions of people to go blind. While on two weeks leave in Ghana, he borrowed a three-ton army truck in order to visit a missionary doctor, Tripp Saunders, who had many blind patients in his clinic. The road to this remote station was blocked by a large fallen tree. As he was about to abort his mission, an identical truck drew up on the other side of the tree. After some negotiation, they exchanged number plates, turned around and proceeded on their respective journeys. Harold spent the next two weeks screening patients and taking samples for subsequent analysis. He examined the eyes of the blind patients with the aid of a slit-lamp microscope, which was powered by the lorry battery carried on the shoulder of one of the native staff. His subsequent paper entitled 'Ocular onchocerciasis' became a cornerstone for future treatments and research.

Harold enjoyed his war years in this remote area. Sir Stewart Duke-Elder had unwittingly scored a home goal: what was meant to be a sentence turned out to be another triumph for Harold. In late 1942, Harold was posted to India and in 1945 to Burma, where he helped in the treatment of allied prisoners of war. At the end of the war, Harold returned to the Hospital for Tropical Diseases, and later he received his most cherished appointment as ophthalmic consultant to St Thomas'.

Fortune smiled on him again one day as he was travelling back from a weekend with his family in Wales. His children had begged him to take the later train, but he persisted in leaving early as he had to operate on the Monday morning. The later train to London crashed, and the sleeper compartment that Harold would have been in was totally destroyed. If he had been in it, he would almost certainly have been killed.

The Ridleys spent most of their weekends in a tiny thatched cottage by the River Wyle in Stapleford, where Harold enjoyed fly-fishing and later retired to this retreat. There we would often reminisce about our lives and careers. He once told me that his children found this constant shift from the Harley Street house in the city to the country quite difficult, as they were always missing out on parties. Harold was conscious of the debt he owed Elisabeth for bringing up his family and regretted that he had not spent enough time with his children during their development. As so often happens to those who are totally dedicated, the job comes first and the children suffer. Yet despite this, all the Ridley children have made their mark in life.

Harold Ridley's contributions to ophthalmology might have ended here had it not been for a chance encounter with a medical student on a ward round of St Thomas' Hospital in 1947. He was discussing a patient who had just had the cataractous lens of the eye removed, when the student asked: 'Sir, why don't you replace the cataractous lens with an artificial lens?' Harold looked at the student and said: 'A good question. I don't know why.' This simple remark triggered a chain reaction in Harold's mind. Why indeed not put a new lens implant over the empty lens bag, behind the pupil, after the cataractous lens had been removed? The concept seemed simple and Ridley already knew that the acrylic plastic he'd seen in the airmen's eyes, during World War II, had remained inert. Harold sought the help of John Pike, an optician from Rayner Optical Company, in East Sussex.

The story goes that they sat in a car in Cavendish Square, London, and brainstormed the principles of a new operation. Their initial thoughts were that implanting a lens into the eye would be too complicated for many surgeons and that the technology available could not support the procedure (at the time, many ophthalmic departments were still equipped with nineteenth-century instruments and medications). Nonetheless, they contacted ICI, which had manufactured the plastic canopy for the Hurricane and Spitfire fighter planes. Dr John Holt of ICI was very supportive of the project and produced a 'clinical quality' modification of the polymethyl methacrylate (PMMA) material, which remained the principal substance used for implants for the next 40 years.

Throughout 1948, these three men developed the first artificial lens implant. Harold had a considerable problem finding patients who were prepared to allow him to use their eyes for his first experiments. Eventually, one woman and one man volunteered, and we owe to these two brave Londoners deep gratitude. It was evident from the beginning that this revolution, rather than evolution, in cataract surgery would meet with serious criticism from the established medical community.

Two decisions were made to improve the chance of the new procedure being accepted. First, it was resolved to keep the project secret for two years to establish long-term success. Second, it was decided to make the work purely scientific and non-commercial. This demonstrated, once again, Harold's high altruistic ideals. In the early years of lens implantation, the three originators kept to their pledge and none of them received any financial gain. Rayner produced the implants at cost price, and the operations were performed without fee under the umbrella of the British NHS. The first implant operation was performed at St Thomas' on 29 November 1949. The operation was performed in two surgical stages to allow the eye to heal after the initial procedure. In the first instance, the cataractous lens was removed using the extracapsular technique. Some weeks later, a biconvex lens implant was inserted through the pupil and placed on the capsular bag of the old lens. To ensure total secrecy, even the theatre book was not properly written up.

Throughout 1950, Harold proceeded with extreme caution and only implanted a further three lenses, although during the year he devised a means of calculating the required dioptic power of the lens implant, which had caused earlier patients' vision to be overcorrected. The secrecy of this project lasted 18 months until, in 1951, a happy patient decided to have his other eye done privately. Inadvertently, he made an appointment with Frederick Ridley instead of Harold, who disclaimed any knowledge of the 'marvellous operation'. He redirected the patient to Harold Ridley with the comment 'a truly beautiful result' and at the same time strongly advised Harold to publish his results before someone else heard of the technique. Harold was thus forced to proclaim his research, and he read his first paper entitled, 'Intraocular acrylic lenses', on 9 July 1951 at the Oxford Ophthalmologic Congress. At the presentation of the paper, which should have been entitled 'The cure of aphakia' (aphakia meaning without a lens), two of Harold's patients attended to demonstrate their delight with artificial lenses. One eminent British ophthalmologist, whom Harold had hoped would support him, famously refused to even look at the eyes, and a leading American surgeon rushed out of the room in indignation. The reception was generally hostile. Harold was distressed to hear the same verdict delivered at meetings in Chicago and later in Buenos Aires. Despite his good results, he was told that the operation was reckless and 'should never have been done, as it offended the first principle of ophthalmic surgery, that a foreign body should not be inserted into the eye.'

In spite of the criticism, the project continued, and a small number of surgeons started testing Harold's technique. These included Peter Choyce in the UK, Edward Epstein in South Africa, Cornelius Binkhorst in Holland and Joaquin Barraquer at the Barraquer Clinic in Spain. Fredrick Ridley, the man who inadvertently forced the early publication of Harold's results, was also among the early pioneers to implant these lenses, which at this time cost one guinea. In 1951, John Winstanley joined Harold Ridley at St Thomas' Hospital and worked with him for the next 30 years, progressing from house officer to senior registrar, followed by a period as his chief clinical assistant at Moorfields Eye Hospital. Finally, for the past 10 years of this period, he was with Harold Ridley at St Thomas' Hospital as a consultant ophthalmic surgeon. During this time, John Winstanley was able to witness, at first hand, the trials and tribulations Harold Ridley underwent, with his colleagues, in trying to perfect his invention.

At the Chicago Ophthalmologic Society meeting in March 1952, Harold met Warren S Reese, one of America's most illustrious surgeons. Warren, after serving in the Army Medical Corps, had joined the Wills staff in 1920 and became a 'chief attending surgeon' in 1939. The Wills Hospital 'for the relief of the indigent blind and lame' had opened in 1934 and is named for

James Wills Jr, a Philadelphia grocer, whose legacy established the hospital. In the early 1950s, the unofficial management of this hospital was in the hands of a group of these 'chiefs,' each of whom was in charge of his own service and not answerable to anyone. Having been given a few lens implants by Harold Ridley, Warren Reese immediately flew back in his private plane to Philadelphia. The next day, 18 March 1952, with the assistance of his colleague Dr Turgut N Hamdi, he became the first American to perform a cataract operation with the insertion of an implant. His operation was identical to that of Harold's. Thus started a programme at Wills Eye Hospital that would continue for the next 15 years. The following weekend they implanted the second intraocular lens, on live television, at the fourth annual conference of Wills Eye Hospital. During most of the subsequent operations, Hamdi would be at the patient's head and Reese at the side, constantly talking to the patient in a very soothing voice.

It was at the American Association of Ophthalmologists' meeting in Chicago later that same year that Harold had received the criticism from his American colleagues – after he had presented his work on lens implantation and produced a film of the procedure and a patient who had had the operation. At this same meeting, Hamdi presented the results of the nine operations performed up to that time at Wills. The American and British results were very complementary to each other: 63% of Harold's patients achieved 20/30 vision or better compared with 64% of Reese's. Hamdi reported excellent results in the Reese/Hamdi operations in eight out of nine patients. Following this meeting, Harold and Warren struck up quite a relationship. They communicated regularly and met on several subsequent occasions. It must have meant a lot to Harold to have an ally such as Warren Reese in America. While several other American surgeons ordered Harold's lenses, most implanted only a few and some none. Warren Reese was, like Harold, an exceptional individual. They were able to challenge the establishment of their profession if right seemed to be on their side. Both had incredible surgical dexterity, with the ability to perform, by the standards of the day, a near-perfect cataract operation before the insertion of the implant. When Warren Reese took up the banner of lens implantation in America, he was already aged 60. Some two years later in 1954, his active operating career came to an end when he became blind in one eye from a central retinal arterial occlusion. From that time on, he could only act as assistant at any operation. His partner Hamdi continued to insert the original biconvex Ridley–Rayner PMMA lens until 1957, when he decided that: 'the weight of the lens was a sufficient disadvantage. Some 25% of implanted lenses dislocated, at some time in the postoperative period, through the posterior capsule into the back of the eye. On account of that, a different style of lens is required.' Hamdi chose an alternative path, along with many other surgeons, by changing to other designs of implants. Walter Reese remained faithful to Harold and his original lens and had his later surgery performed by Dr Cyril Luce, who continued to use this lens until 1967.

When good results were reported in Harold's practice in the UK, many patients were keen to have the operation and many elected to have surgery on both eyes. Over the next few years, many hundreds of implant operations were performed. As with any new surgical procedure, complications could occur. In the early days of lens implantation, the lenses were stored in cetyltrimethyl-ammonium bromide (cetavlon). Although these lenses were irrigated with saline before their insertion into the eye, some of the cetavlon could remain adherent to the surface of the implant and cause a severe postoperative inflammatory reaction in the eye. Frederick Ridley again came on the stage by formulating a safe sterilizing solution, which resolved this situation. Another problem that could occur with these lenses was that, being some 10 times heavier than current models, they at times broke through the posterior capsule of the lens bag to drop back into the vitreous cavity of the eye. Harold Ridley felt that modifications would have to be made with the operation, particularly with reference as to where the implant should be secured in the eye. In Harold's original operation, the simple biconvex lens implant was placed in the position from which the cataractous lens had been removed.

During the latter part of the 1950s, Harold Ridley, along with other pioneering implant surgeons such as Peter Choyce, decided to place the implant lens in front of the pupil rather than behind it. The introduction of the anterior chamber implant caused, in the long term, more problems than it cured. Other early modifications included attaching nylon loops to the lens. These loops fixed the implant in the recess of the anterior chamber of the eye. One surgeon in Barcelona implanted 500 such lenses into the anterior chamber of the eye. After two years, the nylon loops started to biodegrade and many eyes were lost.

Harold Ridley made one other major contribution to science. With the Marconi Company, he assisted in the development of closed-circuit television, so that ophthalmic operations could be viewed on the television screen.

The ophthalmic establishment was still resistant, and by the time I joined him in 1960, lens implantation was in the doldrums, with only a few surgeons in the world performing the operation. In the face of almost universal opposition, Harold had not lost any of his infectious enthusiasm for this operation. By this time, he had reverted back to his original biconvex posterior-chamber lens and, despite the comparatively poor manufacturing capabilities, surgical instruments and operative techniques, he still managed to achieve high levels of patient satisfaction, mainly because of his incredible dexterity.

He was not perturbed if a patient's implant dislocated into the posterior segment of the eye, as the material was inert and little damage would be done to the eye. On one occasion I was assisting him at an operation on a paratrooper. It was important that this patient retained his binocular vision (the vision of the two eyes being used together) so that he could keep his job in the army. Harold had already implanted two lenses on previous operations, both of which were now lying in the patient's vitreous cavity, having been previously dislocated. Harold was now inserting yet another implant. I said to him: 'He will now almost be able to play poker-dice, with his three implants.' Harold was not amused. Despite the magnitude of the surgery that Harold was doing, I cannot recall a single visitor ever attending his operations; yet with every one, I was witnessing history in the making. I learned a great deal about lens implantation at this time. It was apparent that this was the way forward, although it was equally apparent that if a surgeon of inadequate skills performed this operation, problems could occur.

Before one operating session, Harold walked into the operating theatre and strode over to the surgical instrument cabinet. He took out an expensive pair of surgical scissors and started to cut his fingernails, while Sister Sinclair, the theatre superintendent, stood behind him seething with rage but unable to make any comment. On another occasion, when in the operating theatre, Sister Sinclair asked Harold: 'Will you be operating tomorrow?' Harold replied: 'No. I am going to Neil Dallas's wedding.' The cat was truly out of the bag. At the time, Neil Dallas was senior to me on the house at Moorfields, and it was forbidden for residents to marry while serving as interns. Typical of the relationship Harold had with the interns, Neil had turned to him for advice. Harold advised Neil and Gillian to get married in secret to avoid causing trouble with the hospital authorities. In minutes, the whole hospital had heard the good news. As precedence had been taken, Veronica and I made no secret of our own wedding plans, and many of the consultants and staff received invitations.

The consultants often joined the interns for lunch or dinner in the residents' dining hall, made even more enjoyable by donations from the nearby Whit-bread brewery. I think Harold preferred the company of his young residents more than his own contemporaries, who were generally rather antagonistic about his work. Certainly none of his colleagues were doing lens implantation at this time. Sitting at lunch with Harold, after an operating session, we discussed the suitability of the young surgeons waiting to be appointed to the house. He mentioned someone called Ron Fisher, whom he did not think should ever gain a position on the house at Moorfields. I disagreed, saying that Fisher was a hard worker and a very efficient ophthalmologist and had struggled financially to reach his present position. Fisher was the next surgeon to become a resident surgical officer! Ron Fisher was later appointed professor of surgery at the Western Ophthalmic Hospital, a branch of St Mary's Hospital.

CHAPTER 10
Love and partnership

This was an incredible period in my life. I was engaged to a young, outstandingly beautiful and gifted girl, as well as being an intern surgical officer at Moorfields taught by the world's foremost detachment surgeon Cyril Dee-Shapland and the inventor of the lens implant Harold Ridley. With the workload at Moorfields, I had little time to find somewhere for Veronica and I to come home to after our honeymoon.

Our intended flat in Kensington fell through and, with just weeks to go before our wedding, Veronica and I had no idea where we would live. As chance would have it, a friend told me of a new development of houses in Bayswater, just north of Hyde Park. The site had been developed on a derelict area that had been devastated by a German landmine in the Second World War, with tremendous loss of life. There was one house remaining on the market. Veronica and I dropped everything and drove to Bayswater to view it. In a small cul-de-sac of exquisitely built, mock-Georgian terraced houses of red brick, the estate seemed to be paradise on earth. Number 15 Caroline Place was the end-terraced house, two storeys high with a small front garden. It seemed perfect. We made an offer, and that night I hardly slept worrying about whether or not we would be able to afford our new house. Nothing ever changes!

Just three weeks before our wedding, life seemed to have no real problems. How wrong one can be and how temporary and fickle life is. During the first week of November, at the end of my late-night ward round, John called to tell me that my favourite cousin, Johnnie French, had just been found dead in her flat. I was not even given time off a few days later to attend her funeral. Instead, I went alone to her grave in Chiswick, long after the official ceremonies. That night John and I got very drunk. The next morning I got up early and walked around the Round Pond in Kensington Gardens, nursing a monumental hangover and musing about the complexities of life.

Our wedding day was truly memorable: 19 November 1960 was dry and sunny, with a light mist overlying the Thames. My closest friends, John, Francis De Freyne and Hubert Morris, gave me my last bachelor lunch at the St James' Club, Piccadilly. When we arrived at Chelsea Old Church, there was not an empty seat in the church. It was so exciting to see nearly 300 people in the congregation made up of our mutual relatives, friends and medical colleagues. Sadly, my father was too frail to travel and Aunt Vickey was still distraught following the death of Johnnie. Representing the head of my family was my Uncle Tom.

Veronica arrived with Arvid only five minutes late to the accompaniment of *Lead Us, Heavenly Father, Lead Us*. I could not resist turning around to look at her. She wore a full-length white dress with a small train, followed by pages and six bridesmaids in orange silk dresses. Arvid had great difficulty walking at this time, as his war wounds were playing up. Canon Barker, the vicar of Winchfield Church, conducted the service, and John was my best man. Veronica gave all her responses in a crystal clear voice, looking radiantly happy and very beautiful. We walked down the aisle to the strains of the *Grand march* from Verdi's opera *Aida*.

Following the wedding reception at the Basil Street Hotel, Veronica and I went to visit Aunt Vickey. It must have been very poignant, seeing us so happy and with her so sad after the recent loss of her daughter. Later Veronica and I were driven to West Green Cottage. Wiggie Woolford, the cleaner, so-called because of her very obvious wig, had laid on a wonderful dinner for us. A candlelit table had been prepared in the drawing room, and we sat enjoying roast partridge in front of a blazing log fire. At midnight we were driven to Heathrow en route to our honeymoon in Gibraltar. Heathrow was fog-bound, and we spent the first night of our marriage lying back to back on plastic seats in the airport lounge, like a couple of refugees. We finally arrived at the Rock Hotel, Gibraltar, in our rented Austin Mini in time for lunch. Then we went upstairs for a rest. By now we had known each other for more than two years, yet this was the first time we had enjoyed the pleasures of married life together. We were both glad that we had disciplined ourselves to wait for this moment. I had always thought that a honeymoon would be, maybe, a period of some embarrassment, as the couple became adjusted to living their lives together. This was not the case with us. Veronica said she felt only a blissful happiness that we would from then on be living together. She relished every one of her wedding vows and her look of radiance reflected her feelings. We locked into each other's company and renewed our pledges to live together for all time in perpetual love, peace and truth.

Throughout the 40 years that I was privileged to spend with my wife, there was almost nothing that we kept from each other. Our thoughts were so intertwined that at times we almost seemed to think as a single entity. We entered marriage as two young people treading the path of life together and enjoying everything it had to offer – its joys and hardships. On our honeymoon we experienced nothing but pure joy, and later in life when there were troubles, each other's company kept them at bay.

That afternoon we drove as far up the rock of Gibraltar as was possible and climbed the interminable steps to the summit. Despite seeing numerous signs forbidding us to feed the apes, we found no sign of the famous apes themselves. We must have spent too much time on the summit, holding hands and gazing into each other's eyes, as by the time we had descended the steps to the entrance gates, they were locked for the night. We had visions of spending our second night of marriage on the cold heights of Gibraltar Rock. Luckily, we found a gap in the wire enclosure and escaped by passing through the military camp.

The next day we took the ferry to Tangier, before starting the long drive to Marrakesh in our little Mini. It soon became obvious that the car had a cracked gasket, as it was making a noise like a steam engine. In minutes of leaving Tangier, we seemed to be alone travelling through semi-desert roads. Every few miles we encountered checkpoints manned by Moroccan police, who would lower a spiked grill across the road at our approach. At each of these halts we presented our passports and gesticulated meaningfully, not speaking their language. They would peer at us through the window and then wave us on. After a while we found their presence rather reassuring. At least we were not entirely alone on these desolate desert roads.

After Rabat, the road from Casablanca to Marrakesh passes through desert as far as the eye can see. With our faulty gasket, we dreaded the prospect of breaking down. We drove for hours without seeing another person and were so relieved to finally see the palm trees of Marrakech. We stayed in the Hotel De La Menara. We woke the next morning to find the sun streaming into our room. We sat on the balcony, having breakfast, awed at our first real sights, sounds and smells of an Arab town. To enhance the experience, we hired a guide and made for the market.

This Arab market had probably changed little since the time of Christ. The open-fronted stalls were made of wicker. Their displays spilled onto the street – rugs, carpets, poufs and oriental clothing of all colours of the rainbow. Unescorted camels wandered through the streets and were probably responsible for the ever-pervading acrid smell. The market was packed with bartering customers, all looking for a bargain. We bought a carpet rug and a red and yellow leather pouf. We saw an ancient Arab snake charmer mesmerizing a cobra, with its head only inches from the end of his flute.

We drove to Ourika, a lovely mountain valley with medieval farm cottages, where we found a remote spot for a picnic lunch. However far one seemed to be from humanity, whenever we stopped for a rest, an Arab would appear as if from nowhere. In no way were they threatening, but they were always present, like the flies. A little Arab boy joined us for lunch, sitting throughout the meal on a rock immediately behind us.

As was probably inevitable, towards the end of the week, we woke in the middle of the night with a severe stomach ache. The following morning we left Marrakesh to drive towards Oukaïmeden, high up in the Atlas Mountains, on the edge of the Sahara desert. The road up the mountainside was treacherous, with a sheer precipice on one side. We dreaded meeting an oncoming vehicle, and, with our poor gasket, we were terrified there could be other faults in the car. A steering or brake failure would be disastrous at this time. After what seemed like hours of climbing, Oukaïmeden was still 18 kilometres away. With the state of the road, fears about the car and the fragility of our stomachs, we

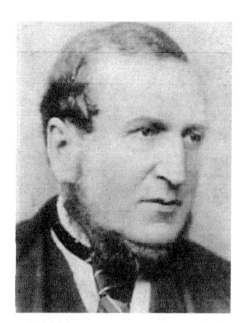

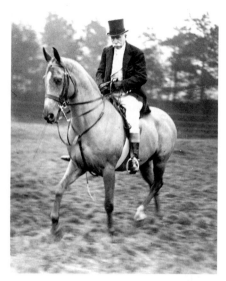

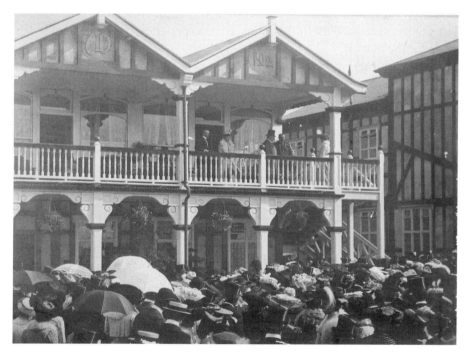

Top left: My great grandfather Sir John Arnott 1st, Bt (1812-1898), MP for Kinsale and a notable Victorian philanthropist who helped to introduce the 'Irish Poor Law Relief Bill'

Top right: My grandfather Sir John Arnott 2nd, Bt (1853-1942)

Bottom: The opening meeting of the Phoenix Park Racecourse, Dublin, 1903. On balcony (left to right), Sir John Arnott, Queen Alexandra, King Edward VII, Lord Enniskillen and Lady Arnott

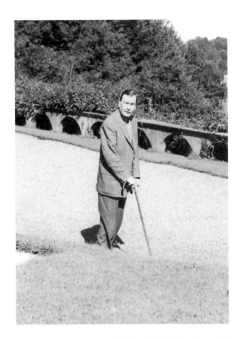

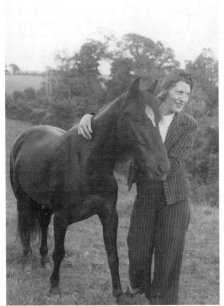

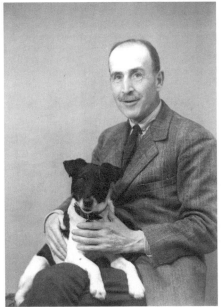

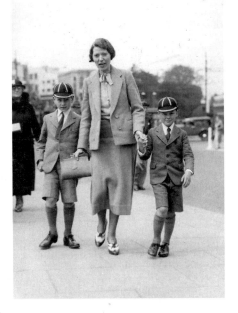

Top left: My father Sir Robert Arnott 4th, Bt, at Ounavarra, Lucan, 1960

Top right: My mother Cynthia with Twinkle, one of the two ponies she used to pull her trap in the war - Swanage, 1944

Bottom left: My uncle Sir Lauriston Arnott 3rd, Bt, with his dog Jester - c. 1948

Bottom right: John and me with our mother on our way to school, Bournemouth - c. 1935

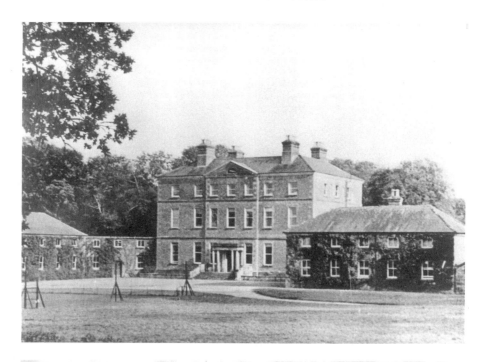

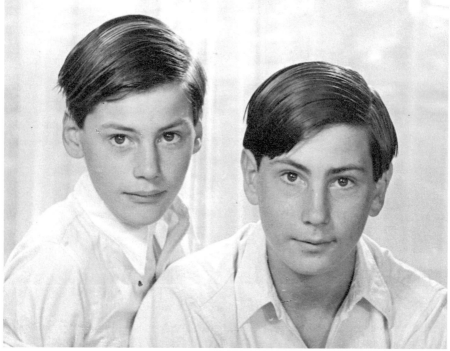

Top: Frenchpark house (built 1667), County Roscommon, Ireland

Bottom: John and me - 1939

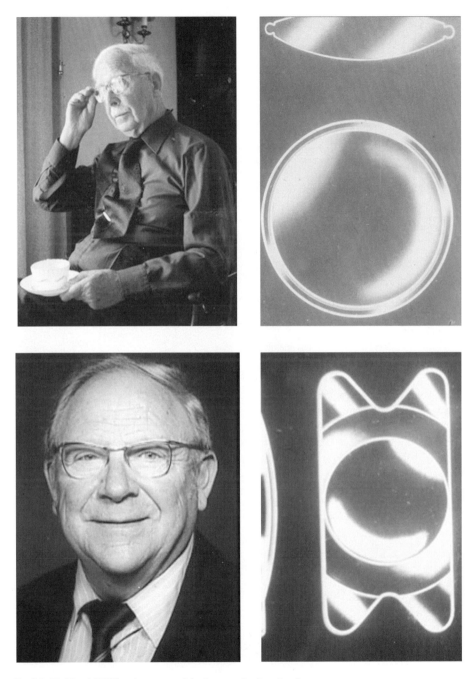

Top left: Sir Harold Ridley, inventor of the intraocular lens implant

Top right: Harold Ridley's first posterior-chamber lens manufactured by Rayner UK -1949

Bottom left: Peter Choyce FRCS, Harold Ridley's senior registrar at Moorfields - an early advocate and inventor of lens implantation

Bottom right: The Rayner-Choyce mark VIII 'gull-winged' anterior-chamber lens - 1963

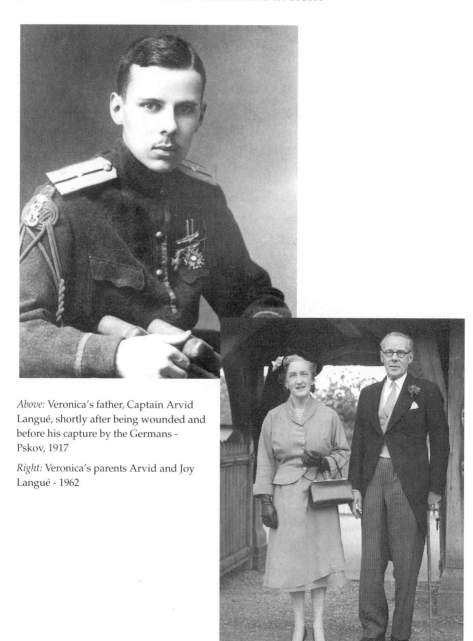

Above: Veronica's father, Captain Arvid
Langué, shortly after being wounded and
before his capture by the Germans -
Pskov, 1917

Right: Veronica's parents Arvid and Joy
Langué - 1962

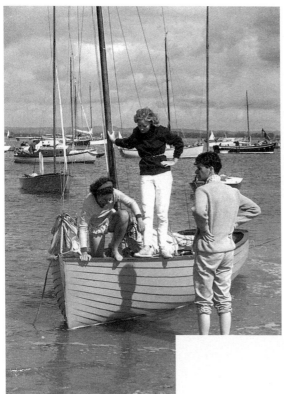

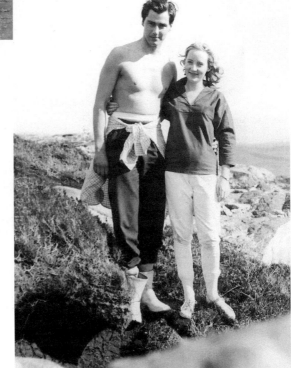

Above: Veronica, Charles and Lelia Orme on 'Siobhan' in Bosham Estuary - summer 1959

Right: Veronica and me on the summit of the Connemara Mountains - summer 1960

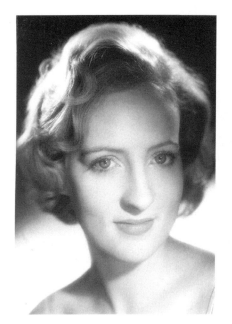
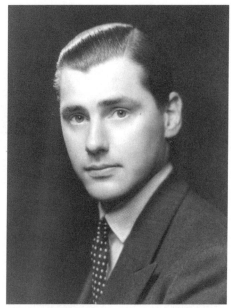

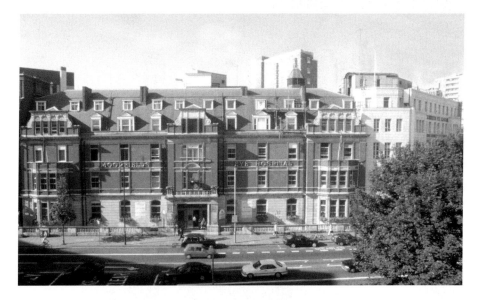

Top left: Veronica Langué, engagement portrait, Leniare Studio - 1960

Top right: Eric Arnott, engagement portrait, Leniare Studio - 1960

Bottom: The world-famous Moorfields Eye Hospital, City Road, London, where I was clinical assistant (1955) and a resident and senior resident officer (1959-61)

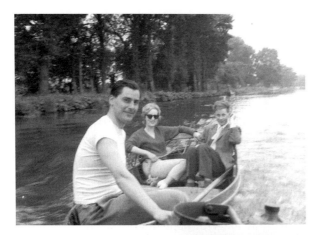

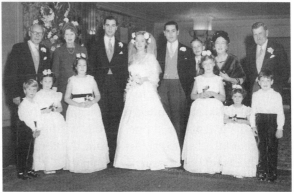

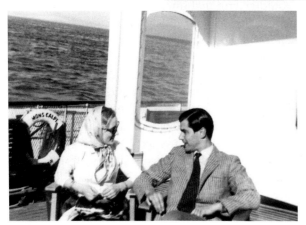

Top: Our engagement day. Veronica and Charles Langué and me boating on the River Thames, Pangbourne - May 1960

Centre: Our wedding in November 1960. (Back row, left to right) Arvid Langué, Lettice Arnott, me and Veronica, John Arnott, Charles and Joy Langué and Thomas Arnott at the Basil Street Hotel, London - November 1960

Bottom: On the ferry from Gibraltar to Tangier on our honeymoon - November 1960

called it a day. We never did see what lay at the top of the mountain, but our failed trip cured our upset tummies.

Our return across the desert to Casablanca did not seem as arduous as the outbound journey. Casablanca was at that time a ghost town. The French had given independence to Morocco four years earlier, and all development had discontinued. The town was littered with abandoned half-finished, high-rise buildings. Nonetheless, the city had a beautiful sea esplanade, reminiscent of Nice, as both were developed under the same French influence. We walked barefoot and hand in hand along the beach, under the perpetual sun, before eating a horrendous dinner, made even more so by the exorbitant prices charged. At least we were well entertained by jewel-bedecked belly dancers!

On the last full day of our truly wonderful honeymoon, we tracked down the local Anglican church and attended the morning service. This was the first of many occasions that we would attend a church service in a foreign country. We always found these services very welcoming and they enabled us to join, for a short time, the community spirit of the local inhabitants.

Veronica was totally supportive to the pledge I had made 12 years before, at my mother's bedside, to serve Christianity through medicine. She made it clear to me that she wanted to participate as fully as possible in my career and, indeed, make it a shared one. Sitting at dinner on our last night of honeymoon, Veronica and I discussed our future. Although she was only 19, she had such strength of character and determination behind her beautiful features and wonderful personality. The adoring young wife of only one week had turned into an equal partner, who would ensure that our future was woven as much by her influence as my own actions. It was this type of unrelenting support and advice that helped me so much throughout my career in ophthalmology.

On this evening, however, I was totally taken by surprise. My cosy idea of returning to Ireland was being seriously challenged. Veronica said: 'I am extremely proud to be your wife and to join you in your profession. I feel honoured to be married to an ophthalmic surgeon who has the ability to help and heal so many people. Nevertheless, I do I feel you should be in London rather than Dublin, where the opportunities are greater.'

'But,' I said, 'my whole training has been based on the assumption that I would eventually return to Ireland to take over from Beecher Somerville-Large.'

'I realize that,' said Veronica, 'but the surgeon I want you to be cannot be confined to the shores of Ireland.' Thus started a discussion that went on well into the night. I felt rather let down and went to bed depressed that my dreams of being an Irish country gentleman, with an Irish ophthalmic practice, were about to be relinquished. I was also desperately worried that I would be letting Beecher down. This was about the only time in our lives that Veronica was so forthright. I realized much later, how she was right and I was so wrong. We did not, in any way, have an argument during that evening, but Veronica was making a point, which she always upheld.

Our honeymoon continued in peace and harmony, as if the issue of our future had never arisen. And after an exhausting trip, we arrived back in London and were driven down to West Green Cottage, where we were greeted with the usual warmth, by Arvid and Joy. Brother John was also there, grinning from ear to ear, like a Cheshire cat. He had just become engaged to Christina Oultram. What a wonderful homecoming and we celebrated until the early hours.

Two days later, the honeymoon was well and truly over! Not only was I returning to Moorfields but also, for the next four months during my final term of office, I would be the senior resident officer. Neil Dallas, the retiring SRO, spent some time explaining my new duties and responsibilities to me. This position held considerable importance in the hospital. Among other duties, the senior resident officer was in charge of the wellbeing of the other residents – six during my time of office – and responsible for the scheduling of weekend casualty and house duties.

Another of the SRO's functions was to attend the examination of any patient who was threatening to litigate, for whatever reason. Marcelli Shaw was the London ophthalmologist who specialized in these cases. He was a short, impressive man, with a thick thatch of grey hair, an aquiline nose and a permanent twinkle in his eye. He and his wife had the unusual hobby of collecting rare teapots.

These patients were examined in his consulting rooms in Harley Street and despite the gravity of the circumstances I always enjoyed attending these sessions. Marcelli's brother was a high court judge and he himself was well-versed in the law. He took great trouble to be impartial towards each party – be it patient, employer or hospital. Most grievances were as a result of industrial accidents, and Marcelli's job was to verify the legitimacy of the complaint and assess the extent of likely damages. I am sure that his expertise was instrumental in ensuring that most cases were settled out of court. One of the patients who we examined claimed to have incurred an injury to the eye that had caused subsequent blindness. The Moorfields' notes of the patient recorded that he had developed a chronic inflammation after receiving a blow to the eye. Marcelli and I examined the eye of the patient and afterwards looked at each other in amazement. One of London's leading specialists had failed to detect a small perforating scar on the cornea and a hole in the underlying iris. The patient had a previously undetected metallic foreign body in the eye, which, over time, had dissolved, causing blindness from the toxicity of the metal. With the judgement of Solomon, Marcelli stated in his report that the blow had destroyed the eye. No mention was made of the metallic foreign body. The patient received substantial damages, and the honour of the famous surgeon who had examined him at Moorfields was preserved.

Some years later, I put into practice the knowledge I acquired from Marcelli Shaw. I had a patient who was suing his employer, as he had fallen off a ladder and subsequently developed a retinal detachment. After examining the patient, I satisfied myself that the retinal detachment was as a result of the fall. The case was to be judged at Lincoln's Inn Fields. Nothing fills me with more dread than having to attend a court of law and, in this case, one of the highest in the country. On the evening before the case, counsel for the defence contacted me and asked if I could act for the employer as well as the patient, as their advising surgeon had no knowledge of ophthalmology. I agreed and entered the court wearing two hats. Following Marcelli Shaw's teaching, I tried to be as impartial as possible. It was obvious that the patient would win the case, but I was a little disturbed when I later received a letter from his lawyers thanking me for my excellent participation. The damages were considerably higher than they had anticipated!

One of the perks of being senior resident officer was that the most junior intern, known as 'Number 6', was assigned to be one's assistant and had the tedious and time-consuming task of writing up the admission, surgical and discharge notes of all patients. Fortunately there was considerably less paperwork than there is today. I am constantly amazed at how administrators now interfere with the medical management of patients and highly skilled doctors and surgeons are expected to waste hours of their precious and valuable time form-filling.

My assistant intern was an Aussie called Dickie Galbraith, who had all the easygoing attributes of people who live 'down under'. He had a tremendous sense of humour and found it difficult to understand the class system, which was still prevalent in England at that time. One morning he raided my bedroom cupboard and pinched my Old Harrovian school tie. He wore it constantly for the next four months, at first as a joke intended to ridicule 'Pommy' authority, but after a while I think he secretly enjoyed looking as if he was part of the 'establishment'.

It was a constant pleasure working with Dickie. Despite our different cultural backgrounds, we made a great team and had a good laugh together. He later returned to Australia and became one of their leading ophthalmic surgeons. He was awarded an MBE for his work and research in ophthalmic diseases of the Aborigines.

As senior resident ophthalmic surgeon, it was my duty to assist the three most senior surgeons of the hospital. These three surgeons were all eminent in their own way, but I had left behind me the world-class pioneers.

Magor Cardell had joined the staff of Moorfields at the time when several of London's eye hospitals merged to form the Moorfields Group. He was a wonderful character, the epitome of Captain Mainwaring from *Dad's Army*. He was a small authoritative man, with a round, almost bald head, and a product of Edwardian Britain.

Despite the fact that microsurgery, intricate suturing and refined instrumentation were just beginning to become available, he continued to operate in the manner that had held sway for the previous 100 years. His cataract surgery was very similar to that still performed in some of the eye camps of India. An operation would seldom last for more than five minutes.

After a single quick, but large, incision into the eye, a pair of toothed forceps was used to grip and tear away the anterior capsule of the underlying cataractous lens. Through this opening into the lens, the hard nucleus of the lens was coaxed out of the lens bag and then from the eye. The residual lens debris was irrigated from the lens bag. The wound into the eye was gently stroked to ensure that the edges were in some form of contact and then sutured. Both eyes were padded for 48 hours, and the patient stayed in hospital for some 10 days before a further six months of convalescence. Partial sight was restored by the use of thick aphakic 'pebble' lenses.

Each operating session took place with military precision. He would arrive in the operating theatre on the stroke of 2 pm each Tuesday afternoon and expect to see his registrar, house surgeon, theatre sister, technician, anaesthetist and nurses enter the surgery in order of seniority. Eight to ten operations would be performed in two hours and all would leave the theatre in the same order and congregate in the surgeon's room for afternoon tea of cucumber sandwiches.

It was enlightening and pleasurable to see one of these grand old men of surgery still performing. On another occasion, I had great pleasure seeing him put a leech onto the lid of a poor patient who had an infection around the eye. Leeches were still kept in the pharmacy at Moorfields but had not been used for some years. All of the residents turned out to watch this extraordinary spectacle. The leech, obviously out of practice, was extremely reluctant to suck, and a full 20 minutes went by before it attached. Amazingly, two days later, the patient's condition seemed much better.

Another of the surgeons I worked with was Edgar King, the most outstanding medical physician in City Road at that time. His knowledge of ophthalmic medicine was phenomenal. He was a living encyclopaedia of ophthalmology. I was lucky enough in later years to inherit his private practice in Harley Street, at which time I was able to truly appreciate his knowledge through reference to his old patient notes. He was a lifelong bachelor and a rather retiring gentleman. As a student some two years previously, I had spent many months attending his clinics soaking up his knowledge. His surgery was slightly odd, as when operating he would prop himself up with bolsters. Once seated, the theatre sister would dutifully stuff these bolsters between Edgar and the operating table. He would then sprawl over these pillows and start his operating session. On one occasion Edgar King returned from holiday to find that his intern had cleared his cataract list. When he had demanded an explanation, the brash intern replied, 'For the simple reason that you were on holiday.'

On another occasion, Edgar King was summoned to relieve high pressure (glaucoma) in the eye of a Saudi Arabian prince. If untreated, this will lead to blindness, but it can be treated satisfactorily by medicine or by surgery. The Saudi prince took over a whole floor of the Dorchester Hotel, and a suite of rooms was converted into an operating theatre, using the same operating table that Prince Charles had recently used when having a tonsil operation. After days of preparation, the prince was wheeled into the theatre, and placed onto Prince Charles's trolley. He weighed more than 20 stone, and his massive body overhung the sides. Edgar King and I scrubbed our hands and put on our sterile operating gowns. With due pomp and ceremony, Edgar walked into the converted operating theatre and sat down at the head of the table. Sister Sinclair, as usual, 'buttressed' Edgar, but as soon as he leant over the patient there was a resounding crack. The operating table had collapsed under the prince's weight and his head landed up in Edgar's lap. Luckily, the sleeping prince was oblivious to the situation and another table was quickly found!

The third surgeon I assisted was Frank Law, who had originally been appointed as a pathologist. I saw little of him during my last four months at Moorfields, as he took sabbatical leave in Australia. During that time I performed all of his surgery with the assistance of Dick Galbraith.

Three days after becoming senior resident surgical officer, Veronica and I went with John and Christina Oultram to the 400 night club in Leicester Square to celebrate their engagement. Sadly, it was an unfounded celebration, as in weeks the engagement was broken off. It would be many years before John finally married.

Veronica and I were still living in our bachelor surroundings, including staying with Veronica's cousin Natalie Lady Hare, before finally returning to Old Court Mansions while Caroline Place was prepared. One evening just before Christmas, Harold and Elisabeth Ridley invited Veronica and me to have dinner with them in their house in Harley Street with Neil and Gillian Dallas. It was typical of Harold's fastidiousness that, when we said goodbye and Veronica kissed him on the cheek, he said: 'That dirty habit should never be repeated.'

We spent that Christmas with Joy, Arvid, and Charles at West Green Cottage and were invited for the first time into their bedroom early on Christmas day to open the Christmas stockings. As a joke I gave Veronica a posy of crêpe-paper flowers made by one of the nurses in my hospital. She was not impressed and burst into tears. Happiness was restored when I gave her a silver powder compact.

Later that day I went for a very long walk up to the common and then down through Hazeley Bottom, smoking a massive Cuban cigar given to me by the Langués. I walked for miles, under the light of a full moon, and contemplated the many blessings that God had given us.

The next day I took Veronica and Charles with me to do a ward round of my patients in Moorfields. By tradition, the SRO had to dress up as Santa Claus for the children's Christmas tea party. I was drawn on my sledge by the other residents wearing reindeer outfits. Many of the children were from the poorer parts of the East End of London and had never seen anything like this! Their eyes popped out of their heads as I gave them presents from my sledge.

A few days after Christmas, Veronica and I attended the annual residents' dinner. Despite the rigid Moorfields' rules forbidding girls in the residents' quarters, most of my colleagues were already married. One night on duty, I sneaked Veronica in to spend the night with me, but the sound of the matron's footsteps outside made her hide in the wardrobe! At this residents' dinner were Gordon Krolman, Peter Rycroft, Rolf Blach, Tom Avril, Peter Watson, David Watson, Dickie Galbraith and Bruce Crawford, accompanied by their wives or fiancées. The only female resident on the staff at that time was Anthea Connel. We had an extremely jovial dinner, rather akin to an army officers' mess evening, and later retired to the boardroom for roulette.

Part Four. The way ahead

CHAPTER 11
The Royal College of Surgeons

Now that we were married Veronica's ballet career came to an abrupt end – not to be realized until some 20 years later, when our daughter Tania joined the English National Ballet Company. Veronica's last appearance was a small part in the 1961 film, *The frightened city*, made at Shepperton Studios. The film was singularly unremarkable and would have been relegated to total obscurity had it not been the first film in which Sean Connery had the lead role alongside Herbert Lom and Alfred Marks.

Filming went on for some weeks and, towards the end, Alfred Marks invited Veronica up to his dressing room, where he tried to impose upon her. An ageing Marks chased an agile Veronica around the room until finally his trousers slipped to the ground and trapped him around the ankles. He had stupidly loosened his belt before trying to capture his prey. On her return to our flat that night Veronica and I had our first tiff, as I felt that this budding film career would inevitably lead to trouble. As an alternative to filming, Veronica later joined Edward Sturges in his gymnasium in Knightsbridge, teaching fitness classes.

Edward had served as a major in the Royal Marines and fought with distinction behind the Japanese lines in Burma. Despite his above-average size, he had the ability to creep with the stealth of a cat and was responsible for almost single-handedly waging a sustained guerrilla campaign, behind enemy lines, for many months. He was an accomplished oarsman who twice won at Henley Royal Regatta – first as a member of the 1938 Radley College crew in the Ladies Plate and then, in 1947, the Silver Goblets and Nickalls Cup with his London Rowing Club partner JH Pinches. He was also at one time the British Amateur Rowing Association sculling champion and many years later the national veteran sculling champion, despite being the oldest competitor by more than 10 years. Edward was an obsessive fitness fanatic and after the war established a very successful gymnasium in Pavilion Road, long before fitness clubs became fashionable. Over four decades he taught generations of young children, including all four of Queen Elizabeth II's children. Veronica worked for 20 years with Edward, during which time he became a great personal friend of the family and godfather to our son Robert.

In February 1961, Veronica and I finally moved out of Old Court Mansions and into our new home in Bayswater. Uncharacteristically for central London, the development was akin to a country village community, where everyone knew everybody else. We made many interesting new lifelong friends at Caroline Place: Huw Thomas was, in the mid 1950s, one of the original Independent Television News presenters, with Robin Day and Ludovic Kennedy.

Two other friends in Caroline Place were Michael and Antonia Gibbs. Many years later, I performed Antonia's cataract and implant operations and, when we celebrated the 50th anniversary of Harold Ridley's implant operation in 1999, Antonia was interviewed for the BBC news.

The Renwicks, who were much older than the rest of us, had one of the few detached houses in Caroline Place and everyone looked upon them as 'the squires' of the community. We gave a cocktail party attended by Lady Brabourne, the mother-in-law of Lord Louis Mountbatten's eldest daughter, who sadly perished with him when the IRA blew up his boat in County Donegal in 1979. She was going on to a dinner party and was wearing an evening dress with an abundance of jewellery. A rather 'merry' Papa Renwick also joined our party and, swaying on his feet, went up to Lady Brabourne and said: 'Lord luv, you're all decked up like a Christmas tree!' She had kindly been responsible for making me the medical officer to the railway division of the St John Ambulance, a crack unit that won nearly every paramedical contest it entered. I did not have to do much except attend the odd ceremonial parade, such as the Lord Mayor's Show, wearing my smart uniform, with four pips on my epaulette. I attended their meetings to learn rather than teach. Nevertheless, its members were always very polite to me and I was sorry when they were transferred to York.

Some years later, Papa Renwick came to my consulting rooms. Sitting opposite me he said: 'I've only come to see you as I want to talk about my cataract with an old mate.' Not the best criteria for choosing a surgeon! Thankfully he received a perfect result thanks to the help of Neil Dallas, my old associate from Moorfields, who assisted at the operation and inserted a Binkhorst 'iris-supported' implant. At this time, only a very few British surgeons were doing lens implantation.

One of the couples that lived next door to us had friends to stay. The wife went into the bathroom and caught 'her husband' as he was pulling his shirt over his head. She gave his 'manhood' a big pull and said: 'Ding-dong, dinner's ready darling.' When the shirt was pulled down, she found to her utter horror that she was staring at a very shocked guest.

Two bachelors, Desmond Briggs and John Salt, shared one of the houses in Caroline Place. Each house had its own garage, but despite this luxury many residents parked their cars outside their house. Desmond woke one morning to find that his car had been stolen. After several months, with the car still not found, he received a settlement from his insurance company and ordered a replacement. Just before the arrival of the new car he was having drinks with his next-door neighbour, when she commented: 'Desmond, I dearly love you, but how much longer will I be garaging your car?'

Veronica and I did have a genuine burglary shortly after moving into Caroline Place. Returning from a weekend with Veronica's parents, we were unable to open our front door. We entered via the back door, lying by the side of which was one of our silver candlesticks. The burglars had made a hasty retreat by the front door, taking with them all of Veronica's jewellery, a silver clock and other wedding presents. We were lucky not to have been bludgeoned by our own candlestick, but Veronica was terribly upset at losing so many sentimental possessions.

Having been in our new home for only a few days, we found out how we had been able to acquire this house so easily. On the Friday evening, we were enjoying a whisky and soda, when suddenly the whole house started to vibrate. We initially thought it was an earthquake but soon realized that we were hearing the deafening sound of Irish music. Behind the brick wall, on the other side of the narrow road from our house, was a casino that played live Celtic music on Friday and Saturday nights. We suffered this stupendous noise every weekend for some months, until finally Huw Thomas contacted the Noise Abatement Society to suppress them.

Another mild problem was that opposite our back door was the 'official' United States Army brothel, and once a young girl from the club was stabbed to death in the Bayswater Road. Despite these setbacks, we really loved our first home.

Some weeks after moving into Caroline Place, Aunt Vickey asked if she could come to tea to inspect our new house with her cousin, Lady Poultney. I was working, so Veronica had to entertain them alone. She awaited their arrival with joyful anticipation. It was a very hot sunny day and our nextdoor neighbour, the local rabbi, was sitting in his front garden with his sleeves rolled up, wearing no jacket or tie but sporting a pair of braces. As they approached Veronica overheard Lady Poultney say: 'Isn't it awfully suburban.' A rather chastened Veronica welcomed them into the house that she so much cherished.

My final two months as senior resident officer overlapped our first few weeks in Caroline Place. During that time, two of our senior surgeons retired – Henry Stallard and Magor Cardell. By now I was doing a considerable amount of major ophthalmic surgery without supervision. I had to do one tragic operation on a child who had bilateral retinoblastoma, a malignant tumour of the retina, which, if left untreated, would have spread throughout the body. I had to commit the poor boy to blindness by removing both his eyes. This was the only operation during my time there that I hated doing, but it was essential to preserve his life.

In February 1961, I performed the last operation I would do at Moorfields for many years. I now had to eke out an existence doing outpatient sessions at Moorfields and focus my attention on passing the final fellowship exam. I was by now in my mid-30s and married, holding down a full-time job and studying every evening.

At Easter, Veronica and I took her parents to Ireland to meet my father for the first time. We were fortunate that their visit coincided with a race meeting at Phoenix Park, and like so many people before, they were amazed at the hospitality we extended to our friends and wondered how it was possible to make a profit from the meeting with such heavy outgoings.

On Easter Sunday, Veronica, John and I went to one of Eileen Guinness's notoriously extravagant parties at Luttrellstown Castle. More than 40 guests were invited to dinner and afterwards we all played 'sheets' in the drawing room. Everyone watched while one couple at a time swapped their clothes under the cover of a sheet. Two guests took particularly long under the sheets – but then the Indian Ambassadress appeared from under the sheet wearing a dinner jacket and the British Ambassador her sari!

After our return from Ireland, Veronica and I went to Manorbier, South Wales, to stay with Gwyneth Taylor at Greenala House, where she had lived since her childhood. Lying in a valley, it had an uninterrupted view of the sea, with on one side the medieval Church of St James and on the other the castle, which was owned by Veronica's cousin, Sheila Dunsany. Manorbier Castle was originally built as a fortress during Norman times and is most famous as the birthplace of Gerald of Wales. Although it was sacked during the English Civil War by Oliver Cromwell's troops, much of it remains intact to this day, including the outer walls, the turrets and the banqueting hall. In a corner of the castle, adjacent to one of the turrets, is a Victorian caretaker's house with its own resident ghost. Legend has it that during Elizabethan times the Lord of the Manor's daughter planned to elope with a soldier billeted in the outside garrison. He was shot with an arrow as he approached the castle and in her distress the maiden threw herself off the battlements.

Veronica and I rambled along the stunning Pembrokeshire coastal paths. A couple of miles outside Manorbier was a derelict cottage that lay snuggled in the undergrowth of the encircling cliffs. We had great fun scrambling down the overgrown path to this hidden cottage totally revelling in each other's company. In all our activities – walking, driving, shopping, playing golf, swimming, travelling or entertaining – we developed an understanding and total unity of purpose. We shared our thoughts and actions, and living with her was a time of harmony and constant happiness. In exploring this cottage, our companionship was typical of how we spent our lives – we played together like two children in a world of our own.

Later that month, Veronica and I went to stay with Eric and Hester Cattley, Joy Langué's brother and sister-in-law, in Devon, on their smallholding where they had established a successful market-garden business selling flowers, fruit, vegetables and early potatoes to Covent Garden. They were also actively involved in the local community: Hester was a magistrate and Eric chairman of Kingsbridge District Council.

Their house, Robins Farm, was on the edge of Kingston Village and only a short distance from the sea. Veronica had spent many happy childhood holidays here, and her favourite beach was Wonwell in the Erme Estuary. It was here that she took me on my first visit. At the head of this estuary are three spiked rocks that look like nuns, where I spent a whole morning 'studying' my Duke-Elder's volume IV of *Neuro-ophthalmology*, as Veronica walked along the coast with her cousin Susie.

Veronica and I were in the main spare bedroom, which had a gigantic four-poster bed and a mattress that must have been at least 100 years old and had a hump in the middle, affectionately known as 'the Welsh mountain'. It was probably here that our son Stephen was conceived.

In July I went to University College Hospital, London, to be interviewed for the senior registrar appointment by two ophthalmic surgeons, Cyril Dee-Shapland and Desmond Greaves, who I already knew. It was a huge relief when Cyril rang me to say I had been appointed: this position is an essential stepping-stone to becoming a consultant and the posts were few and far between. On my first day at UCH, Bill Thornhill showed me around and thus started the next three years of my medical career. Compared with Moorfields, which had a consultant staff of 16, there were just the two ophthalmic consultants, who held only one operating session on Wednesday mornings. The ophthalmic inpatients department and operating theatre were in an annex in Devonshire Street, which was shared with the psychiatric department. The cataract surgery at UCH did not have the benefit of modern technology, and postoperatively the patient was confined to bed for four days, with a week's stay in hospital.

Our first son Stephen was born on 19 February 1962 after a long night's labour, during which I had sat by Veronica's side studying. I felt a wonderful deep happiness to hold my first son. Some days after his birth, we took him for his first walk in our new Silver Cross pram. We must have been the last generation to use this type of vast royal-blue Victorian contraption, suspended by 'car' springs above four large wheels with white tyres. It had cost us far more than we could afford, and certainly the Norland nurses in their smart uniforms would not be seen in Hyde Park pushing any other make of pram. But we did feel rather conspicuous on our country weekends, pushing one of these smart London vehicles in the middle of the countryside.

Our nurse left us after two weeks and we were immediately filled with apprehension about how we would cope with our new responsibility. But our lives rapidly adjusted and the love we had together poured out into a total commitment for the baby, which created an even greater bond between us. Veronica devoted her whole time to looking after Stephen, as I was still studying for my fellowship exam.

On Veronica's 21st birthday we had our first break from our new daily routine. We invited closest friends and relations to Caroline Place for 'Black Velvet' cocktails and then dined at the Savoy Hotel on the Strand, where we were entertained by an excellent cabaret.

Stephen was the perfect baby, with undemanding nights. I studied as hard as possible until the day of the fellowship exam. At Easter, we drove down to West Green Cottage for the traditional Russian Easter breakfast of cold hard-boiled eggs dyed rich golden with onion skins, red with cochineal or green and yellow. Cracking the eggs together like conkers, this Russian Easter breakfast became an annual ritual. For the remainder of that weekend I did little else other than revise for my impending exams, the first of which I sat on the following Tuesday at Queen Square. When I later failed the exam, thanks to misreading a question, I was in good company, with five of my friends who also had to resit.

For my birthday weekend in June, Veronica, Stephen and I drove down to West Green Cottage and spent the first part of it alone in the house. There was glorious sunshine, and Veronica and I spent most of the time lying in the sun. Our second child Tania was certainly a West Green baby. Veronica gave me a large tome on ocular pathology written by Professor Zimmerman.

Later that month, the Langué's old friend, Canon Barker, christened our son 'Stephen John,' at Winchfield Church, Hampshire. Before the ceremony he took us to an ancient yew tree some yards away and with pride showed us a hole in its trunk, which had been used for many years as a nest for wrens.

In the late autumn of 1962, I retook the second part of the FRCS exam with my colleagues John Cairns and Neil Dallas. For two days we answered gruelling questions on anatomy and physiology. There then were eight days before the clinical part of the exam. No doubt the examiners would by then have known which candidates were wasting their time continuing with this ordeal.

Alex Cross, who I knew well from Moorfields, supervised the oral part of my exam. Bertie Nutt, from Sheffield, was the senior examiner. The main topic was the discussion of 'perforating injuries of the eye'. I didn't think I made a good impression on my examiners. Later I returned for the major part of the exam – the examination of patients with Bertie Nutt. I examined a patient with a tumour in the eye, a boy with muscular weakness and, with the neurologist, Dr Earl, patients with vascular conditions affecting the brain. I left Queen Square with little idea whether or not I had passed or failed. The re-do exam had been less traumatic than the original – maybe we were all conscious of impending call-up, as it was the time of the Cuban missile crisis, a conflict that almost started a nuclear war between the US and Russia. The world held its breath, and at the 'eleventh hour' the superpowers saw reason and conflict was averted.

One week afterwards, Veronica and I attended the annual dinner in the Savoy Ballroom for the medical staff of UCH. All the hospital consultants and professors from the various different specialties took tables for their staff. We arrived well-fortified, having first had drinks with Cyril Dee-Shapland and his wife, where the only drink offered was Harvey's Bristol Cream Sherry.

Our ophthalmic table of 12 was situated in the centre of the ballroom. Veronica was glowing with the early signs of her second pregnancy. We had left Stephen in his cradle to be cared for by the hotel's cloakroom staff. In the middle of dinner I was abruptly summoned to the telephone, not knowing why. It was Rolf Blach, who had been asked to tell me that we had both passed the fellowship. It was a brilliant moment to share this news with my wife and ophthalmic friends. I was in a daze throughout the after-dinner speeches and did not listen to a single word. In this magnificent ballroom, with its line of overhead chandeliers, opulent decor and surrounded by hundreds of my medical peers, I marvelled at my good fortune. After more than 14 years of intensive studying, I had at last completed my final exam. How typical of Alex Cross to have told his protégées the results before they were officially listed.

A few days later, Peter Rycroft came with Rolf and Elizabeth Blach to have drinks with Veronica and myself at Caroline Place. Peter had also passed his fellowship but tragically died in a car crash some months later. Rolf went on to become a consultant at Moorfields, specializing in the retina, and was later appointed dean of the Institute of Ophthalmology.

In November, the most important degree of my whole career was handed out in a most simplistic ceremony to which I brought Veronica and my mother-in-law Joy at the Royal College of Surgeons in Lincoln's Inn Fields. There were not many of us, as only nine out of 36 entrants had passed the exam. Little wonder that, at the present time, there is such a shortage of senior surgical consultants. The stakes were always raised far too high for the average individual to be able to complete the course – in a way like the Grand National, in that many start, but few finish. The Royal College Macebearer, with his thick silver rod, ushered in the examiners, who heavily outnumbered the successful candidates. We faced each other like two football teams preparing to play the final cup match at Wembley. We listened in hushed silence as our charge of obedience to the college was read out. After the signing of our diplomas, the examiners all stepped forwards to shake our hands and we were accepted as equals. Some of us would soon become examiners and would instil the same fear into the next new batch of surgeons.

Veronica threw a party at 15 Caroline Place to celebrate: 40 of our great friends demolished 25 bottles of champagne. Our list included many who had supported us in our formative years: Tony and Paddy Woolf (Tony being my senior registrar colleague at UCH, who brought all our children and grandchildren into the world); John and Ger Powell, our closest friends (he a solicitor who guided us through so many troubles in our life); Hubert Morris (who had given me free accommodation in his very expensive flat when I first started out); and Gerard Dent (a lifelong friend, who always instilled such optimism when times seemed hard).

Some two weeks later I again attended the London dinner of the Adelaide Hospital, where I had trained for four years, in the Martinez restaurant, London. It was almost the last time I met Nigel Kinnear, to whom I owed all my general surgical expertise, and David Mitchell, with whom I had been taught practical medicine as their pre-registration medical house officer. These colleagues had spread their wings, not only in the profession, but, as the Irish always do, they took their knowledge and expertise to the far outposts of the world. One of my friends at this dinner was a Nigerian, Ransom-Kuti, who after qualifying had returned home to become the professor of medicine in his home university and Minister of Health.

On the way home, I gave a lift to one of the doctors who had qualified with me at Trinity. David Spencer was a very special general practitioner, practising in a small village just outside Reading, Berkshire. When one of his patients had been dying from kidney failure and no donor was available, David Spencer donated one of his own kidneys.

CHAPTER 12
The British NHS heritage

That Christmas, in 1963, we had heavy snowfalls, which made driving difficult but country walks a delight. As Veronica was again heavily pregnant and virtually housebound, I went for long walks through the magical countryside, with the snow lying thickly on the ground and icicles hanging from the trees. When spring finally arrived, so did our second child, Tania, in such a rush to make her appearance that I very nearly missed her arrival.

We employed a part-time nanny to help Veronica. Nan Peacock stayed with us on and off for the next 20 years. To our children, she and her companion, Joan Hartley, became like other mothers, and she adopted us as her family.

In the spring, Professor Barrie Jones and Professor Perkins were awarded the first two academic chairs at Moorfields.

That year the British Ophthalmologic Society's annual meeting was held in London. Beecher Somerville-Large was the president and decided to hold the presidential dinner in Boodles Club. As we were both members of the Dublin Kildare Street Club, we enjoyed overseas privileges to use this famous club in St James's, Piccadilly. When I went to Boodles to make the appropriate arrangements, I was told that, as honorary members, we were only allowed to entertain two guests at any one time. I used all my powers of persuasion, and the manager very graciously bent the rules and the dinner went ahead with more than 100 guests, including innovative Irish ophthalmologists Tom Casey and Dermot Pierce. It was a magnificent affair and Beecher, as always, displayed his great Irish hospitality.

Tom Casey was one of my colleagues at the Royal Victoria Eye and Ear Hospital, Dublin, and had just been appointed consultant at the East Grinstead Hospital, the position that Peter Rycroft had so dearly wanted to fill after the retirement of his father, Sir Benjamin. Despite having a slight tremor when operating, he was without doubt the most outstanding British corneal surgeon of his time, alongside Noel Rice of Moorfields.

Following the lead of Professor Harmsworth, of Germany, Dermot Pierce was the first person, in the early 1960s, to introduce into the UK the concept of using a surgical microscope when operating on the eye. Thereafter, with Jack Hoskins, an engineer, he designed a range of titanium surgical instruments that could be used in conjunction with the microscope for ophthalmic surgery. His contribution to ophthalmology was enormous and many years later he was appointed President of the Royal College of Ophthalmologists. Ophthalmology was the first surgical specialty to use the microscope, which is now the accepted way to operate on any part of the body that requires precision surgery.

At this time, Professor Dent, one of the pathologists working at UCH, was researching a hitherto undiagnosed genetic disorder, which he had named 'homocystinuria' on account of the fact that affected patients have an abnormal presence of homocystine (an amino acid that forms proteins) in their urine. I was asked to examine the eyes of these patients and discovered that, among other genetic abnormalities, a significant percentage of them had dislocated lenses. In most cases, surgical intervention was not warranted, although in one instance it was necessary to perform emergency surgery. The surgery proceeded without complications, although I was fortunate, as it was later established that these patients present an anaesthetic risk and should not be operated upon unless it is absolutely essential.

My findings were written up and published in 1964 under the title *Ocular involvement in homocystinuria* in the *British Journal of Ophthalmology*. It is unusual to be able to introduce a new condition into the annals of a medical specialty and even Professor Ashton, the pathologist at the Institute of Ophthalmology, wrote a letter of congratulations to me, telling me that he had learned from this article.

To supplement my meagre income, I bought some basic ophthalmic equipment so I could examine private patients at the weekend in Caroline Place. Veronica acted as my secretary, nurse and receptionist. One day a young lady came to be examined in my improvised rooms. Veronica had written on her patient notes that she was complaining of an 'eye discharge'. On taking the girl's history, I realized that my efficient secretary had misinterpreted her condition. She was in fact suffering from 'vaginal discharge'. Both patient and doctor were a little embarrassed.

While Beecher Somerville-Large was in London for the British Ophthalmologic Society's annual meeting we had various discussions about my future. I was still keen to return to Ireland, but Beecher suggested that I should look for a temporary consultancy in London, as the openings that he had anticipated in Dublin had not yet become available.

One day Joy Langué called us in great excitement to say that she had seen an article in the London *Evening Standard* discussing the proposed merger of the Fulham, West London and Charing Cross Hospitals into a single group. This was a Labour Government project under the chairmanship of Lord Inman, which was to be based in totally new premises alongside the old Fulham Hospital in Hammersmith. Although the hospital was not scheduled to open for another 10 years, Veronica and I agreed that a consultancy in this new teaching hospital would be ideal.

Some months later, following the untimely death of Mr Moffat, who had died of a heart attack after the day's salmon fishing with Cyril Dee-Shapland, a vacancy for a consultant ophthalmologist became available at the

West London Hospital, which was part of the Charing Cross Group. I duly applied and, having attended a preliminary interview, my name was included on the shortlist.

At the final interview I discovered that the other candidates were Wally Bains, David Abrahams and Doreen Birks – all of whom I knew. The chairman of the selecting committee was, once again, my senior colleague Alex Cross. He was assisted by Mr Milner, the ophthalmic consultant at Charing Cross Hospital; Mr Higgitt, the ophthalmic consultant at the Fulham Hospital; and two others. The interview was fairly relaxed but somewhat lengthy. It seemed like an eternity waiting in the corridor for the final verdict, but I was thrilled to hear that the position was mine.

I rushed back to Caroline Place to find Veronica outside the front door eagerly anticipating my arrival. She could hardly believe the good news. We hugged for a long time, realizing that we had arrived at another milestone in our lives.

My first impressions of the West London Hospital, Hammersmith, were mixed. On arrival, Mr Taylor, the senior manager of the hospital, courteously escorted me around. I was immediately struck by the exemplary relationship that he had with the medical staff and his understanding for the needs of the different competing factions in the hospital. At the outpatient department, Mrs Bedowes, the sister in charge, greeted me. She was wearing a Florence Nightingale-style dark blue uniform with starched white collar and headwear. She had an air about her, with her slim rigid body and aquiline nose, that commanded immediate respect. She ushered me into the clinic to introduce me to my 'junior assistants'. The senior of these assistants, Dr Morton Palmer, was nearly twice my age. He approached to shake my hand and said: 'Welcome, Arnott, to our clinic.' Realizing I had to establish seniority, I replied: 'You can call me doctor, Eric or Mr Arnott but not plain Arnott.' Thereafter he addressed me as Mr Arnott. The other ophthalmic assistants were Joan Haythorne, otherwise known as Mrs Smout, who had been a medical student at the West London during the days when it had a medical school, and Alex Tomkin, the junior house surgeon, whose father had been one of my teachers at the Royal Victoria Eye and Ear Hospital, Dublin.

Our workload was light at first, but the arrival of a young consultant with new ideas naturally led to a marked increase in referrals from local general practitioners. In weeks we found it difficult to cope with the number of patients. After some initial reservations at having such a young consultant in charge of their clinic, Morton Palmer and Joan Haythorne gradually accepted my position, and it was not long before we were working closely together as a team.

As it was a general hospital, we were often asked by colleagues from other specialties to give ophthalmic advice, and conversely we were able to seek their opinions when necessary. This was one of the great advantages of working in a general hospital rather than a specialist ophthalmic hospital, and a sound knowledge of general medicine was required. Morton Palmer was a general practitioner as well as an ophthalmologist and was particularly skilled at dealing with patients with back problems. It was an incongruous sight seeing a patient spread out on the floor of the ophthalmic department while Morton gave back manipulation. Over the years, he eased many an ache in my own back.

Sister 'Tiger' Monk ran the operating theatres at the West London. Despite her jovial personality, she was a strict authoritarian who made it quite clear to everyone that she was the boss in the theatres. At first she also thought that I was too young for the job, but after a while she seemed to accept me, and we developed a mutual respect for each other. Although I did my paediatric surgery, such as squints and tear ducts, at the West London, as there was an excellent children's ward in the hospital, I tended to do most of my major surgery at the neighbouring Fulham Hospital, where the facilities were slightly better.

With the planned merger of the various hospitals into the New Charing Cross Group of Hospitals, it was inevitable that some fixed operating sessions would have to be rescheduled from one hospital to another while the New Charing Hospital was under construction. One such surgeon, who had to temporarily move his surgical sessions to the West London, was Professor Harding-Rains, one of the foremost general surgeons in the country and author of a standard textbook on surgery.

No doubt Professor Harding-Rains felt that it was demeaning having to operate in a semi-suburban hospital that had lost its teaching status. As always, his surgery was quite flawless, but his manners were deplorable. Throughout his first surgical session he had one tantrum after another. Sister Monk suffered this humiliating experience without saying a word, but as soon as the surgical list of operations had been completed, she took the great professor to one side and said: 'I have never witnessed such a disgraceful performance as this in my whole working career. If you ever behave like this again, I will ban you from my theatres.' For the first time in his distinguished career, the professor had met his match. 'Tiger' Monk was subsequently put in charge of overseeing the furbishing of the operating theatres in the New Charing Cross Hospital. Two such dominant personalities were bound to have an affinity and forge a great friendship. Some years later I performed bilateral cataract and implant surgery on her eyes, and it was Professor Harding-Rains who took her back to his home to convalesce with him and his wife.

During my first year as a consultant at the West London Hospital, Veronica and I were invited to present the awards at the nurses' annual prize-giving ceremony. We really had been admitted to the bosom of this hospital, with its old-fashioned intimacy and friendship, the equal of which, I would never experience again.

During this year, I was introduced to the concept of private practice when Keith Lyle invited me to help him in his practice in Chesterfield Street, Mayfair. He was a fine surgeon and it would have been impossible to find a better master.

He showed me how to merge a busy NHS commitment with a successful private practice, while ensuring that both sets of patients received the same compassion and quality of care.

In 1968 Keith Lyle was elected President of the Ophthalmologic Society and chose me to be Secretary, a position that would enormously influence my own career and lead to monumental changes in European Ophthalmology in general.

Veronica would occasionally travel to Ireland to help John host important functions at the Phoenix Park Racecourse, such as once entertaining Prince Rainier and Princess Grace of Monaco (best remembered as the actress Grace Kelly). Veronica was surprised to see the society beauty wearing thick glasses and making little effort to preserve her famous good looks.

In the play *As you like it*, Shakespeare talks about the seven stages of man, and so it was we found our children changing on an almost daily basis. After months of babyhood, our children were now old enough to reciprocate our love, and suddenly they became a more personal and present part of our lives. Although Veronica and I shared the major part of their upbringing, we were incredibly fortunate to have Veronica's mother, Joy, who was always prepared to help, as well as Nan Peacock and Joan Hartley. We were thus able to travel at any time knowing that our children were well loved and cared for.

Veronica and I were asked by the Dunsanys to join them for a late summer holiday in Grasse, France. On our way we stopped in St Tropez, a beautiful ancient fishing village that had not yet been 'exposed' to the world by Bridget Bardot. Their daughter Bibi was with them, as was Randal's son Eddie Plunkett, who at the time was living in Paris. Eddie is now a very capable and renowned artist but then was still searching for his own unique style. Veronica and I drove him almost every day to an abandoned viaduct that he painted from numerous different angles, each emphasizing other characteristics and light, but none of the finished paintings pleased Eddie. On his return home he was so dissatisfied that he destroyed them all.

On one evening, Randal and Sheila took us to dinner with the Pleschs in their villa just outside Monaco. After an uneventful dinner the ladies retired to the boudoir for coffee and liqueurs. Arpad Plesch left the dinner table with the ladies and invited Veronica to see his collection of paintings. When they reached his picture gallery on the top floor, Arpad lost all interest in his paintings and began to divert his attention to Veronica. Veronica was reliving the scene she had had with Alfred Marks some few years previously in the Shepperton Film Studios. Once again she had to run around and around the room to escape these unwanted advances and was mercifully rescued by the telephone, which rang just as she was becoming really scared. This momentary distraction allowed Veronica to escape to the safety of her fellow guests.

The male guests, including David Niven (who in subsequent years would become my patient and a great personal friend), were having an equally exciting time in the dining room. Arpad had the world's foremost collection of 'butterfly' and pornographic books, which he kept on high shelves in the dining room. As soon as the ladies had left the room, the gentlemen leaped up from their chairs and mounted the ladders to examine the contents of this library, which included many illustrated first editions. It was a memorable sight witnessing David Niven, perching at the top of a ladder, fumbling through these 'classics'. Randal Dunsany had his monocle up to his eye and was leering with obvious pleasure at some precious manuscript.

On our way home at the end of our holiday, we drove via Dijon to visit Professor Philippe Moreau. Philippe was an eminent ophthalmic surgeon, as well as being a wine connoisseur of repute, who owned his own vineyard and marketed his produce in the name of J Moreau & Fils. During the morning, we watched him perform two cataract operations, two retinal-detachment operations and one corneal graft. In the UK, these operations would have taken about five hours, but Philippe completed this surgery in less than four hours with great precision. But the greatest surprise came when he opened bottles of champagne for us all before lunch. In the UK, midday drinking was certainly not on the menu.

I asked how his afternoon's patients would react to the smell of alcohol on the breath of their examiner and was politely told that most of his patients would also have had a glass of wine at lunchtime to assist their digestion. I also told Philippe that it was unusual to perform a corneal-transplant operation on a routine surgical list in the UK, as we sometimes had to wait weeks before a suitable donated cornea became available. Professor Moreau said that there was no shortage of cadaver donor material, as every night there were fatal car crashes on the neighbouring Route National, whereupon the bodies of the victims became state property! Suddenly my champagne tasted a little less appetizing.

The following summer, Veronica and I went to Ireland to help my father move out of his beloved Ounavarra House to the small bungalow he had built in the Liffey Valley alongside the river. At the time my future was still undecided, and there remained a possibility that Veronica and I would return to Ireland should the correct ophthalmic appointment become available. One evening while staying with the De Freynes in Cork Little in Bray, we went to dinner with Quentin and April Agnew-Somerville. After an alcohol-fuelled dinner, during which we all became more and more enthusiastic about our possible return to Ireland, the Somervilles told us that there was an ideal property to be bought in the local area. Arth Con Castle, in West Meath, was some 20 miles from the centre of Dublin and could be the perfect place to live in and bring up our family.

At around midnight we drove to the castle. It was a cloudless night and the Irish countryside was illuminated by a full moon. We had to park our car some distance from the castle, as the drive was inches deep in mud. We walked up to the castle, every stone of which could be seen under the light of the full moon. The outer walls were intact, with its four turreted corners. We had no difficulty entering, as there was no front door. The whole ground floor was filled with cattle. The stone staircase ended halfway up to the gutted first floor and there was no roof. While we were squelching our way across the hallway, groping our way between the cattle, we were disturbed by the presence of a very irate farmer.

'What the **** are you doing on my land in the middle of the night,' he said. With great aplomb Quentin replied: 'I have brought over some guests from Somerville, who may be interested in buying this property as a family home.' The farmer obviously considered us quite mad and rapidly ushered us off the castle grounds. This was the end of our house-hunting in Ireland.

Without realizing it, it was almost the end of our connection with Irish ophthalmology. Beecher and Sammy Somerville–Large invited us to Brooklawn, where he told us that at last an opening was coming up in the Royal Victoria Eye and Ear Hospital, Dublin. I had waited more than five years for this appointment, but by now I was fairly well established as a consultant ophthalmologist in London. We were on the horns of a dilemma. I had spent years under Beecher's tutelage, being groomed for the takeover of his consultancy and private practice, but now I was not sure whether or not to accept, especially as another consultancy was about to come up at the Royal Eye Hospital in Lambeth. I asked Beecher if I could defer a decision until I knew where I stood with the appointment at the Royal Eye.

The Royal Eye Hospital was situated on London's South Bank, near to the Elephant and Castle. It was a hospital that did not have the same traditions as Moorfields and had always been considered second best. There was tremendous jealousy between these two hospitals, which centred upon the two dominant personalities of the hospitals: Sir Stewart Duke-Elder, Head of the Institute of Ophthalmology, and Professor Arnold Sorsby of the Royal Eye Hospital. It had always been a bone of contention to the Moorfields group that the first professorship in London ophthalmology had gone to a surgeon at the Royal Eye Hospital. Professor Sorsby was, however, extremely well qualified – an exceptionally gifted author of textbooks and a world authority on genetics.

I applied for the post of consultant ophthalmic surgeon but felt that, as a Moorfields graduate, I would have little hope of achieving the position. I did, however, have one trump card up my sleeve. I had recently supported the neurologist Dr Frank Rose with his application to join the staff of the Charing Cross Group, and, as he was on the staff of the Royal Eye Hospital, he had promised to help me with my own application.

I had to compete against a number of my equally well-qualified erstwhile colleagues, all of whom wanted the position as much as I did. Professor Arnold Sorsby and eight other consultants conducted the interview, most of whom I didn't know. As well as Professor Sorsby, there were Dermot Pierce, Mr Philpott, Doreen Birks, Peter Clover, Miss Savory, Noel Moore and an anaesthetist, Dr Goldsmith. I was, however, a little relieved to see that I had two friends on the committee, Frank Rose, the neurologist, and Alan Higgitt, my ophthalmic senior at the Charing Cross Group.

Despite the strong opposition, I obtained the consultancy and thus acquired an appointment in an ophthalmic hospital, as well as one in a London teaching hospital, Charing Cross. I was devastated at having let down Beecher Somerville-Large, but, despite his obvious disappointment, he realized that the long delay in an opening becoming available in Dublin had inevitably encouraged Veronica and me to look elsewhere. This must have been a great sadness for him, as he had spent 10 years grooming me to take over his practices in Dublin and I was now absconding to the larger pastures of England. It says much for Beecher's depth of understanding that he never once tried to question my judgement.

On my first day at the Royal Eye Hospital I was summoned to see the administrator Joan Barber. She was known to have a rather low opinion of doctors, and I found her absorbed in the obituary column of the *British Medical Journal*. She looked up and said: 'I have a good laugh every Friday reading about the saints who have passed on.' Having completed the necessary paperwork, she gave me a tour of the hospital. As well as being triangular in shape, its main staircase wound around the solitary lift, which was too small to hold a full-length theatre trolley – so if a coffin had to be taken out of the hospital, it would go down in the lift in the upright position. It was always said that a ship's architect had planned the building.

As in the West London Hospital, my clinics were staffed by ophthalmologists who were all considerably older than me. Ted Smith, with whom I formed an immediate rapport, managed the outpatient department most efficiently. I was equally blessed in the operating theatre.

The hospital had an annex in a large Victorian edifice of a house in Surbiton, in the outskirts of London, which had been financed by the NHS and was almost exclusively used by one of the senior surgeons from the Royal Eye Hospital, Timmy Tyrrell, who looked upon it as his own personal fiefdom. When examining patients, he would bind the patient's chair to the examining desk so they could not get away from him. Shortly after I started, Timmy had a severe heart attack, which forced his retirement, and, unwillingly, I inherited the twice-weekly responsibility of the annex in Surbiton. Sister Margaret Umpleby, the theatre superintendent, and I totally reorganized the operating theatre. Bruce Mathalone introduced the microscope. We brought in one of the first operating microscopes to be used in the UK and upgraded the ophthalmic equipment. Although we had not as yet reached the sophistication of current ophthalmic surgery, we were certainly on our way. It really was most enjoyable working and operating in this country house with its relaxed atmosphere, and we carried out a huge workload. My clinics were shared between the main hospital in Lambeth and the annex in Surbiton. Most of the patients chose to have their operations in Surbiton, as it gave them a week's holiday in the country.

As a young consultant surgeon, my immediate junior, the senior registrar, was little younger than myself and would treat me as an equal. The first time

I used the operating microscope was with my senior registrar, James McGrand, at the Royal Eye Hospital in 1966. We looked through the tubes of the microscope and found a whole different perspective of the operating field. All we could see was the eye we were operating upon and the distal portion of the operating instruments. Our hands were out of view but seemed to be in a different dimension. Together we explored the mysteries of the microscope and carried out the operation, which was a success, but it took three times longer at first. In weeks we would have found it difficult to operate without the visual aid of the microscope, and we had climbed another pinnacle in the advancement of ophthalmic surgery.

Most of my senior registrars ended up as senior surgeons in different parts of the world, teaching and practising the skills they had acquired during their final training in the UK. Over the years I have had senior registrars from Australia, New Zealand, Africa, Mauritius, Nepal, India, Pakistan, South America, Europe and the Middle East. As well as training them in surgery, I always tried to instil the importance of realizing that, as surgeons, we are merely performing a few deft manoeuvres on our patients. The whole of the healing process is carried out by nature and we are but the catalysts.

One of my Egyptian registrars, Mr Ahmed, was a real character. On one occasion I was doing a plastic operation on the eyelid of a patient who was suffering from trachoma, a condition that was the scourge of the Middle East and causes massive scarring of the lids and cornea of the eye. Halfway through the operation, he told me that he knew a simpler and more effective procedure than the one I was doing. I asked him what experience he had had with this condition and he casually replied that he had performed this surgery on more than 700 patients. I bowed to his superior knowledge and allowed him to show me the more practical way to do it. From then on, this became my standard technique for this operation. On another occasion, one of my patients was a friend of King Hussein of Jordan. After surgery, his young wife, Princess Muna, came to visit this patient, but when leaving the hospital, she was sidetracked by Mr Ahmed, who spent the next three hours discussing Middle Eastern politics with her. Ahmed eventually became the senior ophthalmic advisor to the Egyptian Armed Forces.

One of my tragedies at this hospital was the treatment of a seven-year-old Irish child, who required a straightforward squint operation to correct the deviation of his eyes. Before surgery I discussed the procedure with the boy's young parents, who had misgivings about any operation being performed on their only child. I reassured them that it was a routine procedure that would give their child an improved quality of life. The surgery proceeded without complication and after its completion, while having tea in the surgeons' sitting room, the anaesthetist rushed in to say that the little boy had suffered a cardiac arrest. Resuscitation treatment was immediately applied and by the time the paramedics arrived with the ambulance, the child's pulse had been restored. I accompanied the child and his parents in the ambulance to the Fulham branch of Charing Cross Hospital with sirens blaring and lights flashing, and we made the journey from Surbiton to Fulham in less than 15 minutes. Having seen the boy admitted to the hospital I made my way home. The next day I went to visit the child and, on entering the intensive-care unit, was told that the little boy had died 10 minutes earlier. There was little comfort I could give the distraught parents. This tragedy made me realize that undue optimism should not form part of the surgeon's armoury. That afternoon Veronica and I took our two children to see Julie Andrews in *The sound of music*. I sat through this magical film thinking about nothing but the child and his parents.

I had not as yet begun to subspecialize in cataract surgery. One of my patients with retinal detachment was treated with one of the first silicone explants available in the country. My colleague John Ayoub of Moorfields had brought a few of them back to England after a visit to the continent and he kindly gave me one. I was most impressed with the simplicity and success of this operation and ordered my own supply of explants from Europe. The procedure was very simple. A silicone tube was sewn onto the outer coat of the eye in the area overlying the retinal hole. This explant indirectly plugged the retinal hole and affected a cure. Over the next few years, this operation phased out Cyril Dee-Shapland's procedure, which had so helped those with this condition over the previous years.

One of the patients I treated at this hospital was a young man of 22 who was blind in one eye and had developed a retinal detachment in his only seeing eye. Martin Highland had a growth condition and was under five foot in height. Despite his physical disabilities, he was a very accomplished drummer who played in a successful pop group. It was obviously imperative that he regained his sight so that he could continue with his chosen career. His retinal detachment was very complicated, and I was apprehensive as to whether or not we would be able to cure his condition. I performed the operation assisted by my ever-faithful Sister Umpleby and my senior registrar, Paddy Condon from Waterford, Ireland. The operation took more than two hours and required the combined skills of all the team. On the next day, the Royal Eye Hospital held its annual summer fête, to which all the patients were invited. The grounds were filled with marquees and the tables laden with home produce for the hundreds of guests and staff. I couldn't enjoy the festivities until I had checked on Martin, and I found him lying quietly in bed: I was expecting a pessimistic outcome, but when I took off the dressing, it was such a thrill to see that the operation had been a success.

In the framework of the Royal Eye Hospital was the need for a charitable vehicle to fund Arnold Sorsby's professorial unit and the supplementary needs of the hospital, which could not be supplied by public finances. Colonel and Mrs Digby Jones ran the hospital's charity trust, assisted by the secretary Joan Hamilton Price and a volunteer helper David Inglefield. Veronica was co-opted into this group. This was the start of Veronica's charitable works, and she could not have found a better place to gain valuable fundraising and administrative experience. The team worked efficiently together in an atmosphere of constant gaiety and companionship, and I always enjoyed breaking off from my duties in the hospital to join them. Throughout the year they organized various events, such as the Christmas party and the summer fête.

Their most ambitious project was the annual Iris Ball, which was one of London's best-known charitable dinner dances, held at the Hyde Park Hotel. For many years, a very young Veronica was chairman of this ball. It was a wonderful way of enjoying a sophisticated evening with our friends, made even better in the knowledge that all proceeds went to help the hospital, its staff and the patients. Veronica soon realized that the financial success of the event was determined not by the ticket sales but by the added trimmings, such as the raffle, tombola and auction, which added a huge amount of fun to the proceedings. Veronica was a very good chairman and, with her 'Irish' adoption, knew how to create a carefree and relaxed party. There was never any difficulty selling the tickets for the ball or finding generous sponsors.

CHAPTER 13
A link to private practice

Within weeks of starting at the Royal Eye Hospital, we had another stroke of fortune. I bumped into Edgar King at church one day, and he asked if I'd like to take over his private practice in Harley Street. He was about to retire and had only approached one other young ophthalmologist, David Abrahams.

David was a friend and a colleague who, many years later, asked me to do the cataract and implant operations on his mother. I called David to discuss our predicament and with great largesse he said that he was still undecided but suggested that we should both compete for it and let the best man win.

Edgar King met both of us several times but was totally unable to decide. In desperation, he sought the advice of his landlady, Mrs Smith, who had acquired a long lease on the property from the superior landlords – the Howard de Walden estate. The Smiths were Irish and very keen on horse racing and with my own connections in this field, they voted for me.

Mrs Smith's husband had been an outstanding general surgeon, who had practised from this address. 82 Harley Street is a four-storey terraced house situated in the heart of London's private medical sector. As their private house, the ground floor comprised the drawing room and ladies' boudoir, which doubled up as a waiting room for the patients and an office for the receptionist. On the first floor was the dining room and pantry, which were later converted into the consulting room suites to be used by Edgar King. In the passage between these two rooms, there was a dumb waiter – a small lift shaft used to bring the meals up from the kitchen in the basement.

Edgar King sold me all the fixtures and fittings of his consulting rooms for £500. Although this was a princely sum, it was outstanding value. The contents included an oil painting by Fred Taylor, the artist who had painted the posters for the Great Western Railway at the turn of the century. There was also a fabulous suite of Art Deco furniture.

So in early 1966, at the age of 37, I had finally consolidated my two part-time NHS appointments, and to add to these I could now include Edgar King's private practice. Before moving into Harley Street, Edgar gave Veronica and me lunch in the Bucks Club, with his secretary, Diana Rigall, to discuss the final details of the handover. Diana was the cousin of one of our colleagues, Jimmy Doggart, and had been Edgar's devoted secretary for some years. Edgar had acquired an enormous practice, and there were some 30,000 patient notes in his files. His most eminent patient was undoubtedly Sir Winston Churchill, who he had seen no fewer than 45 times. Sir Winston suffered from in-turning lower lids that caused tears to run down his cheeks, which added to the appearance of his already overcharged emotions. All he required was a simple corrective plastic surgical procedure to these lids, which would have given him instant and permanent relief, but the great man fluffed the issue on every occasion – hence his numerous attendances. When Edgar finally retired, the only thing he took with him were the notes of his old friend and patient Sir Winston Churchill. I had inherited his very capable secretary, the rooms, a mews garage and all his equipment, including the very ophthalmoscope with which he had examined Sir Winston Churchill. This most important historical instrument will one day have to be bequeathed to a museum.

My first private, non-paying, patients were Sir Francis Dashwood, his wife Victoria, who had been one of my previous girlfriends, and their young daughters Emily, Georgina and Caroline. Of all the thousands of patients I acquired, Edgar reviewed only three sets of notes with me in advance. These belonged to men of prominence, each of whom had a particularly difficult ophthalmic condition. All three patients remained in my practice, and over the ensuing years became personal friends.

One of these was Victor De Rothschild, a member of the famous banking dynasty and one-time head of the government's Central Policy Review Team under Edward Heath's premiership. Victor was totally blind in one eye and having trouble with his other. Although only in his early 50s, he had an obscure degeneration of the retina. After an extended examination, I told Victor that his ophthalmic condition was caused by a more generalized condition in his body. He was suffering from a fat dyscrasia. Indignantly, he rose up and said I was talking rubbish, having had numerous previous opinions from the most eminent consultants in the country, none of whom had even mentioned this diagnosis. He left my rooms in a rather agitated state, and I thought I had probably lost another of Edgar King's former patients. After several weeks, Victor returned, and with good grace he apologized for his former attitude. He had just spent several weeks in the Mayo Clinic in America having extensive diagnostic tests that had confirmed my opinion. From that time onwards, Victor became one of my most supportive patients. On one occasion at a dinner party, he was sitting next to a lady who was rapidly going blind in her only seeing eye. She had been told that an operation on this eye would be hazardous and could cause total blindness. Victor referred her to me.

Another of these patients was Sir Ronald Edwards, the former chairman of what is now GlaxoSmithKline. He suffered from extreme short sight, and his examination was always prolonged, as I had to explain and discuss with him every detail of his condition. With him, I felt like a medical student giving his findings to a senior colleague who would then decide how best to treat the condition. He and his wife were great lovers of the ballet, and Veronica and I were invited to join them at Covent Garden Opera House on many occasions. He was asked by Harold Wilson to become chairman of British Leyland. His doctor had refused to let him accept this appointment, as he considered it could adversely affect his vision. When I inherited Ronny as a patient, I strongly advised him to take the job to actively employ his very alert mind. He became an outstanding chairman, and during the years that he held this office, British Leyland prospered – free from the industrial action that later crippled the company and heralded the demise of the once-mighty British car industry.

The final patient discussed with me was Sir Ronald Milne-Watson, deputy chairman of British Steel. Both he and his brother had severe glaucoma. Ronald had already lost the vision in one eye, and was rapidly losing sight in the other. Despite being on the strongest medication possible, I checked weekly that the pressure in his eye was within reasonable limits. Unlike the other two 'special' patients he had a very placid temperament, and although a very busy man, he endured the inevitable wait in the reception area with great patience. He came into my consulting room on one occasion, full of merriment. While dozing in a very crowded waiting room one very elderly patient, who happened to be the penultimate survivor of the Titanic disaster, said to her friend in a loud voice: 'Do you think that man sitting opposite us is dead, he hasn't moved for some time.' It eventually became impossible to keep Ronald's ocular pressure under control and it was essential to perform a decompression drainage operation. The operation exceeded all expectations and the pressure in the eye became normalized. Thereafter his visits became six monthly.

The practice in Harley Street naturally diminished after Edgar King's retirement. Edgar was an 'elder statesman' who was well known for his sound medical judgement, whereas, I was young, relatively inexperienced and totally unknown. Despite these shortcomings the practice survived, with much thanks due to the continuing services of the secretary Diana Riggall. One patient in particular did not approve of my youth. She had diabetic changes in both her retinas and I personally took her for a physician's opinion regarding her general treatment. She subsequently required cataract operations but felt that I was too young to perform the necessary surgery, and instead she had the operations carried out by a more elderly colleague. He performed outdated surgery that confined her to bed for a week, with the result that she developed a fatal clot in her lung. Surgery by a younger surgeon and a shorter convalescence may well have produced a different outcome.

Edgar King had many patients in the theatrical world, and after his retirement I attended the needs of several well-known film stars. Alistair Sim, of *The Girls of St Trinians* and other Bolton films, was one of these. He was a truly lovely patient to examine, but his condition required several lengthy tests in my consulting room. On one occasion, I apologized for the time and cooperation he had to give me for this examination. Raising his bushy eyebrows, he exclaimed: 'Dear boy, I am enjoying every minute of this.' Another of my patients from Edgar's theatrical contacts was Ava Gardner, who took some umbrage when

I challenged her about her age. Her only problem was that she needed glasses for reading.

A year later, Cyril Dee-Shapland invited me to take over his private practice, which markedly increased the numbers of my patients. I felt very honoured and pleased that this would enable me to keep in touch with Cyril and his wife. Cyril's patients mainly reflected the skill for which he had been most noted – namely the treatment of retinal detachments. One patient I inherited was a distant cousin, Willie Van Cutsem, who had undergone a failed retinal-detachment operation, as a result of which he had sight in only one eye. Despite the failure of his own surgery, he would visit the ophthalmic ward of UCH every Tuesday evening to give comfort and hope to the patients who were scheduled to have their surgery on the following day. Although Cyril Dee-Shapland was a brilliant surgeon, his life's dedication had been to his wife and ophthalmic career, so he was extremely vulnerable to the forces of the 'real world'. Desmond Greaves, his colleague at UCH, was very supportive to 'Shappy' at a time when his advancing years and innate naivety made survival difficult. Des Greaves supported Cyril in such a loving manner that he could almost have been his son.

I also inherited Sir Neville Cardus, who in his day was the world's most noted ballet critic and cricket correspondent. He became a very great friend, and it was he who introduced us to the Garrick Club. On our first visit, we went together up the winding front stairs leading from the hall. Halfway up, a horrified porter intercepted us and politely informed us that ladies were required to use the back staircase! Neville would always make Veronica smoke a black Russian cigarette after dinner, which in those days was still fashionable. He was fascinated by her Russian background. He suggested that I became a member of the club, which wasn't easy – especially as most of the members have a theatrical background. A little black book in the hall lists the names of prospective members, and each name is expected to get support from 30 existing members before being considered. Shortly after my name was put down, Neville Cardus passed away. I received a letter from the Secretary notifying me that I had lost my sponsor, but adding that, in honour of Neville, if any member of the club could sponsor me, I would be automatically admitted. As far as I know, Prince Charles and I are the only two members of the club who were elected without a ballot – such was the affection in which everyone held Neville. Our evenings spent with him were always full of wit and anecdotes.

CHAPTER 14
BBC TV and a boating fracas

In May 1967, Veronica and I went for a fortnight's holiday to Italy with my brother John. We first spent a memorable couple of days in Rome soaking in the treasures of the city and joined thousands of pilgrims in Vatican City, where we were rewarded with a glimpse of Pope Paul VI waving to the crowds from a second-floor window. It really was a wonderful time of year to be there, with the late spring flowers still in full bloom and the sun enhancing the beauty of its ancient buildings.

After a magical few days in Rome, we drove south with our Irish friends, Peter and Sally Jury, to the small village of Priano. Our villa was perched on a cliff and was owned by Nanky Morehouse, an elderly relative of Denny Wardell. During the war, Nanky and her late husband had managed the Anchor Bleu Inn in Bosham, East Sussex. Before the D-Day invasion, they had billeted several army officers – one of whom was the well-known artist, Rex Whistler. Whistler spent his last evening doing a sketch of a gnome sitting astride a wooden cask of brandy, which Nanky now had hanging in her drawing room. The day after drawing this picture, Rex Whistler was killed in action.

Soon after our arrival our other friends, Dennis and Hillary Wardell and John and Sheila Wilson-Wright, joined us. Later that night Veronica and I received the devastating news that Beecher Somerville-Large had died in a Dublin hospital the day before. I had lost a true friend, a second father and one of the most influential mentors of my life.

The next day we woke to find that Veronica had developed mumps and had a high fever with a temperature of 103°F. For the following six days I sat by her bedside, only joining our friends for meals in the nearby Continental Hotel. She eventually recovered after I gave her a massive injection of tetramycin. The evenings we spent in Positano were always quite boisterous, and on one occasion everyone went for a midnight skinny dip. Swimming was illegal in Italy after nightfall and we had some difficulty retrieving our clothes, as we had to circumnavigate the police, who had heard our laughter and were waiting for us on the beach.

After some days we befriended a young Italian, who spent most of each day with us practising his English, but when the Angelus bell was rung at midday he would run off. At first we thought that he must have been going to the church for prayers, but we later discovered he was enjoying an illicit hour with a young schoolmistress at the local school.

When Veronica was sufficiently recovered, we were able to enjoy the latter part of the holiday in Priano. Our most memorable day was an excursion in a rented boat to Capri, where we took a ride through the Blue Grotto, a natural cavern that is filled with an ethereal and eerie light reflecting on the blue water. We joined the rest of our party for lunch and between us all demolished some 20 bottles of wine, which the waiters took great pleasure in lining up along the balcony. That afternoon we walked up the steep hill to San Michele to visit Dr Axel Munthe's house. This celebrated Swedish physician has always been one of my role models in medicine and his book, *The Story of San Michele* was one of my favourites. His ideals and philosophy, which I have always admired, are summed up in this short passage:

'When the eagle's eye flashed down the list of officers proposed for promotion to Generals, he used to scribble in the margin of a name 'is he lucky?' I had luck, amazing uncanny luck with everything I laid my hands on, with every patient I saw. I was not a good doctor. My studies had been too rapid, my hospital training too short. There is not the slightest doubt that I was a successful doctor. What is the secret of success? To inspire confidence? What is confidence? Where does it come from? From the head or from the heart? Does it derive from the upper strata of our mentality or is it a mighty tree of knowledge of good and evil with roots springing from the very depth of our being? Through what channels does it communicate with others? Is it physical to the eye? Is it audible in the spoken word? I do not know. I only know that it is neither acquired by book reading nor by bedside manner. It is a magic gift granted by birthright to one man and denied to another. The doctor who possesses this gift can almost raise the dead. The doctor who does not possess it will have to submit to the calling in of a colleague to a patient in the case of measles.

'I soon discovered that this invaluable gift was granted to me by no merit of mine. I discovered it in the nick of time when I was beginning to become conceited and very pleased with myself. It made me understand how little I knew and made me turn more and more to Mother Nature – the wise old nurse for advice and help. It might even have made me become a good doctor in the end had I stuck to my hospital work and to my poor patients, but I lost all my chances. I became a fashionable doctor instead. If you come across a fashionable doctor watch him carefully from a safe distance before handing yourself over to him. He may be a good doctor but in very many cases he is not. First because as a rule he is far too busy to listen with patience to your long story. Secondly because he is inevitably liable to become a snob – if he is not one already. To let the Countess pass in before you, to examine the liver of the Count with more attention than that of his valet. To go to a garden party at the British Embassy instead of to your last born whose whooping cough is getting worse. Sadly, unless his heart is very sound, he will soon show unmistakable signs of precocious hardening of that organ. He will become indifferent and insensible to the suffering of others like the pleasure-seeking people around him. You cannot be a good doctor without pity.

You are always trying to explain to your patients what you cannot even explain to yourself.

'*It is all a question of faith not of knowledge, like the faith in God. The Catholic Church never explains anything and remains the strongest in the world. The Protestant Church tries to explain everything and is crumbling to pieces. The less your patients know of the truth, the better for them. It was never meant that the workings of the organs of your body should be watched by the mind. To make your patients think about their illness is to tamper within the laws of nature. Tell them that they must do so-and-so, must take such-and-such in order to get better and if they don't mean to obey you they must go somewhere else. Do not call them unless they are in need of you. Do not talk to them much or they will soon find out how little you know. Doctors, like Royalty, should keep aloof as much as possible or their prestige will suffer. We all look our best in somewhat subdued light. Look at the doctor's own family who always prefer to consult somebody else.*'

It gave Veronica and me great pleasure to see the house and garden that had drawn this great man from his medical practice to this retreat on the top of the hill in Capri. San Michele stands aloft as a monument and tribute to his life.

On our return to London we received another blow. My father had been diagnosed with terminal carcinoma of the lungs. John and I immediately travelled to Ireland to be with him at his bedside in the Adelaide Hospital. As his physicians had decided that treatment would be useless, we took him back to his bungalow at Ounavarra, so he could pass away peacefully surrounded by his own possessions. After a few days Veronica took our place in Ireland, and John and I returned to London.

Veronica cared for Father for some weeks before going down to Manorbier Castle to join Arvid and Joy and our children, who were on summer holiday. Early on a Monday in July I was phoned by Joe Sheridan, my father's helper, to be told that Father had passed away during the night. The previous evening the local vicar had twice visited my father. On the second occasion, Father had said: 'You can go now, I am all right.' On receiving the news, I immediately rang up John in Dublin and Veronica, who was staying in Manorbier Castle, but extraordinarily Veronica already knew. She had been given the haunted turret room in the castle, and at one o'clock in the morning she was woken by a raging storm outside, to see my father standing at the end of her bed saying, 'Farewell for the moment.' Father did so love Veronica, in whom he saw so many similar traits as in his own beautiful wife.

Having lost my father and mentor, we realized with much melancholy that we had passed imperceptibly into another stage of life, in which we were now the older generation.

The administrator of the original Charing Cross Hospital in the Strand invited me to join the staff, the jewel of the Charing Cross Group of Hospitals, to work in the hospital for one day a week. The staff of Charing Cross looked on themselves as senior to those in the other hospitals in the group and remained somewhat aloof. The hospital still retained its monthly independent medical board meeting, at which all administrative, financial and medical affairs of the hospital were dealt with. It also had its own exclusive consultants' annual dinner. As a newly appointed member of the staff, I had to make an initiation speech at this dinner, which was well received by my older colleagues in this venerable hospital. I was thus accepted and worked alongside medical colleagues who were the peers of their own profession, including Professor Harding-Rains in general surgery, Lionel Taylor in ear, nose and throat (ENT), Frank Rose in neurology and David Trevor, the orthopaedic surgeon. The atmosphere in this hospital was akin to that of a London club such as the Garrick, which was just around the corner. The staff were intensely proud of its traditions of excellence in healing and the society with which they worked.

Shortly after, the queen came to tea. It was an extremely informal occasion. The consultant staff met her in the boardroom with the two administrators, Frank Hart and his deputy assistant Mr Barclay. I was seated some chairs away from Her Majesty but was near enough to appreciate her intelligence, vivacity and the interest she showed in our work. We witnessed, at first hand, the dedication and service our young queen was giving to her subjects. Meeting her for the first time made me conscious of how lucky we were to have this lady as our Sovereign.

Some 100 years earlier, an officer in the Royal Horse Guards (The Blues) had fallen off his horse, during an official ceremony in Horse Guards Parade. He was admitted to Charing Cross Hospital, where a concerned Queen Victoria later visited him. The queen was so impressed with the treatment her officer was being given that she awarded the hospital her Guards Colours. The Guards Ribbon, with dark blue and burgundy stripes suspending the Charing Cross, made the nurses' badge one of the most distinctive in the nursing profession.

I was always rather proud to be working in a hospital called Charing Cross. Like many other thousands of families, mine is directly descended from King Edward I 'Longshanks' and his wife Eleanor of Castile, who together had 16 children! When Eleanor died near Lincoln in 1290, a grief-stricken Edward ordered that her body should be carried in a sombre procession to Westminster Abbey in London. At each place where the procession stopped for the night, mass was said, after which Edward built a memorial cross in her honour. The journey took 12 days, and crosses were erected in Lincoln, Grantham, Stamford, Geddington, Northampton, Stony Stratford, Woburn, Dunstable, St Albans, Waltham and Westcheap. On the last night of this journey, the entourage camped in a field one mile from Westminster Abbey. The following morning, the king had mass and raised a station of the cross. He said farewell, in this world, to his dear 'Charing'.

A single Matron was in charge of Charing Cross Hospital and under her were a number of sisters, who ran the wards and various departments. Even as a consultant in the hospital I would make myself known to the sister before examining a patient in her ward. A sense of territorial rights and responsibility permeated into every department of the hospital.

Throughout my working career I would go for a swim at 5.30 am in the Royal Automobile Club, Pall Mall. The staff became great friends, and Sam Jabou, the head waiter in the restaurant, is still working there today. One day, while enjoying my early morning exercise, a member of the night staff collapsed with a heart attack by the side of the pool. Having rushed him in my car to Charing Cross, I was castigated by the night sister for not having brought him in an ambulance.

Another formidable member of the staff was Sister Coarser who ran the outpatient department. She had little time for me, as I looked too young to be a consultant, but she idolised David Trevor, the orthopaedic surgeon, who epitomized every characteristic she admired. David was a strict disciplinarian, both to his staff and patients. A small dapper man, he would do his ward-rounds like a general inspecting his troops, while his staff would stand rigidly to attention at the patient's bedside. His eccentricities and insistence on protocol were forgiven by the true brilliance of his surgery. Many years later, he developed bilateral cataracts and became almost blind. I was privileged to have him under my care. This most aggressive and bombastic surgeon was a most docile and cooperative patient. Thank God I was able to restore to him the same type of health that he had given to so many of his own patients.

I found the outpatient sessions at Charing Cross the most trying of my whole career. Local general practitioners referred most of their routine ophthalmic patients to Moorfields, which had inherited the original ophthalmic unit. Patients referred to the unit at Charing Cross were those requiring an ophthalmic assessment for a condition totally unrelated to the eye and would inevitably take a considerable time to examine. With my general medical training I was able to cope, but it did stretch my knowledge of medicine to the limit!

At Charing Cross I worked in close cooperation with my colleagues who specialized in territories bordering the eye, such as the sinuses and the brain. With their help I delved into terrains far beyond the skills of an ophthalmic surgeon. One of my patients had a large tumour behind the eye, so I enlisted the aid of Harry Holden, a great friend and an excellent ENT surgeon. We started the operation together, and after he had made a surgical approach by removing the bone by the side of the eye, he took his leave to the surgeons' tearoom, leaving me to do the delicate dissection of the tissues behind the eye. One hour later I had, with some difficulty, removed the tumour without damaging the nerves and other structures around the eye. Harry Holden was an enthusiastic yachtsman, and as he came into the theatre and reviewed my operative field, he said: 'This is like coming from below decks and witnessing the calm after the storm.' With great aplomb, he replaced the bone that had been removed and closed the incision.

Harry Holden and I did many major surgical operations in this hospital, some of which took hours to complete. Although most of our results were good, we sadly totally failed with one patient. This lady, in her early 40s, was very beautiful, with raven black hair. She had developed a devastatingly malignant tumour in the tear duct between the eye and the nose. The tumour was removed without much difficulty, but it had already spread. Harry and I did endless operations, often involving the brain and sinuses, to try to remove the spreading tumour. Months later she died, with the inadequate results of our surgery imprinted on her face and head. Once again, I learned that as surgeons, we cannot presume to act as the Creator.

In 1967, the BBC produced a series showing the most common conditions in medicine. Originally scheduled for an off-peak slot, they were so well received by the public that in weeks they became mainstream viewing. This was one of the first times that the media was made aware of the avid interest that the public had in the hidden secrets of the body.

A programme on squints, the condition of 'cross-eyes' was thought to be the most representative ocular problem. Sophisticated corrective surgery for cataract and laser treatment for refractive conditions of the eye were still in the future and not even considered for discussion. The BBC approached me to ask whether or not I would be prepared to cooperate in the production of a full-length feature on this subject. I agreed to produce this programme in collaboration with Frank Rose, the neurologist.

Peter Riding, the assistant producer, decided that the best way to master the subject was to have a full understanding of how a squint occurred. He attended my ward rounds and surgical sessions and soon mastered a fair knowledge of ophthalmology. After much discussion, we decided that the best way to present the programme was to study several of my patients with different forms of squint. One of Veronica's cousins, Sarah Lloyd, was an ideal patient on whom to demonstrate, as she had a perfect manifestation of a deficiency in turning the eyes in to read a book. Another of my patients was a beautiful baby with a large-angled squint due for immediate treatment. We prepared coverage of the appearance of the squint before and after surgical correction in five different presentations, each showing a different aspect of the condition.

As filming was about to start, the producer arrived and was amazed that I had been allowed to produce a documentary in five parts, when in the allocated time there was only room for two. I began to feel apprehensive. We set up the five sets for the programme and had two dress rehearsals, during which I had to learn how to read the autocue without moving my eyes from side to side. A great deal had to be learned about television presentation in a very short time.

In the green room, I met the other guests, including the patients who would appear on the show and their relatives. I was advised by BBC staff to have two large whiskies, for 'Dutch courage', but no more! Just before walking onto the set, the director gave me one final piece of advice. I was told that it was imperative that once filming had started, I must carry on irrespective, as any pause would cost the BBC a lot of money.

At precisely 7 pm, the television cameras started to roll. I had completed the first three sets without any difficulty and nimbly stepped over to the fourth when I suddenly lost my place on the autocue. I had blown it! The director leapt onto the stage and shouted: 'Cut!' My embarrassment and shame was quickly relieved when he rushed up to me and humbly apologized that they had run out of film. The remainder of the filming went without any further hitches, and it was eventually broadcast some months later in the evening and again one Saturday afternoon, which we enjoyed watching with friends after a lunch party.

As Veronica and I spent most of our time in London, we thought it sensible not to have a dog, but by the time Stephen and Tania became toddlers, we realized our mistake. While staying with friends, the children became hysterical at the sight of two boisterous Labradors. It was obvious that our children were getting no insight into the ways of domestic pets. We immediately contacted our long-standing friend Susan Constable-Maxwell, who bred Cavalier spaniels, and for Veronica's birthday I bought her a black and white puppy, who we named Titus.

For the next eight years Titus became a part of the family. He had no vices and helped our children to appreciate the real relationship that can grow between our four-legged friends and us. His only fault was that he had no sense of direction and if lost on a walk, would panic and run as fast as he could in any direction. We spent many afternoons chasing a distant black and white speck through Kensington Gardens. Titus accompanied us on all our children's holidays – to the Cattleys at Robins Farm in Devon, Manorbier Castle in Wales or Ireland. When travelling to Ireland, Titus would stay in the car on the overnight ferry and guard it!

Ever since my bachelor days in Ireland, I had always hankered to own my own boat and the fact that I was not a natural yachtsman made no difference. One weekend, Edward Sturges, Veronica's boss, invited Veronica and me to join his wife Jean on their Thames Barge, which was moored at Newhaven. During the afternoon, we visited a boatyard and saw a small yacht that had just been built and fitted out by a New Zealand boat builder called Brad Pittard. Edward strongly advised us to buy it. Against our better judgement we did so, mistakenly thinking that it would be a good substitute for a weekend cottage. She was only 24 ft long and built of plywood. There was a single mast, and she sailed with a main sail and a forward jib. Space was extremely limited, although at a squash it could uncomfortably sleep four. Despite its cramped space, we felt quite snug below decks, even if a storm was raging above us.

We moored Acushla in the marina at Newhaven, before launching her and reeking havoc around the South Coast. Despite her many inadequacies, Acushla did become a sort of second home and we spent many weekends of mixed fortune on her. We would often ask friends to join us for the weekend, although because of the spartan accommodation and our ineptitudes, they had to be very good friends! Veronica's brother Charles was our most regular guest, and he would often sleep in the open cockpit under a canopy suspended from the boom. This was certainly more spacious than our quarters below deck but considerably more draughty!

In the middle of one night, when Veronica was sleeping on the sofa and I was in my quarter berth, Charles descended from the cockpit into our cabin and asked meekly if he could join us, as the canopy in the cockpit could not keep out the rain. Not too pleased with his intrusion, I begrudgingly said he could bring his sleeping bag down and lay it out between the sofa and portside cooking area. For the rest of the night we all slept soundly. The following morning I opened the hatch and could not believe what I saw. There had been an inch of rain over night, and most of the surrounding countryside was flooded.

Against all advice, we left for London that afternoon, as I had a long surgical operating list to do the following day. Making the return journey was like playing snakes and ladders. At every turn in the road we were confronted with another flood. When still 30 miles from London, we gave up and joined dozens of other stranded weekend commuters in a pub. Later that evening, we saw that several cars had managed to break through the floods from the London direction, so we decided to continue our journey. We were making good progress through the flooded roads, until the bow wave from a car coming from the opposite direction flooded us. Charles once again became very wet, as he had to climb out of the rear window of our Rover and push us to dry land. We finally arrived home, but our car had been severely damaged by the floods. It had been a long wet journey to make it to see my patients!

We had some great antics on Acushla, but I cannot pretend that Veronica and I were able or safe sailors. On the contrary, we either disobeyed or were blissfully ignorant of the most basic fundamentals of sailing. We often went out together and wondered whether or not we would manage to return to the safety of our pontoon without causing a major embarrassment.

We got caught out at sea many times, when our nautical skills would become strained to the limit by a sudden increase in the wind or the descent of fog, which so often drifted in over the South Downs. On one occasion, a strong southerly wind forced us to make a rapid retreat to the safety of our pontoon. With great seamanship we negotiated the entrance to the Newhaven Channel, when a sudden gust of wind sent us totally out of control. We roared through the narrow channel and finally came to a halt jammed between the sterns of two boats securely moored on their berths. The surprised owners were enjoying their Sunday lunch. Both parties showed considerable reserve, disentangling their uninvited guests from their mooring.

After numerous mishaps, we soon realized that a small boat, moored in a marina, was not an ideal or safe holiday home for young children. In retrospect we were lucky to have escaped any major accidents, especially as our children seldom wore life-jackets. One weekend, Tania tripped over one of the mooring ropes and fell into the murky waters of Newhaven Harbour. After a few terrifying moments, I managed to tug her out of the water by her hair on the third time that she surfaced, but thereafter she always had a fear of the boat. On another occasion I sailed out of Newhaven in a force six wind with Stephen not even wearing a life-jacket. He clung to the forward railings of Acushla as she plunged up and down in the raging sea. The wind was blowing so strongly that I was unable to turn the boat about. In desperation, I did a jibe and narrowly avoided capsizing. We were extremely fortunate to get back to harbour. I later realized how foolhardy I had been.

Part Five. Into The New World

CHAPTER 15
Charlie Kelman and the phaco sensation

As we were now firmly established in London, we decided to buy a house with a larger garden, where the children could play safely. On the advice of friends we looked at a number of houses in the unfashionable and bohemian area north of Holland Park and although we could not afford it, we decided to buy number 10 Lansdowne Crescent, Notting Hill Gate.

Lansdowne Crescent was on the ridge of Notting Hill, once the site of the former Hippodrome Racecourse. The houses were all semi-detached, well proportioned and had both front and rear gardens. Our house was on the eastern apex of this development, at its highest point. From the front, looking down Lansdowne Rise, we had an uninterrupted view of West London. At the rear of the house, beyond its own garden, was a large semicircular communal garden filled with mature trees, which, in the height of the summer, obscured the opposite houses from view.

It was in this home that our children enjoyed their formative years. They would spend hours bicycling and playing with friends in the enclosed safety of the garden. There was one permanent resident in the communal garden, an elderly lady who had fallen on hard times. Rumour had it that she had once owned one of the surrounding properties, but she now lived in the extremity of this garden under cardboard boxes hidden by shrubs. Nobody knew how she catered for her own hygiene, but she was left undisturbed by all our community. With her unkempt tangled hair, limping gait, bent back and sad expression, she remained one of our neighbours for many years.

This region had previously been a Mecca for artists and painters. At one time the voice of Enrico Caruso was heard resonating over the garden. Our neighbours included the famous cellist Alvin McCall, and the pianist Russ Conway. Rock legend Jimi Hendrix died only a few houses away.

It was at this time that my brother John resigned from the *Irish Times* and returned to Ireland to become managing director and chairman of the Phoenix Park Racecourse, Dublin. He moved into Ashtown House on the edge of the racecourse. Veronica and I now had an ideal country retreat for our children's holidays in Ireland. The racecourse made a wonderful playground for children, with so many exciting places to explore, such as the empty stands and bars and the course itself, with the starting gates as excellent climbing frames.

Riding on the racetrack was allowed only on the Sunday after a race meeting, as, come Monday, the keepers of the course would walk the track, replacing every hoof mark in readiness for the next meeting. I personally only raced once up the straight five-furlong course, after recklessly challenging my cousin Max Morris. Max was a part-time amateur jockey who was spending his gap year working on the course. With the whole family watching, John opened the starting gates and we were off. Max immediately left me in his wake and by the second furlong was at least one furlong ahead of me. Providence was on my side: one of Max's stirrup straps came undone and he came crashing to the ground. For a moment I considered stopping to check that he was unhurt, before my sporting instinct took over and I raced forward on my horse to win the solo sprint – to the great amusement of my family. On a rerun I was of course easily beaten.

On the Saturday of one race meeting, Veronica and I were finishing lunch in Ashtown House, John having already gone up to the course, when a very jovial Irishman burst into the kitchen.

'Is Sir John in?' he asked.

'No,' said Veronica, 'but can we help?'

'I've brought Lester Piggott,' he replied.

With that, he opened a large cardboard box on the table, revealing a bust of a man. It was as if Lester Piggott himself was staring up at us. The bearer of this trophy was sculptor Gary Trimble, who would become one of our greatest friends. The bust was to be presented to Lester, who was due to ride that afternoon in the 1,500 Race, which he fortunately won.

Gary had a fairly typical Irish upbringing. His family was very sympathetic to the Irish cause of independence and, as a boy, he could remember hiding under his parents' dining-room table in Fitzwilliam Square, Dublin, while Michael Collins, one of the great Irish patriots at the time of the revolution, talked to his parents. He later did a bust of the death mask of Michael Collins, which the Collins family considered was the best. He also sculpted Charlie Haughey, then the Prime Minister of Ireland, and many other statesmen. He was commissioned to do a silver bust of Queen Elizabeth II, who was so impressed with the result that she invited him to a private lunch with her at Buckingham Palace. This was the proudest moment of Gary's life.

While sculpting both Veronica and our daughter Tania, he stayed with us for two weeks to 'study' his subjects. On most days he would accompany me to my clinics and operating sessions. On the ward rounds I would introduce him to the staff and patients as Professor Trimble. Gary much enjoyed his time acting as an ophthalmic surgeon. The two busts were beautiful, but Veronica had a rather sad expression, as, while she was sitting, Gary had ceaselessly played Beethoven's last string quartets on his tape cassette player. When finally finished, Veronica's bust fell out of the back of our car when we were bringing it home. Despite clattering down a hill, it remained undamaged. Both bronzes featured the elongated swan neck that is the hallmark of Trimble's work.

Gary Trimble bought the top-floor flat in our medical practice at 82 Harley Street. Despite his upbringing, he became a committed Anglophile, even going so far as to buy a black London taxi to drive around Dublin. Sadly he died in a motor accident in this cab while returning from a Beethoven concert. He is now respected as one of the great Irish sculptors.

From the moment that John became the managing director of the course, he instigated many changes, including the introduction of a six-furlong straight, the construction of a 1.5-million gallon reservoir and watering system and the laying out of a pitch-and-putt course. These changes had come about after Edmond Loder, a respected racehorse owner and trainer, joined John and me on the board of directors. The straight six-furlong track was an immediate success and with its fine springy turf was responsible for some of the fastest six-furlong sprint races in Europe. When the European track record was finally broken at Phoenix Park, the English Jockey Club took notice and arranged for it to be officially measured in case it was too short. It was found to be one metre too long!

John, with Teddy Tighe the manager, worked hard to develop alternative income streams. The area under the grandstands had a massive amount of spare space, in which they built a restaurant, a function hall and a disco. These conversions markedly improved the member's facilities during race days and created full-time employment for many workers. The function hall became one of Dublin's most popular venues for wedding receptions, and the discothèque was one of Dublin's first.

At the 1969 annual meeting of the Ophthalmologic Society of the UK, I was elected Joint Secretary for the next two years. I have no doubt that this appointment was influenced by Keith Lyle, then in his final year as president of the society. It was a great honour, as there were many other young surgeons, of equal status, in the country. The decisions made by the Secretary played a major part in the functions of the society over its immediate future.

Shortly after receiving this appointment, Veronica and I attended the Barraquer Clinical Symposium in Barcelona. At that time, the Barraquer Clinic was the most renowned in Europe, being run by the third generation of that family of ardent ophthalmologists, who put the interests of this specialty before all else. When the elder Barraquer died, he bequeathed his eyes to the clinic, and one of the sons used them for corneal transplantation operations!

The opening ceremony of the meeting was conducted with great pomp. When the hundreds of delegates were seated in the hall, buglers ushered onto the stage a line of elderly colleagues wearing black mortarboards and gold and black gowns. The lectures were unremarkable, but the surgical demonstrations given by the two Barraquer brothers were memorable. The quality of their cataract surgery was brilliant, but it was still old-style surgery, with a large incision into the eye and no lens implantation.

This congress would have been of little importance if I had not, one evening, joined a small unofficial splinter session. I attended out of idle curiosity and joined several dozen other colleagues. Three American surgeons were sitting at a desk debating cataract surgery. The leader of this group, Professor Richard Troutman, of the Manhattan Eye and Ear Hospital, New York, introduced us to one of the two young surgeons sitting beside him. He said: 'This is Dr Charles Kelman, one of the consultants in my hospital, who has invented a cataract operation which will take all the fun out of this procedure.' The young, very sun-tanned ophthalmic surgeon acknowledged his introduction and started to address us.

Charles Kelman had been given a grant of $250,000 to research the feasibility of removing the cataractous lens through a small incision that could only be achieved by breaking up the nucleus of the lens before its removal from the eye. At this meeting in Barcelona, Charlie Kelman said:

'I had tried a number of different techniques to break up this lens nucleus. Attempts to crush the lens or squeeze it within a bag had not been successful. A whole series of drills, punches and other instruments were tried, but failed, as the lens would slip forward out of the way, without being eroded by the punches or rotary instruments. I was almost admitting failure when, while sitting in a dental chair having my teeth cleaned with an ultrasonic toothbrush, I realized that the ultrasonic energy used by this cleaner could be the answer to my problems.'

'Ultrasonic frequency starts at 17,000 cycles per second. I developed a hollow needle that was activated ultrasonically and oscillated at 64,000 cycles per second with an excursion of .001 inch on each cycle. I considered that, when the tip of this oscillating cannula was placed against the lens, its acceleration would be so great that it would penetrate into its substance. The analogy could be made of a soldier's dummy being bayoneted. If a bayonet is placed against the dummy and pushed, the dummy would move without being penetrated. For penetration, a thrust has to be made with the bayonet. This premise proved to be correct; the needle/cannula did penetrate into the hard lens. Once the cannula had plunged into the cataractous lens, trapping a small portion of it within its lumen, it was necessary to remove this particle from the eye. Alongside the ultrasonic tip, which 'emulsifies' bit by bit the hard nucleus, I developed a sophisticated irrigating/aspirating system, which will remove this lens debris from the eye. I used the same company, Cavitron, who manufactured the ultrasonic tooth cleaner to develop my ultrasonic cataract machine. All this operation is performed through a micro-incision into the eye which will only be 3 mm in size.'

I sat spellbound in my seat. I had witnessed, only that day, current cataract surgery performed by world experts, who had to make an incision of 10 millimetres to gain entry into the eye for the removal of the cataractous lens. Now I was listening to a surgeon who had developed an operation that would enable the cataractous lens to be removed through an incision more than three times smaller. This was surgery from a different planet! As with Harold Ridley's invention of lens implantation, I was listening to the birth of a concept that would herald another revolution, not evolution, in cataract surgery.

I left this small, ill-attended meeting, realizing that this was the 'way ahead'. Later that night, Veronica and I decided that Charlie would be our guest lecturer at the next meeting of the Ophthalmic Society of the United Kingdom, which was to be held the following spring in Churchill College, Cambridge.

Veronica and I 'saw out' the 1960s as guests of Jimmy and Margaret Hudson. Jimmy had been a leading influence in forging our ophthalmic profession into the next generation. He was a senior consultant at Moorfields, High Holborn, and was on the faculty of the Royal College of Surgeons and the Ophthalmic Society of the United Kingdom. Their New Year's Eve party reflected his long-time membership of the Garrick Club and included a number of well-known and interesting political, legal, medical and theatrical guests, such as Sir Geoffrey Howe, who would later become one of our most noted Tory chancellors, and Donald Sinden, the actor.

Many of my ophthalmic colleagues who had matured with Veronica and me were also present, including Mike and Thalia Sanders and Barry and Marcelle Jay. Mike Sanders assisted Jimmy in his practice in Harley Street and was for many years our leading neuro-ophthalmic physician, working out of the Hospital for Nervous Diseases in Queen Square, London. He always envied my surgical commitment to ophthalmology, in which a single operation could restore permanent sight, compared to his specialty, in which hours of dedicated examination and treatment could possibly give no release to the patient's incurable condition. Barry Jay was on the staff of Moorfields and in later years became the dean of the Institute of Ophthalmology.

1970 heralded further changes in cataract surgery in Europe: 20 years earlier Harold Ridley had introduced the concept of replacing the human cataractous lens with an artificial plastic one. His invention was still at this time being almost totally ignored. Now the ophthalmic profession was to be introduced to the concept of 'keyhole' micro-incisional cataract procedures.

In April, our annual meeting was held in Cambridge, during the university's Easter recess, for some 400 delegates. The three-hour session process was traditionally rather repetitive and could become tedious, but it was a means of introducing new ideas into our profession.

That first morning, after operating in the London Clinic on the headmaster of St Paul's School, I drove to Churchill College, to make sure everything was ready. Charlie Kelman and I had lunch; then I had arranged for him to have primetime for his address, immediately after the president's opening speech, which was traditional and conventional. Charlie Kelman then gave a 'New World show', the likes of which had never before been seen at a British ophthalmic meeting. Even the oldest members of the society were forced awake from their postprandial slumbers. Charlie's presentation was not a lecture but a film show, with sound, music and caricatures. It started with his three young children, Jennifer, Leslie and David, all with blonde hair, running across a wooden bridge over a river and onto a sunlit meadow full of daffodils to the music of a song called, 'The Butterflies', which had been composed by Charlie.

He then showed a futuristic presentation of cataract surgery, in which mature cataracts, in children, were removed using a needle activated by ultrasonic energy. The whole presentation was brilliant, both in its production and the concept of the development of cataract surgery. Incredibly, this superb and wonderful demonstration fell mostly on deaf ears. The delegates were more aghast at the florid presentation and loud music than the pearls of wisdom contained therein.

Following the afternoon session, I collected Veronica, and brought her to Churchill College. From the moment she was introduced to Charlie, he virtually never left her side.

That evening we attended the presidential dinner, given by Keith and Jane Lyle at the Senate House in Cambridge. The 30 other guests read like a *Who's Who* of ophthalmology: Harold and Elisabeth Ridley, our lens-implant inventor; Sir Stephen Miller, the queen's oculist, Jimmy and Margaret Hudson and Peter Wright, my fellow Secretary.

On Wednesday the council met, and Keith Lyle handed over the presidency to Professor George Scott of Edinburgh. I tidied up and left the college alone, late in the evening. My Ford Cortina estate, which Charlie had used during his stay, had a flat battery. Our American guest, not comprehending our car's workings, had inadvertently left the ignition turned on.

In June, a meeting was convened in the Senate House of London University to discuss the future of ophthalmic surgery in London. Professor Barry Jones, Clinical Professor at Moorfields, was planning to propose that all cataract patients in the London area should have their surgery performed in the two Moorfields Eye Hospitals. In one stroke, this would deprive the other multidisciplinary teaching hospitals in London of their major ophthalmic surgery. Barry Jones was on yet another of his 'empire-building projects,' which, if successful, would have given Moorfields a total monopoly of eye surgery. I arrived fresh from the Derby at Epsom (thrilled to have seen Nijinsky, ridden by Lester Piggott, win an all-time unforgettable race). Wearing my ridiculous race outfit and flushed in the face from a combination of an adequate amount of champagne and frustration at having to attend the meeting, I castigated Barry Jones and his Draconian proposals. The consultants of the teaching hospitals rallied to my cause and we put Moorfields to rout. This particular issue was never raised again, and we maintained the right to do major ophthalmic surgery on our NHS patients in our own teaching hospitals.

Shortly afterwards Charlie Kelman invited us to attend the annual conference of the American Academy of Ophthalmology in Las Vegas. Needless to say, we accepted the invitation.

Little can match the thrill and wonder of visiting America for the first time. The differences between the European and American cultures may have narrowed over the years, but in 1970 the two continents were very dissimilar. The first noticeable difference was the size of the cars; the American ones were vast compared to the average European cars, and the bright yellow cabs seemed to drive so much faster than our staid black cabs. New York with its famous skyline seemed to pulsate with urgency and vitality. Everything seemed to be bigger and brasher. We felt like schoolchildren on a day outing.

Charlie had included us in his group of ten, with his business manager, artistic director and their wives. We were to join up with a further 30 New York surgeons and their partners to fly to Las Vegas. Charlie had given his local travel agent $10,000 in pre-payment for our return flights, accommodation in the Stardust Hotel and a number of tickets for evening entertainment in Las Vegas. At La Guardia Airport, we all made for the American Airlines private lounge to find that our tickets had been invalidated. The travel agent had obviously never handled so much money at one time and had fled to Costa Rica with the proceeds. We each had to pay a second time, but Charlie quickly wrote out another cheque for his team. When we finally met Charlie's wife Joan, she was amazed: 'But you are both so young!' Charlie had prepared her to meet a very elderly couple from England. This light-hearted banter continued for the remainder of the trip. After a delayed departure, our plane dropped down in Kansas City, where we passengers were allowed to disembark and stretch our legs in the terminus. Charlie's name was announced on the tannoy to take an urgent telephone call. After a few seconds on the phone, he said: 'There must be some mistake,' and promptly dropped the receiver, leaving it to dangle at the end of the coiled cable. He rushed to us and said: 'Back to the plane immediately.' Once on board, we asked what all the fuss was about.

'You didn't expect me to pay for the tickets twice, did you? I am not that dumb,' he said. As soon as he had written out his second cheque in the La Guardia Airport, he had immediately phoned his secretary and told her to cancel it. Charlie was the only surgeon in the New York ophthalmic group who eventually managed to negotiate a settlement with the Airline Company.

Las Vegas is a true oasis in the middle of the Arizona desert. The main boulevard is sprinkled with five-star hotels, and overhead the sun burns relentlessly in a cloudless sky. Our hotel was the Stardust, whose darkened lobby contained hundreds of one-armed bandits, most of which were in constant use. We were at once struck by the incessant noise of piped music, mingled with the sound of the machines continuously disgorging coins as the players pumped their handles. This cacophony continued for 24 hours, day and night.

On our first evening in Las Vegas we went to the Landmark, which resembled a large mushroom, for dinner. It had a high concrete tower, atop of which was a large dome-shaped revolving restaurant, from which the diners had an uninterrupted view of Las Vegas. Outside lifts propelled the guests up the tower to the restaurant. Our party was confronted with a long queue of people waiting for a table in a restaurant, which was already full. It was fascinating to watch the way that an affluent man deals with the universal disease of queuing. Our party followed Charlie as he casually walked to the front of the queue and asked for a table for eight.

'Can't you see that there is a queue,' growled the manager. Quietly slipping a $50 bill into the manager's hot hand, Charlie replied: 'I didn't hear what you said, I simply asked for my table for eight.' In minutes we were sitting at the best table in the restaurant.

Nearly 10,000 ophthalmic and ENT delegates attended the meeting of the American Academy of Ophthalmology. There were courses of instruction in every conceivable subspecialty, as well as a huge trade exhibition represented by ophthalmic companies from all over the world.

Las Vegas was the ideal location for this congress, but regrettably it was later moved to Dallas to give it more gravitas. The morning was spent listening to scientific presentations and soaking up new ideas, and in the afternoon the delegates wandered around the exhibition halls or enjoyed the swimming pool or tennis courts. During this time we were introduced to many of Charlie's ophthalmic friends, who would soon become ours as well. One of these was Marvin Kwitko, who became one of Canada's foremost surgeons in pioneering the advances in surgery that were about to take place. Marvin was one of the early American pioneers on intraocular implants and, along with Herve Byron, Miles Galin, Chuck Letocha, Henry Hirschman and Norman Jaffe, inserted his first series of lenses in 1967. I so well remember meeting Marvin for the first time and being introduced by Charlie around the pool at the Stardust Hotel, all of us in our bathing trunks. Many years later, when Marvin was president of the Canadian Ophthalmological Society, he invited me to be one of his guest lecturers. So much is achieved outside the official meetings of any society.

Charlie accurately predicted that by joining him in the pioneering of small-incision cataract surgery, our professional life would be changed forever. Charlie Kelman was himself a most dynamic personality and would have made a success in any profession he had chosen. His father had come out of Europe at around the turn of the century, and when he first arrived in New York, he used to pull a cart through the streets. However, with his fertile Jewish brain, he soon established himself as an entrepreneur and built up his own business empire.

Charlie wanted to become a musician, but his father insisted that he must have a professional degree and pursue music as a hobby. He decided to do medicine and started his studies in Geneva. While studying in Geneva, he auditioned for and was accepted as a member of the Swiss Jazz Quartet. The young musicians in Switzerland were annoyed that a medical student from overseas should become a member of a semi-professional musical band, so a further series of interviews were arranged, and once again Charlie got the job. During his life, he also wrote more than 100 tunes, and Jean Sablon recorded one of his songs, *Le petit dejeuner*. He even gave solo concerts at the world-famous Carnegie Hall in New York. As well as being an outstanding ophthalmic surgeon, inventor, musician and saxophonist, he also flew his own helicopter. He proudly states that when he learned to fly, he did so with a Pan-Am pilot: he went solo at 19 hours, the Pan-Am pilot at 25 hours!

By the time that we met him in 1969, he had made a number of other major contributions to ophthalmic surgery. He designed a cryoprobe, an instrument that, when frozen to −170°C, could adhere to the human cataractous lens, enabling it to be removed from the eye. With his invention of the phaco machine for cataract surgery, he introduced into ophthalmology a revolutionary concept of surgery, the importance of which was both comparable with and complementary to Harold Ridley's invention of the lens implant.

Our relationship with Charlie was rather unique. Despite our different upbringings, religion and nationality, we shared many things in common. Charlie had a young family and was a top surgeon in a New York hospital. These similarities would have been enough to ensure that we enjoyed a good working relationship for the next three decades, but there was much more. We enjoyed each other's company, and over the ensuing years shared many happy holidays together.

After spending a few days in San Francisco and a weekend in Miami with Bob Daroff, a neuro-ophthalmologist at the Jackson Memorial Hospital, we returned to England inspired by all we had seen and learned. We had also had a number of serious business discussions with Charlie Kelman. Charlie was inviting a few top ophthalmic surgeons to help pioneer his invention and was running instruction courses in Manhattan. Cavitron was manufacturing a few of the Kelman phaco-emulsifying machines at a cost of $50,000 and Charlie advised me buy one for the UK. Although Veronica and I were totally committed to introducing this form of surgery into Europe, we had no idea how we could raise even a fraction of the finances to buy the machine.

Two days before our tenth wedding anniversary, fortune came our way. For some weeks previously I had been treating a lawyer called Rex Hyem, who had been suffering from a very unsightly lesion on his right eyelid. He had sought multiple opinions but no remedy had been found. It seemed to me that the most suitable treatment would be to surgically remove the lesion and replace, if necessary, the denuded area of the lid with a skin graft. Surgery proceeded without any complications and he was very pleased with the results. At his final visit he said: 'I cannot begin to express my thanks to you for what you have done. I can now carry out my legal business with confidence. In return for your help, is there anything I can do for you?' Without expecting any reaction, I said: 'Probably not, but we are looking for a considerable sum of money to buy a machine for cataract surgery.' I told him how much it was and he said quite casually: 'You can have it. One of my clients has just died and there are no living beneficiaries. The estate is the Ely Webster Trust. The income from this is £7,000 a year and you can have this interest for the next four years.' He was as good as his word, and we put in a firm order for the phaco machine. It transpired that his mother had been blind from congenital cataracts and he had always hoped that he would be able to help other sufferers of this condition.

A few weeks later, the chief executive of Cavitron, Bob Naven, flew into London from Los Angeles to confirm the financial arrangements for the phaco machine, which was to be the only one exported from America for the next two years. We also received the hospital administrator's consent to allow this 'experimental' technology to be used. This was an example of the decisive leadership that was present, at this time, in the NHS. All had been achieved in a one-hour meeting without the need for other administrative, ethical, medical, social, financial or bureaucratic committees. Together in the Charing Cross Group of Hospitals, we had formulated the future of cataract surgery, which would ultimately involve the whole country.

CHAPTER 16
A changing pattern

In March 1971, Lionel Taylor, the ENT surgeon at Charing Cross, and John Ayoub, my former teacher and ophthalmic consultant at Moorfields, invited me to join the staff of the Royal Masonic Hospital as one of their two ophthalmic surgeons. It was considered an honour to be on the staff of this hospital, which could choose colleagues from any of the London teaching hospitals. The only stipulation was that one was required to be a member of a masonic lodge.

The Royal Masonic Hospital, situated on the edge of Ravenscourt Park, Hammersmith, was built in the 1930s art-deco style. Although anyone could use the hospital, the majority of the patients were Masons and their families. Here we gave equal quality of treatment to all, irrespective of the financial rewards. The patient's expenses met by 'the Samaritan fund' were intended to cover all costs associated with treatment, which included those of the hospital, surgeon and anaesthetist. The hospital would first recover its costs and then pass the residual funds to the medical staff. This led to the bizarre situation that in extreme cases the surgeon could receive as little as £2 for treatment that would have cost a private patient approximately £500. One of my anaesthetists was once paid one penny for an operation.

Despite these financial irregularities, the total aggregate from the Royal Masonic Hospital did help to supplement our still modest income. Virtually every patient referred for treatment required surgery, be it a child with a squint or an adult needing surgery for cataract, glaucoma, corneal transplant or retinal detachment.

One afternoon, I was attending my clinic in the Royal Eye Hospital, Cambridge Circus, when the matron came to tell me that there was an outbreak of dysentery in the wards. As the only consultant in the hospital, it was my responsibility to take appropriate action. I recommended that all the inpatients be discharged as soon as possible and no new patients were to be admitted until the health authorities had given the all-clear. In a year that was to see a number of major changes in our lives, my action was the cause of one. I had unwittingly closed the famous Royal Eye Hospital forever. Inspectors from the Ministry of Health and Safety examined the hospital, and it failed on several points, including having an inadequate number of fire escapes and too few lifts. Some £35,000 would need to be spent before the hospital could be reopened. These funds were not forthcoming, and the hospital never reopened.

I was then left with the option of joining the staff of St Thomas' Hospital, which was to absorb the professorial unit of the Royal Eye Hospital and any of its staff, or remain at Charing Cross Hospital. My choice was to stay with Charing Cross. Like the proverbial 'Pied Piper', I took with me from the Royal Eye all my theatre and outpatient staff. Although my patients were given the option of being transferred to St Thomas,' everyone opted to follow me. Suddenly I had a massive clinic.

The secretary I had inherited when I moved into Harley Street, Diana Riggall, became progressively more ill and had to retire from the practice. She had given me so much support and help in my early years in the practice and I was saddened to see her go. After some months of temporary secretaries, a young girl, called Joy Hughes, came to be interviewed. It turned out that she had no previous medical experience but was prepared to 'give it a go' on a one-week trial. After two days in the position she rang my anaesthetist to find out what a cataract was! The trial period extended to 30 years, and she has continued to work with my successors at the Arnott Eye Associates, in Harley Street, after I retired. Once I failed to recognize her on the stairs, as she had cast off the mini-wig and large false eyelashes that were so popular at that time and I saw the 'natural' Joy for the first time. Joy was totally uninterested in finances, and once, when we were particularly busy, she failed to bill any patients for more than six months. It took me a little time to work out why my overdraft had so markedly increased. She had, however, an abiding interest in all the patients and was very instrumental in developing a truly caring practice. She could never say 'no' to a patient requiring an appointment, with the result that we were always grossly overbooked.

I was lucky to retain most of my staff over many years. When I took over Edgar King's rooms in Harley Street, a very young Hazel Saunders was the receptionist for all the consultants in the building. After Joy's lack of interest in managing the accounts, Hazel took over this responsibility and was still a member of our team on the day that I retired. My orthoptist Carolyn Calcutt, who trained with me at Moorfields, joined me throughout my career in both my teaching hospitals and private practice.

Waiting times were a constant cause of anxiety, yet with the volume of work that we were doing it was very difficult to find a remedy. My main priority with all my patients was to provide them with the best possible treatment. Inevitably, as the reputation of the practice grew so did the waiting problem. Some patients learned how to deal with the system. One of my patients, Lord Porchester, who later became the Earl of Caernarfon, had a recurrent eye condition that required treatment on innumerable occasions. On one of his visits he turned up at the rooms at 5.30 pm for a 4.30 pm appointment and, being one hour late for his appointment, was in the waiting room for only a couple of minutes. Unfortunately, another of my patients, who happened to be one of my in-law's oldest friends, thought that I was giving Lord Porchester preferential treatment and promptly walked out of the rooms in a huff. I had lost my 4.45 pm patient!

During this period, Veronica was pregnant for the third time. We had joined John for the Double Diamond Stakes at Phoenix Park. After the lunch, Veronica decided to rest in bed, as we had a long evening ahead. When the races had finished, John and I walked back to the house with four of our friends. One of them ran in to greet Veronica. By the time I joined her she was doubled up with pain, having been given a big bear hug by our friend.

I thought little of the incident at the time, and we changed and joined the group at the Gaiety Theatre in Dublin to see the Norman Wisdom show. In the middle of the performance, Veronica whispered to me that her stomach felt less distended. But it wasn't until the next morning, driving to church, that I realized with horror that she had burst her placental membrane and was in imminent danger of suffering a miscarriage. I raced back, cursing myself for being such an ignorant fool not to have appreciated the situation earlier. I made an emergency call to the Rotunda Hospital and spoke to the dean of the hospital, Ian Dalrymple, who had been in my year at Trinity College, Dublin. He had always been a friend but now became a saviour. He said that Veronica was to be admitted immediately and we were to drive very slowly into Dublin. Veronica had an uneventful three days in the Rotunda before going to recuperate at Dunsany Castle with Sheila Dunsany.

On 12 August 1971, Tony Woolf delivered for us a totally healthy son, Robert Lauriston John Arnott. There were no signs that he had spent the previous three months cramped in a dry uterus, without the shock-absorbing effects of the amniotic fluid. Tony considered that Robert's survival was because he was a very strong baby.

With the arrival of Robert, Veronica and I returned to the routine of bringing up our family. Stephen was now settled in at his prep school, St Peter's, Seaford, and Tania was at Queensgate in London and attending ballet classes after school. From a very early age, Robert identified himself with our other children and never appreciated the difference in age. His formative years at Lansdowne Crescent mirrored those of our other two children, and he loved the open space of the garden. He was once given a Guards' military uniform, in which he would parade around all day, and it was difficult to make him wear any other clothes. Bob hated going up to bed before the rest of the family, so, night after night, he would sleep on the sofa in our kitchen-breakfast room and after dinner we would carry him, still in his uniform, up to bed.

At this time Veronica's brother, Charles, was working at Christie's auction-eers in London, where, thanks to the patronage of Count Alexis Bobrinskoy, he had become recognized as a leading expert on Russian silver, icons and Fabergé. When still in his 30s, he was appointed as the buyer for the Silver and Russian Department of Asprey's in Bond Street, London. He reached these heights of expertise despite having some difficulties with his early education. Charles's father Arvid, although caring and affectionate, was injured and unable to enjoy outdoor pursuits with him. And at the age of five, Charles was struck down with rheumatic fever, which meant a two-year confinement, and at the age of

12 he was well behind his natural age group. So when Veronica and I married in 1960, it was as if he had a second pair of parents. Charles had become our constant companion. We took his presence for granted and loved having him with us. Other than our honeymoon, he accompanied us on all our family holidays.

In many ways, Veronica and I enjoyed the most perfect relationship possible. We spent most weekends at Hartley Wintney with the Langués. Charles was some 14 years older than Stephen, but they happily grew up together. Veronica would take them all for holidays with her aunt and uncle, Eric and Hester Cattley, in Devon, or in Wales, staying with Gwyneth Taylor or the Dashwoods in Manorbier. There were endless hours of building sandcastles on the beach and exploring rocks and rugged coastlines.

In later years, when my income had increased, we would either rent a villa or charter a yacht in the Mediterranean, and we took great pleasure in watching Charles become a young adult.

We sold Acushla, our treasured 24-foot yacht, and the Langués sold West Green Cottage, where they had lived for over 25 years. This left a huge vacuum in our lives, which was somewhat compensated for when Sheila Dunsany let us use one of her bungalows in Manorbier, yards from the gates of Manorbier Castle. It had a small garden and over the next few years our family enjoyed many visits. Life in Ireland was also changing: John had at last found the girl, Annie Farrelly, whom he would marry.

When Veronica and I had been at the meeting of the American Academy of Ophthalmology in Las Vegas, we had met a Californian ophthalmic surgeon, John Beale, whose family owned a private eye hospital in San Francisco. He invited me to speak at my first New World meeting – the ophthalmic congress in San Francisco. John Beale as a personality was larger than life, standing over six feet three inches in height. He had a wonderful ability to mix a serious scientific meeting with an abundance of hospitality. We met up again with Charlie and Joan Kelman, whom we had not seen since the meeting in Las Vegas the previous year, and Charlie agreed to be Robert's godfather.

John Beale's congress was organized to precede the AAO's congress, which was once again held in Las Vegas. By this time I had been elected a fellow of the society and was among its first British members. During the congress, Charlie hosted a champagne breakfast for the select few pioneers who had started to use the Cavitron phaco-emulsification machine. We were very aware of the obstacles that lay before us, as well as the criticism, hostility and obstruction that we would encounter from the peers of our profession.

On the way home, we took a trip to the Grand Canyon, staying in a log cabin 10 yards from the edge of an 8,000-foot drop. In the morning we joined eight other riders for the famous 'Mule Ride' down the treacherous Angel Trail. The path started gently, but after riding some few hundred yards we were introduced to its true nature. Rounding a corner, the Angel Trail could be seen to zigzag down the side of the bowl to distant plain thousands of feet below.

As it was now too late to turn back, we gripped the saddles between our knees, rigid with apprehension. We were not in control of the mules – they were of us. At each bend our mules would walk to the edge of the precipice and ponderously look over it for several seconds before deciding to continue down the track. We felt totally helpless. The mules seemed so unaware of the surrounding danger and walked with such sure-footedness that, after a time, we became quite fond of them and more confident about our safety. The views were quite spectacular; with the northern side of the canyon some miles away, we were descending into a large plain beyond that was the final vertical drop to the Colorado River. When we reached the plateau with its open spaces, one of the other mules decided to have some less restricted exercise and bolted with its rider. The guides were obviously used to this occurrence and were quick to return the rider and truant mule to our party. Few places can be more peaceful than this, with no sign of any other human being within many miles of us. The sky was cloudless, the air crystal clear and we were at a high enough altitude for the temperature to be moderate despite the severity of the overhead desert sun.

On the return ascent, one girl fainted and fell off her mule on one of the narrower parts of the track, which caused the guides some difficulty getting her remounted. We heard later that she was in early pregnancy and should not have been on the ride. We had one final night at the Bright Angel Lodge before flying to New York, where we again stayed at the Plaza Hotel. By this time we were becoming more seasoned travellers to America, and we had booked a bedroom with a view over Central Park.

CHAPTER 17
Dogs and pigs

In 1971, Veronica and I returned to America to embark on the most important course of my career: Charlie Kelman's fourth on phaco-emulsification of the human lens, which was held at the Manhattan Eye and Ear Hospital, New York.

The term phaco-emulsification is derived from the Greek 'phakos', meaning lens, and 'emulsification,' meaning liquefaction – in this case, of the hard lens nucleus by the ultrasonic needle. In time, the procedure became simply known as the phaco operation.

On arrival, I was presented with an excellent folder that gave a historic review of the procedure, the instrumentation required and a well-illustrated account of how the phaco operation should be performed. Charlie took us very slowly and methodically over the surgical technique. In the afternoon, we operated on 'simulated' eyes made of plastic. Only very accomplished ophthalmic microsurgeons, younger than 45 years, were invited to the course, and it was generally considered that a surgeon needed at least 50 hours' practice before performing the procedure on a patient. To test our dexterity and steadiness of hand, we were all required to insert a fine copper probe through a small electrified coil without touching its inner surface. At this time, only 5% of surgeons who attended phaco courses went on to practice this type of surgery – such was the degree of new skills that were required.

On the second day of the course, we went to the operating theatre to watch Charlie perform the operation live and via closed circuit television. We took it in turns to look down the assistant's eyepiece on the microscope. This was the first time that I had witnessed a phaco-emulsification cataract operation. It was performed under local anaesthesia.

A small clamp exposed the eye for surgery, and methylene blue was applied to the globe, which coloured all the superficial exposed tissues apart from the cornea. This solution was used to increase sterility and reduce the glare from the light in the operating microscope. An incision of 3 mm was then made between the clear cornea and the now bright blue adjacent tissue. Having gained access into the anterior chamber of the eye, an instrument resembling a needle with its tip bent to an angle of 90° was inserted into the anterior chamber of the eye. This bent tip was used to grip and tear an opening in the anterior capsule, a fine membrane that encompasses the lens. Once the tip had engaged this fine membrane, it was withdrawn towards the incision, creating a triangular-shaped tear in the anterior capsule. This torn flap of anterior capsule was brought, still on the tip of the needle, to the incision, where it was cut off with scissors, placed flush to the section. Charlie called it the Christmas tree, because of its shape.

Then the lens nucleus was brought through the pupil and into the anterior chamber of the eye. This was the most complicated part of the procedure. With an instrument called a cystitome (again, in essence, a bent needle but with a broader base) the nucleus was gaffed in its mid-periphery. Rather like a fisherman trying to bring his catch from the river onto the bank, the surgeon had 'to play' the nucleus and rock it out of the capsular bag and ease it through the pupil. At any time the grip on the nucleus could be lost and it would drop back into its original position. With extreme caution and care the nucleus could usually be coaxed into the anterior chamber. Once trapped in this compartment of the eye, it was in a position where the surgeon could readily attack it, with the ultrasonically activated tip of the phaco machine.

As the oscillating tip entered and gradually eroded and emulsified the hard nucleus, the debris was removed from the eye by a sophisticated irrigating and aspirating device. The probe was surrounded by a silicone sleeve, which allowed fluid to enter the eye, before being aspirated out of the eye with the emulsified particles of lens. Simple aspiration, using vacuum pressure, without ultrasonic energy, removed the final soft lens material, which had been retained in the capsular bag. This bloodless exquisitely beautiful operation was now finished.

During the morning we saw this same operation performed on four patients, all of whom ended up with a perfect result. In the afternoon we had to attempt to emulate Charlie's operation by operating on pig cadaver eyes. When not attending lectures, we would spend many hours over the next few days in the 'wet lab', improving our operating skills, with Charlie in the background giving us helpful advice. We got through buckets of these pig eyes. When they were fresh we had a good chance of doing a reasonable procedure, but with time the pig eyes would dry up and the cornea would become opaque, which made the operation considerably more difficult. We were all aware of the need to become familiar with this equipment, which was totally different to anything we had previously handled.

I realized that although I was an accomplished ophthalmic surgeon, there was a long way to go before becoming a good phaco operator. At the Kelman's Long Island home, I had never been more pleased to see Veronica, who, with her usual perception, at once appreciated the difficulties I was experiencing trailing so far behind Charlie in a technique that he had been developing over the previous two years.

By the end of the week I had operated on dozens of pig eyes and was beginning to feel that I had at last mastered the basic principles of a technique that would in time render current methods totally obsolete. Irrespective of the fact that surgeons, such as Dick Troutman, were now using fine sutures to close the previously large incision, a long period of postoperative convalescence was still required. With the conventional incision of 10.5 mm, the patient's sight undergoes a changing pattern of instability for at least two months after surgery. The wound is subjected to strain and can rupture with even the smallest knock for some considerable time after the operation. With 'phaco', the situation is totally changed. As in other 'keyhole' operations, postoperative convalescence is virtually eliminated and patients can resume normal activities almost immediately.

A few days after this course, Bill Freeman, one of Cavitron's senior executives, arrived with the first phaco machine in the UK, which were delivered to the old Fulham Hospital, where I worked while Charing Cross was being built. By modern standards this first-generation Cavitron phaco machine was very large and unsophisticated. It looked like a tea trolley, the top of which was filled with tubes and taps, but to us it was a beautiful 'wonder machine'.

The following evening the two administrators of Charing Cross Hospital, Frank Hart and Mr Barker, organized a cocktail party/press reception in the operating theatre. Public relations were not their forte, and only one newspaper journalist came to the reception. He was from our local *West London Observer* and wrote a major article entitled 'revolutionary cataract surgery' for its next edition.

Our guests had to change into operating garb before attending the party. John had kindly flown over from Ireland for this memorable occasion. He had never before been into a theatre and looked quite out of place with his green scrubs open over his abdomen and the trousers riding above his knees. Despite the paucity of his apparel, we greatly appreciated his support at this important time in our lives. Once again the administrators of Charing Cross Hospital, all two of them, had been totally cooperative.

We were now in charge of only the fourth Kelman Cavitron machine in the world and many thousands of miles from either technical assistance or moral support from the few other, all American, pioneers of this form of cataract surgery. It was a huge responsibility to bring this as yet totally unproven surgery into Europe. We did not have the approval of either the Ophthalmic Society of the United Kingdom or the American Academy of Ophthalmology, both of whom were, as yet, blissfully unaware of the phaco procedure. In retrospect, we were possibly remiss in not having alerted the Royal College of Surgeons, the General Medical Council or the Medical Protection Society of our intentions to start this totally revolutionary surgery, but, in those days, medical litigation was not an issue of concern.

My prime concern was for the welfare of my patients and at no time was I prepared to do anything that would put the patient under any added risk. This I achieved by initially only doing a small part of the operation using the phaco machine and then reverting to conventional surgery if any difficulties presented. Of secondary importance was the reputation of the hospital and my own practice.

A few days later, Veronica and I were walking up Portobello Road when we saw a dog being pushed up the road in a wheelbarrow. On being told that the dog was totally blind from cataract, I knew that I had found my first British patient. Mr Ward was very grateful that I could treat his pet the following day in the animal house of Charing Cross Hospital as a NHS patient. The operation took some considerable time to complete, but at its end the eye seemed to be in a satisfactory state. On subsequent occasions we saw the dog still being pushed in the wheelbarrow, but whether out of habit or lack of success with the operation we never discovered. Another of my early patients was a poodle owned by Peter Phillips, the senior urologist of Charing Cross Hospital. Two months later Peter turned up with a large basket of apples to thank me for restoring his beloved dog's sight. Sadly the poodle later escaped onto the road and was run over.

Within a month of taking ownership of my new phaco machine, Cavitron had appointed Mike Kennedy as their agent for the UK. Along with Alan Macmillan, the chief executive of the parent company Synergistic, they visited me, in the theatre of the old Fulham Hospital, on Tuesday 27 October 1971, to witness my first phaco operation on a human patient. The surgery was uncomplicated, and apart from a small nick in the iris of the eye, which was of no clinical significance, the result was perfect. The first patient outside of America was able to appreciate the full benefit of this form of surgery.

That spring I joined Charlie Kelman in Italy for a congress in Bologna. Veronica stayed at home looking after Robert, but, even in this relatively early period in our life together, I was becoming very dependent on her company and always felt rather lost when I had to go to meetings without her.

Charlie read a paper on phaco-emulsification and followed up by operating on the Lord Mayor of Bologna's pet monkey, who was totally blind from bilateral cataract. No surgeon in Italy, for fear of the consequences of failure, would take on this responsibility. Charlie's presence in Bologna seemed providential, as he could demonstrate his new form of surgery on the monkey and resolve the problem. I was invited to the operating theatre to watch the surgery, which was completed without any problems. Some minutes later a panic-stricken anaesthetist informed Charlie that the monkey had failed to survive the anaesthetic. Legend has it that Charlie, racing out of Bologna on the motorway to Milan, was overtaken by only one car – that of the anaesthetist!

After the congress in Bologna, Charlie and Joan Kelman came to stay with us for the weekend in London. On Saturday morning Charlie watched me perform two phaco operations. I felt very proud at being able to demonstrate two perfect results. By a cruel twist of irony, later that day we heard that Rex Hyem, the solicitor who had donated the £27,000 for the purchase of the phaco-emulsification machine, had died. In reply to my letter of condolence to his wife, she had written to me saying how Rex had felt that his donation for the machine had been one of the most worthwhile projects in his life.

For the summer holiday in 1972, Veronica and I took Stephen and Tania to Greece to stay with our very old friends Dick and Maria Musgrave in their villa perched on a cliff top on the island of Syros. As usual, Charles accompanied us, but Robert stayed home with friends of ours – Tom and Beris Laidlaw. This was the first time that our eldest children had been abroad, and it was a holiday to remember, most notably because during our stay an almighty storm hit the island, blew away all the outside furniture and sank Dick's speedboat.

In Syros, news travelled fast, and it took little time for the locals to realize that an international eye surgeon was staying on the island. As in any other part of the world, one's work is never far away. Every day locals would come up to the Musgrave's villa, Komito, seeking ophthalmic advice. Some of these patients I could help, and several came to England for surgery. In those days, the NHS was freely available to patients from overseas.

On our last night on the island, we went to a small restaurant, as Dick wanted me to examine the proprietor, who was totally blind. Unfortunately I was unable to help, as his optic nerves had been irrevocably destroyed by an infection. I felt like a maestro lacking a baton and was very humbled about my inadequacies in being unable to help a fellow human being.

After dinner, Veronica and I walked, hand in hand, along the cliff path, guided by the light of a full moon. With all the changes in our lives, we were once again able to experience the bond between us. We didn't talk – we just walked along that majestic coastline, so thankful to be together.

John Beale invited me to join a course teaching microsurgery to conventional ophthalmic surgeons in America. The introduction of the microscope heralded major advances in ophthalmology, particularly in glaucoma and corneal-transplant surgery. Total proficiency in the use of the microscope was a necessary prerequisite of performing phaco.

New skills and instruments are required when doing ophthalmic surgery using the microscope. I designed a whole set of microsurgical cataract instruments and for my 60th birthday Veronica gave me a set made of gold plate. Many surgeons found it difficult to adapt to the microscope, but the teaching course really helped, and the one at the San Francisco Eye and Ear Hospital was one of the most popular in America. I became a permanent member of John's faculty and would join his course annually for many years.

The students spent hours practising on pig eyes and increasing the dexterity of their hands, as they were taught surgical procedures that could not be performed without the use of the microscope, such as the finer dissection of the tissues and the use of micro-needles and suture material. Corneal transplantation, in which the patient's cornea (the 'watch-glass window' at the front of the eye) is replaced with that of a donor, was transformed by the introduction of the microscope, as the donor cornea could now be very accurately positioned. The trabeculectomy glaucoma operation perfected by John Cairns, Peter Watson and myself required the use of the microscope for the delicate dissection to the outlet channel of the eye. All of these procedures were demonstrated to the surgeons on John Beale's very intensive course, who returned home with a totally new concept of what could be achieved with ophthalmic microsurgery.

During time off from these courses, I was introduced to the keep-fit regimens adopted by many of America's top professionals. On one morning, after a very late night, we were roused for the next day's activity at 5.30 am. John Beale, with 65 others, was to take part in a triathlon, which included a seven-mile run, a three-mile swim across Lake Clare and a trek 3,000 ft up and down a mountain. Fortunately I was not asked to participate in this trial of endurance and instead spent the morning in a rowing boat on the lake.

On one of my annual visits to these courses I had to undergo a particularly severe test. My flight from London had taken even longer than usual and I did not arrive in my hotel until 11.30 pm San Francisco time. I had no sooner entered my bedroom before the telephone rang. It was John Beale.

'Eric, be ready for me to pick you up at 4.30 in the morning, as I have arranged for you to do a solo Alcatraz swim.'

'You must be joking,' I replied, 'I am exhausted and need a good lie in tomorrow morning.'

'Go to bed now,' he insisted, 'and you should be able to get a good four hours' sleep.'

Promptly, at 4.30 the next morning, John collected me in his golden convertible Rolls Royce Corniche. At the Dolphin Club, we were taken by rowing boat to Alcatraz Island, the notorious former-prison situated in the middle of a very cold, shark-infested bay, which has very dangerous currents. San Francisco Bay was a scene of extreme beauty and I momentarily forgot the cold and the hazards of the swim which lay ahead. Behind us was the city, lit up by lights in the thousands of houses that spread up the hills. To the west, a full moon was just dipping between the two pillars of the Golden Gate Bridge and to the east there was a gentle red glow in the sky, as dawn broke over the Berkeley area of the bay.

The official rule of the event, supervised by the Bay Watch Patrol, was that the participant had to be within five metres of the shore of the island before starting the one-and-a-half mile swim back to the mainland. Wearing only bathing trunks, I jumped overboard and was instantly 'paralysed' by the extreme cold of the water. I surfaced, gasping, and tried to grasp the side of the boat.

'Keep away from the boat,' yelled John Beale. 'If you touch it you are disqualified.' He waved a finger towards the city, which seemed to be a great distance away, and told me to head off in that direction. This I did and was amazed at how quickly the body can adjust to extreme conditions. In minutes the acute coldness became bearable, and I was determined to complete this most formidable swim. A string of barges gave me yet another handicap as they passed in front of me, forcing me to tread water for several minutes. Ninety minutes later, I finally reached the beach in front of the Dolphin Club. Totally jet-lagged, hypothermic and exhausted from the longest swim in my life, I eased myself up the shallow beach on all fours. On standing up I collapsed like a jellyfish in front of the Lord Mayor of San Francisco, who had risen early to witness yet another person 'escape from Alcatraz'. I can still visualize him standing on the beach, with outstretched hand, while I lay totally incapacitated on the ground. I was later presented with a large silver trophy of a swimmer about to dive into the sea. Inscribed on it was 'Eric J Arnott, Swimmer No. 242, another conqueror of Alcatraz'.

Later in 1972, I joined Charlie Kelman at a congress in El Paso. Phaco was now beginning to slowly gain momentum in the US, and at this meeting I was introduced to several well-respected American ophthalmologists who had adapted to this procedure. These included Gerald De Voe, Alsten Callaghan, Richard Kratz and Charlie's brother-in-law, Don Praeger. Dick Kratz from Los Angeles, already a relatively elder statesman in our profession, with his expertise and dedication, made a major contribution.

After the congress in El Paso, Charlie and I flew to New York. That evening Charlie drove me out to his home in Roslyn, where I delightedly but unexpectedly found Veronica waiting for me. It was a revelation to watch Charlie at work: the way he examined his patients was something I had never seen before in private practice. In England, an ophthalmic surgeon would carry out the whole examination by himself before expressing an opinion about the patient's condition. The consultation would take up to half an hour and a consultant would normally see no more than 12 patients in one session.

In the Kelman practice, ancillary staff carried out the whole of the examination. Each patient would then be ushered into the consulting room with a folder containing the patient's details and a resumé of the whole examination. Charlie would quickly examine the patient to confirm the diagnosis and then clearly explain the problem and how it could be treated. In the course of half an hour Charlie had given an opinion to 10 patients. I was most impressed with the orderly running of this clinic and over the years incorporated many of its features into my own practice.

At the end of the week's work, the four of us went for a weekend in the Bahamas, meeting up with John and his fiancée Annie Farrelly on the way. Some months previously, during a routine ophthalmic examination, I had made a diagnosis of dyslexia in the son of our friends the McCloreys. Kevin McClorey was a film producer married to Bobo, a member of the Seigrist family. They were very grateful to me for having alerted them to their son's condition early enough for him to get treatment. They very kindly lent us their house 'Pieces of Eight' on Paradise Island, a bridge away from Nassau.

At the entrance we found that their long driveway had been blocked by tons of boulders. The McCloreys were having a boundary dispute with the local mafia and we had to carry our luggage up to the house on foot. After a long walk we arrived at 'Pieces of Eight', which could have been taken out of a Tennessee Williams' play. The house lay within a few feet of the ocean and the exterior was almost English Victoriana, with its austerity and gabled windows. Inside was deep American South, with dark wooden panelling. When Veronica and I went down to the drawing room for cocktails, Charlie was playing the Sinatra song *Softly, as I leave you* on the Steinway piano. This had been one of our special songs, and we felt enormous joy at the devotion between us all.

Kevin McClorey had produced the James Bond film, *Goldfinger*, and in one of the outhouses on the property we found many of the props used in the film. There was a model of the delta-wing Vulcan bomber that is shown in the opening scene, crashing into the sea and dropping to the seabed. The yellow mini-submarine was also stored in this shed.

CHAPTER 18
The New Charing Cross influence

Despite our frequent visits to America, we did manage a social life with our friends in England, as well as giving sufficient time to our children. Stephen was at boarding school in Seaford for much of the year, and Tania was becoming ever more involved with the ballet. Tania had been dancing from the moment she could walk, and, although never pushed, she chose to follow in her mother's footsteps. She took classes at the Junior Royal Ballet School in Hammersmith and also at Madame Betty Vaccani's in Knightsbridge. Robert had not as yet started school and was looked after by Veronica and our au pair Cézanne. We were incredibly lucky with our au pairs, who invariably became members of the family and often joined us when we went on holiday.

Veronica and I spent many evenings with friends at Covent Garden or the Festival Hall. We saw Margot Fonteyne and Rudolf Nureyev on many occasions. Veronica liked front-row seats in the dress circle, from where she could study the dancer's footwork. Often I would arrive exhilarated but fatigued after a very long day in the operating theatre. We'd sit holding hands and, through the vibrancy of her touch, I was able to experience the beauty and expertise of the ballet, while with closed eyelids planning the next day's surgery.

Many of our friends were also my patients. On one occasion after a late-night session with Charles and Lelia Orme in their country home, I was puzzled to see an older version of Charles in my Harley Street clinic – I was examining his father. Charles's younger brother Anthony also came to see me with bizarre visual symptoms, which I eventually diagnosed as being caused by a small lesion in the brain. I sought the opinion of Mike Sanders, a leading neuro-ophthalmologist at Queen's Square. Further tests confirmed that the lesion was associated with a very rare but fatal manifestation of disseminated sclerosis. I had the most unpleasant job of breaking the news to Charles that his kid brother had only six months to live. The prognosis proved correct, and the Ormes were at least grateful that they had advanced warning of the sadness that was to follow.

Towards the end of 1972, all the hospitals I was practising in had closed one by one. These included the Royal Eye Hospital in Lambeth, the original Charing Cross Hospital in the Strand and the West London and Fulham Hospitals in Hammersmith. It was nostalgic seeing these old established hospitals being phased out, but the authorities of the time were doing a good job consolidating London's medicine into compact modern units. We were gratified to know that we would be taking our entire ophthalmic staff into the New Charing Cross Hospital.

In December of that year, the contractors allowed us to enter this new hospital in Fulham Palace Road, Hammersmith, to examine our state-of-the-art operating theatres, inpatient ward and outpatient department. It was better than any that I had previously visited throughout the world. The buildings were beautifully landscaped, with a water garden, well stocked with perch and goldfish, and fountains. Over the front porch was a large blue clock with a golden dial and hands. The vast airy foyer had shops down one side of it and the outside walls were essentially glass. The hospital was constructed in the shape of a cross, the two arms and head of which contained the wards, while the services were housed in the main body. There were eight lifts and 15 floors. The ophthalmic inpatient department was on the 10th floor, the operating theatres on the 14th floor and the private patients' wing on the 15th. There was no 13th floor, so even superstitious patients would be happy!

The hospital had a non-sectarian octagonal-shaped chapel. No ward had more than four beds, and several wards were single. The examining facilities were excellent and spacious enough even for the 25 inpatients I found waiting for me one Saturday morning. There were 12 operating theatres, and each specialty had their own. In the planning and development of the hospital there was no shortage of money and, within limits, each surgeon could equip his theatre as required. My colleague Alan Higgitt and I spent hours going over our surgical needs, and we ended up with by far the most advanced ophthalmic theatre in London. We also had the only phaco unit outside America. This was every surgeon's dream! We also had a very experienced, loyal and dedicated staff, including Sister Anna Amadian from Ireland, who was in charge of the inpatient ophthalmic ward. Anna was most supportive in our revolutionary cataract surgery and would do anything to help. We looked upon her ward as a home from home, and any member of our family requiring an operation was admitted to 10 North. It was in her ward that I treated Victor de Rothschild as an emergency, when he had suddenly lost his sight. He later made a generous donation of £75,000.

I did my first outpatient clinic in the New Charing Cross Hospital on Monday 15 January 1973. It did not take long for doctors around the country to realize that we had a unique facility. With the micro-incision into the eye, made possible because of Charlie Kelman's phaco, a whole new dimension of safety was introduced to cataract surgery. We were getting referrals from all over the country, and our department became classified as a subspecialty unit for cataract surgery. Over the ensuing few years, more than 400 cataract operations were performed on patients who had, for one reason or another, only one good eye. These patients were naturally very apprehensive in case anything should go wrong and what little sight they had would be lost. Our team genuinely felt that we had the safest means of restoring their sight, and we were usually able to bolster up their confidence before they underwent surgery.

One of my patients, Mr Cook, was totally blind, with a mature cataract in his only 'good' eye. He came in for surgery several times, but his nerve failed him every time. Eventually we managed to sedate him before he once again changed his mind and I was able to perform the surgery. I had hoped that he would stay in hospital for a few days after his operation, but that evening I saw him sitting in the foyer, fully dressed and wearing his blue overcoat with a bowler hat perched on his head. After thanking me for his sight, he could not leave the hospital quickly enough.

Another of my young patients had lost the sight of her other eye after a haemorrhage, following conventional large-incision cataract surgery, one year previously. She reluctantly entrusted to us the surgery on her remaining eye. The phaco cataract operation went totally according to plan. The next day on her drive up to the north of England she suddenly lost her vision when halfway up the M1 motorway. I was immediately alerted but could not believe that this could have happened. Upon her return to Charing Cross I examined the eye and found that all was normal. On being told this good news, the patient's sight immediately returned. She had been so afraid of losing her sight, her brain had made her worst fears come true. Fortunately she was fine.

Of these hundreds of 'only-eye' patients who we were able to help in our unit at Charing Cross Hospital, one other stands out. She was a very beautiful red-haired girl of 18, with dark blue eyes that saw nothing. She had suffered from juvenile rheumatoid arthritis, a condition that can cause devastating inflammatory damage to the joints of the body and the eyes. One eye was beyond redemption and the other had severe scarring and a dense cataract. Even with the aid of Charlie's phaco machine her surgery presented a real challenge. I recorded the operation on video, and it later became a very useful teaching aid. Against the poorest of odds, she regained the sight in her one eye and was able to return to the life of a normal teenage girl.

Although our results gave me enormous satisfaction, I was very aware of the inadequacies of what was being accomplished in the overall picture of ophthalmic cataract surgery. In the rest of the country, in Europe and most of the remainder of the world these advances were as yet unknown. We realized that we would have to cooperate closely with our colleagues in America, and particularly with Charlie Kelman, in teaching and promoting this form of surgery.

Our desire to promote these advances was realized much sooner than we had hoped. At another Barraquer Congress in Barcelona, I hatched a plan with two of my British ophthalmic colleagues, John Cairns from Cambridge and Tom Casey from East Grinstead Hospital. We decided to organise at the New Charing Cross Hospital a congress to which we would invite top international ophthalmic surgeons to perform live surgery on my patients. A television camera attached to the operating microscope would relay the picture of the surgery to 300 delegates. This would be the world's first live surgical international congress.

On arriving back in London, I found that my consulting rooms in Harley Street had been decorated, and I hardly recognized them. One of my patients on whom I had performed surgery was Sir Frederick Hoare, chairman of Messrs Hoare & Co and my bank manager. He had just completed his tenure as the Lord Mayor of London. At Eton College he had not particularly distinguished himself, and in one of his reports his headmaster had written: 'This boy will never set the Thames on fire.' In later years Frederick would love to joke about this and say: 'I might not have set the Thames on fire, but at least I went down the river in the mayoral barge.'

Some weeks previously he had tripped over a hole in the threadbare carpet in my consulting room. He took in the dilapidated state of the décor: the walls and ceiling had not been decorated since the 1930s and part of the ceiling had collapsed.

'I am your friend, patient and bank manager,' Frederick said, 'and I will allow you as large an overdraft as you wish, but you must get these rooms refurbished.'

A few days later I examined an interior decorator who worked for Courage Breweries. He kindly agreed to undertake the task of 'smartening up' my rooms to complement the existing Art Deco furniture. The final effect was quite stunning and not too dissimilar to Harry's Bar in New York.

Although the New Charing Cross Hospital had been fully functional for some months, Her Majesty Queen Elizabeth II did not officially open it until May 1973. This was the same year that the supersonic British and French 'Concorde' completed its maiden flight.

The opening of the New Charing Cross coincided also with the centenary of the New York Eye and Ear Hospital, which had been fashioned on Moorfields Eye Hospital. To celebrate this occasion, the staff at Moorfields Eye Hospital hosted a party for a number of their American colleagues in the Café Royal. Here we met two Americans, Arnie and Marion Pearlstone, from Connecticut, who become lifelong friends, and in later years Marion flew to London to have her phaco and implant cataract operations performed by me.

That autumn we went to America to once again teach at John Beale's course in San Francisco, following which we flew to Los Angeles to join Irv Kalb and his wife Barbara. This was my initial introduction to the small but very elite band of ophthalmic surgeons who were now performing this cataract surgery in their own hospitals. Irv took me to his hospital, the Lions Eye Institute in Santa Monica, Los Angeles, and we watched one of his colleagues, Robert Sinskey, perform perfect phaco surgery. Bob was wearing an extraordinary headpiece: not a sterile green cap but a hat on which was stuck a toy white chicken that waggled its beak every time Bob moved his head. I was witnessing the relaxed and professional attitude of a surgeon who was advancing the frontiers of his profession despite stiff opposition from the ophthalmic establishment. It was as if by wearing this ridiculous cap, Bob was sticking up two fingers to the establishment and saying 'I'll do it my way'. From that first moment, I knew that he was a kindred spirit. The Sinskeys, like our other American colleagues the Kelmans, Pearlstones and in later years the Apples, became among our greatest friends. Over the next decades, Veronica and I shared some of the happiest times of our lives with these four families.

Bob had served as an officer in the US Navy and had been sent to Japan to study the effects of the atomic bombs that had been dropped on Hiroshima and Nagasaki. His experiences and findings had a profound influence on his life and turned him into a dedicated surgeon determined to correct some of the injustices inflicted on mankind. Bob would later develop one of the best lens implants of the latter part of the twentieth century. We spent the evenings with the Sinskeys, Kalbs, Kratzs and also Jim Little, who had flown in from Oklahoma.

This small group of surgeons brought in the first modifications to Charlie Kelman's classic phaco operation. No changes were made at this time to the incision into the eye, but the 'Christmas tree' opening in the anterior capsule of the lens was modified into the 'can opener'. This involved making small continuous nicks into the periphery of the surface of the anterior capsule, which, when completed, would leave a relatively large circular serrated edged opening in the capsule. It was now possible to emulsify the nucleus through this new opening in the anterior capsule while it still lay in the capsular bag. This obviated the need to dislocate the nucleus of the lens into the anterior chamber of the eye but made the removal of the nucleus in the posterior chamber a more difficult procedure. They also produced an instrument to polish and clean off residual debris left on the fine posterior capsule of the lens.

That time in Los Angeles was an important training ground for me. We then flew from Los Angeles to Oklahoma to stay two nights with Jim Little, his wife Margarite and their children. Jim was well over six foot tall, a giant of a man with ginger red hair that stood vertically out from his scalp like a thatch of hay. He spoke in a soft southern drawl. Despite being a very gentle person, he had an abiding love of hunting and shooting. I attended surgery with Jim and saw him do five phaco operations. I was most impressed with the very apparent admiration that his patients held for him. During a round of his patients, he said to me: 'Every patient on whom I operate will bring in eight others.' Over the years, I realized that this would equally apply to my own practice.

Jim Little flew his own twin-engined Cessna jet and we went in this from Oklahoma to Dallas, which was the new venue for the annual meeting of the American Academy of Ophthalmology. After this congress, Veronica and I stayed in New York with Charlie Kelman. By now we were entrenched into this small circle of surgeons dedicated to small-incision cataract surgery, and I was often asked to lecture on this subject.

I was invited to speak at Yale University in Connecticut, some 80 miles from New York. The talk was scheduled for 3 pm, but at 1.45 pm I was still in Charlie's consulting rooms in 58th Street, New York, and becoming a little anxious about my time schedule. Thankfully, the last patient was seen shortly afterwards, and then Charlie flew me up Long Island and across the Bay to Connecticut Airport in his helicopter and left me on the perimeter of the runway in Yale airport. It was by now only half an hour before the time for my lecture but I was at the wrong terminal and forced to hitch a ride with a kind fuel-truck driver to the correct terminus, where I was met and taken to the University by Arnie Pearlstone. I met my host, Professor Fasanella Savat, just five minutes before my lecture was due to start. While speaking to the ophthalmic interns in this most venerated American university, I became acutely aware that they had never before heard of phaco. Such was the extraordinary ophthalmic world in which we were living.

On my return to England, I spent a great deal of that Christmas writing a thesis for the Treacher Collins Ophthalmic Prize, in which I elaborated on the equipment in Charing Cross and described the modern microscopic phaco-assisted surgery, which could be performed with it. Treacher Collins had been a renowned ophthalmic surgeon of the previous century and had left this bequest. The prize was eventually awarded to a surgeon who described the way to perform a conventional old-style cataract operation on a child. The elders in our profession were still blind to the advances that were occurring in the ophthalmic world!

Part Six. A Time to Practise

CHAPTER 19
Rebirth of lens implanting

Early in 1974, I travelled to Gröningen, in the Netherlands, to attend a course of instruction on lens implantation. Although I was now an expert phaco surgeon and had originally been taught lens implantation by its inventor, Harold Ridley, I was still not up to date with the recent advances. Until this time, the majority of my patients were fitted with contact lenses after phaco cataract surgery.

The eye has several compartments. Behind the clear cornea, there is an area known as the anterior chamber. The iris of the eye, that beautiful diaphragm which gives the eye its colour, is the posterior limit of this chamber, and in its centre is the open space of the pupil. Although 3.5 mm in depth at its centre, the anterior chamber of the eye becomes progressively shallower towards its periphery, where the cornea almost comes into contact with the base of the iris. This recess at the periphery of the anterior chamber contains a spongy meshwork of tissue, within which are outlet channels for the exit of the circulating fluid within the eye. Behind the iris diaphragm lies the posterior chamber, where the lens is suspended by a circular ligament to the inner surface of the eye.

These two compartments, the anterior and posterior chambers, which are separated by the iris diaphragm, form the anterior one-third of the eye's structure. Behind the lens is a cavity, the vitreous chamber, which is filled with an inert fluid and lined on its posterior surface by the retina, which transmits the visual image to the brain.

When Harold Ridley invented the lens implant to optically replace the lens that had been removed with the cataract operation in 1949, it was designed to fit into the posterior chamber of the eye, in exactly the same position as the previously occupied human lens. Although by modern standards his surgery was outdated (as the size of the incision required in removing the cataract necessitated months of postoperative convalescence) his concept was quite brilliant. Problems did arise, however, as his original biconvex acrylic lens, similar in shape to the human lens and with no fixating elements, was some 10 times heavier than later contemporary intraocular lenses. In some cases, this relatively heavy lens broke the posterior lens capsule and dropped back into the posterior vitreous cavity of the eye. Although the only problem that this caused to the patient was the instant loss of discriminative vision, Ridley felt that modifications to the operation were necessary. He therefore changed the placement of the lens implant from the posterior chamber of the eye to the anterior chamber and radically altered its design. Three legs were added to the periphery of the optical portion, and these new anterior chamber lenses were fixed with little legs in the narrow recess between the posterior surface of the cornea and iris. This positioning of the implant in the anterior chamber would be the cause of one of the major disasters in ophthalmic history and would set back the development of lens implants by at least 20 years.

The cornea and the lens are the only two transparent tissues in the body. This transparency is maintained by active metabolism. When the metabolism of the lens breaks, down the patient develops a cataract. In the case of the cornea, the front 'watch glass' of the eye, the main metabolic process occurs in a single layer of cells that are spread over its posterior surface. These cells, each some 14 microns in diameter and vital for transparency of the cornea, actively draw fluid out of its substance and if damaged are not replaced. Lying on the back surface of the cornea, they number some 4500 per cubic millimetre at birth but gradually become reduced by wear and tear over the years. If the number of cells becomes fewer than 1400 per cubic millimetre, they cannot maintain the integrity of the cornea, which becomes waterlogged and opaque. If one of these cells on the posterior surface of the cornea is destroyed, neighbouring cells will spread into the vacant space.

The problem with early models of the anterior-chamber lens implants arose from the fact that the distal portion of their legs, lying in the narrow recess of the anterior chamber, in some cases touched the posterior surface of the cornea and rubbed against these cells. These endothelial cells were then destroyed one by one, which reduced their number until the remaining ones could no longer maintain the vitality of the cornea. This would lead to the cornea becoming waterlogged and cloudy. Complications were compounded by the fact that many of these lenses had nylon legs that dissolved, causing the implant to dislocate. In one European clinic, nearly 500 eyes were damaged or lost because of corneal problems associated with anterior-chamber implants.

During the 1950s, early pioneering European surgeons such as André Baron, Strampelli, Dannheim, Barraquer and Boberg-Ans developed several styles of anterior-chamber implants. As these implants could be in the eye for many months or even years before the cornea became destroyed, it was not until the latter part of that decade and the early part of the next that these manmade problems became truly apparent.

Throughout this time, a British surgeon, Peter Choyce, designed various modifications to Strampelli's original three-point fixated anterior-chamber lens. Peter was an ardent follower of Harold Ridley and had worked with him at Moorfields Eye Hospital. In 1963, he produced the Choyce Mark VIII lens, which overcame the inherent defect of 'corneal touch' in these anterior-segment implants and provided greater stability and fixation. He achieved this by modifying the footplates at the distal end of the legs to a 'gull-wing' configuration, so that they touched only the root of the iris in the narrow recess of the anterior chamber. As the cells on the posterior surface of the cornea were not destroyed by this implant, the cornea remained viable and the long-term results of this implant were excellent. Both the Choyce Mark VIII and subsequent Mark IX (1978) anterior-lens implants remained in production for many decades, and I implanted hundreds of them with good results. Peter Choyce made a huge contribution to lens implantation and will be forever remembered for these anterior-chamber implants, as well as for the unstinting support that he gave to his mentor Sir Harold Ridley.

The catastrophic results of lens implantation in the 1950s and 1960s led most surgeons to reject the concept. During these two decades, only a small band of surgeons continued to perform this form of surgery. After briefly experimenting with anterior-chamber lenses, Harold Ridley reverted back to his original posterior-chamber implant, which he was still using when I was his house officer at Moorfields Eye Hospital in 1959–60. By the mid 1960s, virtually the only two safe lenses to implant were Harold Ridley's original biconvex posterior-chamber lens and Peter Choyce's Mark VIII anterior-segment implant – both of which were made by the world's first manufacturer of lens implants, Rayner of England.

In the early 1960s, two Dutch ophthalmic surgeons, Cornelius Binkhorst and Jan Worst, produced an alternative style of lens implant known as the 'iris-supported clip lens'. Edward Epstein originally proposed this concept in 1953, but his 'collar stud' lens was quickly abandoned after it was found to cause a series of problems, including glaucoma and depigmentation of the iris. Binkhorst developed a lens in which the optical portion was overlying the pupil in the anterior chamber and the fixating loops hugged the margin of the pupil. The anterior haptics were placed in front of the iris in line with the optical portion of the lens, and the posterior loops passed through the pupil to lie behind the iris. The effect was similar to a lady's 'cameo' brooch, in which loops from the brooch pass through the buttonhole of a coat's lapel to grip both of its surfaces. After the insertion of the iris clip lens, it was essential for the pupil to remain constricted, because if it dilated beyond the width of the loops, fixation could be lost with dislocation of the implant. To avoid this complication, Jan Worst had modified the design of his lenses by removing the anterior loops and, in their place, creating two suture holes, so the lens could be stitched to the iris. This lens was known as the medallion lens and was the forerunner of the Platina (1973) and the 'lobster claw' (1976).

It was to learn about the use of these intraocular implants that I travelled to Gröningen. Jan Worst met me at the airport, full of enthusiasm about his new lens. Jan had the knowledge of an optician and engineer, as well as being an excellent ophthalmic surgeon. He worked with his wife in his own building, which doubled up as his workshop and consulting rooms. He loved inventing gadgets, and one of these was the 'Worst' lens for examining the rear of the eye.

After a disturbed night, as the church clock outside my hotel window struck every quarter hour, I joined the three other delegates – one from Antwerp, one from Germany and John Sheets from Odessa, America. John Sheets and his beautiful Native American wife, Rebecca, would later become our very good friends. Following this course of instruction in Holland, John became extremely interested in lens implants and subsequently developed his own lens and instruments – notably a simple strip of plastic that could facilitate the insertion of the lens into the eye, which John likened to a bridge over troubled waters.

The first day of the course was taken up discussing the merits of these new iris-supported implants. The fact that this course attracted only three surgeons from around the world was reflective of the total lack of interest in lens implantation shown by the ophthalmic profession at that time. During the course, Jan described the loss of cells on the rear of the cornea caused by the rubbing of anterior-chamber lenses. To illustrate this effect, he used the analogy of the occupation of Holland by the Germans in the Second World War. Dutch resistance fighters would kill individual German sentries stationed in small villages throughout Holland in the night by cutting their throats. Their replacements would suffer the same fate, as would the next, and so on, until eventually the elimination of these German sentries would so deplete the numbers of the invading army that control of the country was lost. The analogy was apt, but we felt extremely sorry for our innocent German colleague, who had to hear about the slaughter of his fellow countrymen during the Second World War.

A major contribution to the advancement in ophthalmology was made at this meeting. Jan Worst reported that if the iris was damaged during cataract surgery, it could release a fluid that would pass into the posterior segment of the eye and cause an inflammatory water-logging of the retina, thus seriously compromising the patient's vision. I had recently attended a general medical symposium at which the subject of prostaglandins was discussed. These were fluids originally described as being released from the male prostate gland after trauma, which caused inflammation in the surrounding tissues. Other parts of the body, if damaged, could release a similar fluid. I suggested that the fluid Jan was talking about could be a prostaglandin. Some 10 years later our hypothesis was proved to be correct. The next day we watched Jan perform several operations using iris-clip lenses. After lunch, John Sheets left the dining hall for a few minutes and returned to report that he had looked at the patients who had had surgery that morning, and one of the patient's intraocular implants had dislocated. John Sheets was joking: he had only gone to the 'loo' and had not been to the patient's ward. We all laughed as Jan rushed out of the hall to see his patients. The crazy thing was that one of the lenses had in fact dislocated! Before we left the congress to return to our various countries, we watched as Jan repositioned the dislocated implant.

In February, I returned to Los Angeles to join Bob Sinskey and Dick Kratz, who had organized their own course of instruction on small-incisional cataract surgery and phaco-emulsification of the cataractous lens, having been trained by Charlie Kelman. Charlie was not initially impressed at having to compete against a rival course on phaco in Los Angeles, as up to this time he had had a total monopoly in the teaching of this form of surgery. In time, it was realized that the two courses were complementary.

Whereas Charlie Kelman virtually ran a one-man show with his course in New York, Bob Sinskey and Dick Kratz had a faculty of several leading phaco surgeons. I was invited onto the permanent faculty of this course, and my visit to Los Angeles in February 1974 was the first of many. I helped with the teaching of the delegates and attended the surgery of Bob Sinskey in the Lions Eye Hospital, Santa Monica, and Dick Kratz in the Presbyterian Valley Hospital just down the coast.

As a 'Brit', I was not insured to operate in the US, but I enjoyed watching these two superb surgeons. On the final evening of the first course, Bob and Annie Sinskey invited the teaching faculty back to their beach house in Malibu for dinner. This included William Vallerton, ophthalmic professor of Charleston University, West Virginia, Professor Frank Hurite from Pittsburgh and me.

Later that year, I returned to America to once again teach at John Beale's microsurgery course in San Francisco, before going on to Dallas for the annual meeting of the American Academy of Ophthalmology. On 28 August 1974, Henry Hirschman, an ophthalmologist from the mid-west, chaired the inaugural meeting of the American Intraocular Implant Society, which he had formed with the help of Ken Hoffer. Ken was an innovative phaco surgeon who had some problems keeping up with his 'jet-set' colleagues, as he could not sit in an aircraft and had to travel to all the congresses by train, car or ship. As was the American custom, it was a satellite meeting within the annual academy meeting, and a small conference room was booked for a working breakfast, at which scrambled eggs were served. Seating was for only 200 or so founder members, but the organizers totally misjudged the interest that this society would attract, and hundreds of surgeons failed to get either breakfast or a seat. I was lucky enough to sit next to Dick Kratz from Los Angeles and Malcolm McCannel from Minneapolis. Malcolm was a large jovial surgeon who would make a success of any social function. He often visited me in Charing Cross and was best known for a stitch bearing his name, which was used to keep in place an insecure ocular-lens implant.

Most of the founder members of this society were still unaware of the importance of phaco, and the emphasis at this first meeting was on conventional cataract procedures with lens implantation. From these small beginnings, this society has thrived over the years, and as a remodelled society called the American Society of Cataract and Refractive Surgery now has more than 10,000 members.

Returning from this inaugural meeting in America, Veronica and I decided that it was time to demonstrate the phaco technique in our own country. Later that year, we gave our own course of instruction in the new Charing Cross Hospital – the first to be held outside the US. Its style was similar to

Charlie Kelman's in New York and the Sinskey/Kratz course in Los Angeles. These three courses were, at that time, alone in teaching and introducing a technique of surgery that is now the norm throughout the world.

I had no other surgeon to assist me on this first course, apart from my colleague, Alan Higgitt, who, although supportive, had no knowledge of phaco. We did, however, have the back-up of Rusty Rogers of Cavitron, who had flown over from Los Angeles, and Mike Kennedy, the British agent. As usual, we had the full support of our theatre staff and the technician Mike Haddingham. Mike had been a drifter, never able to hold down a job until he joined our staff, when his attitude to life changed, and he became a valued and dedicated member for some years. His mission on this first course was to go to the abattoir in Abingdon to collect a bucket of pigs' eyes, on which our delegates could practise their phaco surgery.

Throughout the first morning of the course, Mike exaggerated the horrors he had experienced in the abattoir. He relished telling everyone how he had waded, with blood up to his ankles, in the slaughterhouse, while the pigs were having their throats cut. At lunch that day, only one Polish delegate asked for the pork chops – she couldn't understand why there was so much mirth at her order!

Of all our assets in life, the family was the most important. Our three children were rapidly growing up. Stephen was about to start at Shiplake College on the riverbank of the Thames near Henley. Tania had left Queensgate and, after an unhappy year at More House, where she was bullied because of her passion for ballet, had moved to Nesta Brookings School – a specialist ballet school in Marylebone High Street. Robert was now four and at Wetherby, a kindergarten in Notting Hill Gate.

As one generation blossoms so another passes on. In September 1974, I went over to Dublin for the wedding of my brother John to Annie Farrelly and to say goodbye to my beloved Aunt Vickey, Lady De Freyne, who had so lovingly looked after us all after my mother's early death. She was now well into her 80s, very frail and almost totally blind with cataract and degeneration of the retina. Sitting by her bedside in the nursing home, I remembered the time in 1947 when she had visited Swanage to tell Mother that she would always care for Father, John and I. During her stay, I took her for a ride in the sidecar of my very old BSA motorbike. She claimed to have enjoyed this strange journey, sitting only two inches above the road, despite getting covered in oil from the exhaust pipe!

Aunt Vickey died some weeks later. On the day of her funeral, I took the early morning flight to Dublin and joined my family and other mourners at Howth Church, before she was laid to rest in the last of the vacant family graves in Sutton Hill Cemetery on the Hill of Howth. I had planned to be in my rooms by 2.30 pm to spend the afternoon seeing my patients. Waiting for my flight to be called, I was shocked to see engineers peering into one of the engines of my plane. I had problems! I managed to change my flight, but I did not arrive in my consulting rooms until five o'clock in the afternoon and found the waiting room still full of patients. I had hoped that my patients would have made alternative appointments and that I, at this late hour, would only have to look at my post before going home. Such was not to be. David Niven, the actor, had been booked in as the first patient of the afternoon. With his characteristic charm, on being told of the reason for my delay, he expressed sympathy and decided to stay to see me – no matter how long the wait. Eight of my other patients decided likewise, and David entertained them with a 'one-man show'. My patients had had a thoroughly enjoyable and memorable afternoon.

A few days after Aunt Vickey's service, we hosted the first international congress on 'concepts of microsurgery' at the New Charing Cross Hospital, London. This meeting was sponsored by the International Society of Laser and Phaco Surgery which had most of Europe's leading surgeons, including Jean Jacques and Danielle Rosen, Philippe Sordille, Patrice De Large and Philippe Crozafon from France; Hans Witmer, Jorg Draeger from Germany; Fabio Dossi and Lucio Borato from Italy. This was the fulfilment of the meeting that John Cairns, Tom Casey and I had envisaged during lunch in Barcelona the previous year. This really was a world first.

The congress took an enormous amount of preparation and, as so often happened, Veronica took responsibility for organizing the meeting, with the assistance of Bob Sinskey. Our senior administrator, Frank Hart, was very cooperative and 'rubber stamped' our use of all the facilities that we required – for no charge. Pat Turnbull, head of medical illustrations, enlisted the help of her counterpart, Peter Hansall, of the Institute of Ophthalmology. Peter had good contacts in the BBC and quite unbelievably was loaned one of their new specialist television cameras. This had to be fixed vertically onto the side of the operating microscope and linked into its optics, so that the operation could be relayed to a large screen in the Wolfson Hall. We were at the frontiers of discovery, and none of the technicians had any idea how the BBC camera would survive from overheating while recording for many hours in the vertical position. Throughout the surgical sessions, the camera performed perfectly, and the delegates were treated to a professional BBC-quality presentation.

As well as seating our visiting ophthalmic colleagues in the Wolfson Hall, we had also decided to include a trade exhibition of ophthalmic companies, whose stands were placed around the periphery of the hall, so that their representatives could participate in the viewing of the procedures.

We had invited international ophthalmic surgeons who were pre-eminent in their particular subspecialty of microsurgery, and every one accepted our invitation. Our faculty included four other British surgeons, two American, one German, one Frenchman, a Dutchman and me. This symposium was not restricted to cataract surgery but also demonstrated corneal and glaucoma operations, as well as an operation to remove a tumour from behind the eye. All patients were on my own NHS waiting list, and it was imperative that they understood the situation. They had to be prepared to have their surgery performed by an international surgeon, under the glare of television lights and viewed by an audience of over 250. They all seemed to enjoy the experience, most people relishing being the centre of attention.

On the day before the opening of the congress, Jan Worst operated on Arvid, Veronica's father, removing his cataract and inserting one of his Medallion lens implants. At the time I did not feel that I should perform the operation myself, although some years later I did acquire the confidence to do a phaco and implant operation on his other eye and a similar procedure on my mother-in-law, Joy. I must admit that operating on my in-laws was among the few times in my career that I felt more than anxious during the surgery, but fortunately there were no problems.

On the opening day of this international meeting, I had my usual morning swim in the pool at the amenity centre of Charing Cross Hospital. Holding my swimming goggles in my hand and still with wet hair, I went up the stairs from the pool and into a packed hall. It was a splendid sight to see the instrument stands and their representatives lining the congress centre, filled with delegates, all waiting for the programme to commence. They were seated before a vast screen on which the live surgery would be shown. Sir Stephen Miller, the chairman of the session, sat at a desk to the side of the screen. Leaving the hall in my wet condition, I met Michael Ham, the Keeler's representative, who expressed amazement that I should have found time for a swim before the start of such an important meeting. It said a lot for our staff, and the organization in general, that my presence as director had not been required.

I did a hasty change into my green surgical gown and went into the operating theatre. The relaxed atmosphere, which was our usual norm when operating, had changed to one of tension, intermingled with anticipation and excitement. Tom Casey, my co-director, was the 'opening batsman' and was scheduled to do a corneal transplant. He was already seated at the head of the operating table looking down on my patient. In front of him was the operating microscope, which looked slightly unbalanced by the large vertically strapped BBC camera. On one side of Tom was Sue Shayler, our theatre sister, standing behind a trolley of surgical instruments, and on the other the moderating ophthalmologist, who would commentate on the operation that was to be performed and viewed on the big screen. Also in the theatre were the anaesthetist, Eric Emery, other nurses, the technicians and a few observers. They were all 'frozen' in their place, like actors on a stage waiting for the curtain to go up. Once the live surgery started, our staff worked with clockwork precision. We hosted the congress banquet that evening at the Apothecaries' Livery Company in the City of London.

The congress was not only highly praised by all the attending delegates but also made a small profit, so we treated the staff of 40 to a dinner dance in the Villa Elephant overlooking the River Thames. It was a wonderful evening, enjoyed by everyone from the senior surgeons to the junior technicians, and all around there was an atmosphere of enormous friendship.

CHAPTER 20
Spreading the news

At around this time, Charlie Kelman gave the first of several solo concerts in Carnegie Hall, New York, which was filled with his patients and friends, including the famous jazz pianist Lionel Hampton, who was invited onto the stage. The only other amateur artist in this two-hour show was Charlie's son David, and together they dressed up and sang *We're Just a Couple of Toffs*.

It was now my turn to sing for my supper. With Mosha Lazar from Jerusalem, I joined Charlie in teaching his phaco course at the Manhattan Ear, Eye and Throat Hospital. The phaco operation was now officially known as the Kelman phaco-emulsification, or KPE for short. I gave a lecture on how to bridge the transition from conventional intracapsular cataract surgery to KPE. After the course, we drove out to the Kelman's home in Roslyn, with Mosha driving Charlie's brand new Jaguar. I could not believe my eyes as I saw Mosha reverse the car straight into the side of another car, only to then move forward and hit the other side against the exit barrier of the car park. We arrived at the Kelman's house with a rather battered 'new' Jaguar car.

Whenever possible, Veronica and I tried to attend the Chelsea Clinical Society dinners, which were held three times a year in the Berkeley Hotel, London. This is an old medical society meeting at which guest speakers are invited to talk on any subject except medicine. Most of London's medical practitioners were members, and Stanley Rivlin was for many years its secretary. Stanley was probably the best-known varicose vein surgeon in the country, and, along with me, was mentioned in the introduction to the first edition of *The Good Doctor Guide* – as the two highest earners in Harley Street. Would that it had been true in my case!

The society attracted an incredible list of speakers, and, on one occasion, I proposed David Niven as guest speaker. That evening he sat next to Veronica, who could not help noticing that this famous actor was sweating profusely throughout dinner. Before standing up to speak, David turned to Veronica, opened his mouth and asked her if there were any remnants of spinach wedged between his teeth. Throughout his address he stood erect and entertained his audience of some 300 guests with a memorable talk about the history of Hollywood. We later learned that the cause of David's anxiety was associated with his terminal motor neurone disease.

I was later appointed chairman of the Chelsea Clinical Society and as my guest speakers had Princess Anne, Sir Ranulph Fiennes (the polar explorer) and General Sir John Hackett (author of the *Third World War*). Ran spoke about his experiences in the Antarctic and how he had spent six months living alone in an ice cave, surfacing twice a day to make weather checks. This extraordinary explorer held his audience spellbound as he related his experiences in this cramped winter accommodation, admitting that he had never been busier in his life.

My second guest, General Sir John Hackett, was of a very different ilk. He lectured us on the possible scenarios should war be declared between the North Atlantic Treaty Organisation (NATO) and the Warsaw Pact countries. Up until this time, he was the only speaker to be paid. His expense was well merited.

As chairman of the society, one of my roles was to introduce the speaker to the assembled diners. While introducing Princess Anne, I rose to speak without any prepared notes and thus made one of the biggest gaffes in my life. In all innocence, I said: 'This is only the third time in the history of our society that we have been oversubscribed and unable to accommodate all those wishing to attend. The first occasion was when Alistair Cooke, famous for his *Letter from America*, was our guest, and the second time when David Niven was invited to speak to our society. We do not expect tonight to be entertained with the intellect of the former or the wit of the latter.' When Princess Anne stood up to make her address she replied: 'This is the first time that an excuse had been made for my ineptitude as a public speaker, even before the speech has been given.' Everyone erupted with laughter, and from then on she had a captive audience. Her talk was on her work for Save the Children, an organization devoted to creating a lasting change for disadvantaged children. Her address was voted as one of the best that the society had heard.

Some months after Baroness Margaret Thatcher had ceased to be our prime minister, she was invited to speak to the society. The 'Iron Lady' gave an incredibly insightful address, at which she discussed the special relationship between the UK and the US, bemoaned the fragmented nature of Europe, lambasted the weakness of NATO, predicted the fall of communism and colonialism and envisaged the rise of Islam. Looking back now, her predictions were startlingly accurate.

Having had a phaco machine for some years, I could now use it like a concert pianist would his piano. By this time we had upgraded to the Model II, which closely resembled a dalek from *Doctor Who*. The chief engineer at the Royal Masonic Hospital, Dick Patmore, or his wife, Ruth, used to transport the machine to each of the hospitals in their truck! All my patients reaped the benefits of the machine, be they private, amenity, Masonic or NHS. In the confines of Charing Cross and the Masonic hospitals, which were my own domains, its use was taken for granted. In the private nursing homes that I shared with my other ophthalmic colleagues, the theatre staff was incredulous that I seemed to be so alone in my field of surgery.

Four years after introducing phaco at Charing Cross, other surgeons eventually began asking to be taught the procedure in their own hospitals. The first hospital I attended was in Newcastle, at the invitation of Neil Manson, who was extremely 'go ahead' in his thinking and ordered a phaco machine after watching the surgery. This was the start of a new format in my teaching that continued until the mid-1980s. I would travel with the Cavitron representative, Mike Kennedy, and my theatre technician, Mike Haddingham, and spend a day in the hospital, doing phaco surgery in the morning, with lectures in the afternoon. I found these days quite trying – operating in strange surroundings and being watched by the ophthalmic staff, many of whom I did not know. Our team must have looked like travelling salesmen trying to sell a product, but we had a great responsibility, particularly towards the patients who had placed their faith in our procedure. The second of my hospital visits was to Manchester as a guest of Emanuel Rosen.

Another hospital to which I was invited was the Bristol Eye Hospital. The morning surgery was uncomplicated, and, as usual, I lectured the ophthalmic staff in the afternoon. Seated in the front row was the hospital's senior surgeon Philip Jardine, who seemed to be fast asleep the whole way through my address. He truly seemed to be totally disinterested in my technique. How wrong I was. A few days later he wrote to me, saying how very impressed he was with this small-incisional cataract surgery. He himself had dense bilateral cataracts and wished me to perform his operations. Nobody in his hospital was to know that he had cataracts, and on the day of each of his operations he would tell his colleagues that he was going to London for an ophthalmic meeting. I did his first KPE operation on a Friday morning and he returned to normal hospital duties the following Monday. It was a testament to this procedure that no one realized that he had had major eye surgery only three days previously. Charlie Kelman performed surgery on his other eye during the second phaco course that we gave at Charing Cross Hospital a few weeks later. He was the first ophthalmic surgeon in Europe to have this form of surgery and would have been a good ambassador for this procedure – had it not been for our vow of secrecy!

Despite the excellent results we were achieving with phaco, we were still uncertain of the best way to replace the lens that had been removed from the eye. By 1975, the atraumatic removal of the human cataractous lens had developed technologically far beyond its replacement by an artificial lens implant.

It was against this background that I had another stroke of luck. John Pearce, the consultant ophthalmologist at Bromsgrove Hospital, visited me on several occasions to watch and learn how to perform extracapsular cataract surgery. It transpired that his interest in extracapsular surgery was to enable him to place an intraocular lens, of his design, into the posterior chamber of the eye. For a lens to lie in this position, the posterior capsule of the lens has to be retained after removal of the cataract. Harold Ridley's first implant procedure was combined with an extracapsular operation, with the nucleus of the lens being removed through a large opening into the eye. The phaco operation is essentially an extracapsular cataract procedure, with the lens nucleus being broken up and removed through a small incision. In both procedures, the posterior capsule is retained.

After 26 years, John Pearce was the first surgeon in the world to follow the lead set by Harold Ridley and produce an artificial lens that could be positioned in the same place as the removed cataractous lens. His bipolar lens looked rather like the propeller of an airplane. From the optical portion of the lens, two 'legs' were positioned at the 12 and six o'clock meridians to aid the fixation of the implant. Whereas the optical portion of the Ridley lens was 10 mm in diameter, in the Pearce lens it was only 5.5 mm. With this reduction in the size, its weight was reduced by 90%. In one stroke, the main defect of the original Ridley lens was rectified. Like the Ridley lens, the Pearce lens was made of PMMA and manufactured by Rayner of England.

After watching John insert a few of these lenses, I realized that the design of the fixating legs could be improved. Thus started my interest in lens design, which occupied a part of my career over the next 25 years. Veronica and I asked Ernest Ford, the production manager of Rayner to lunch and explained how we could have better fixation with three legs rather than two. Ernest Ford told us that John Pearce had already reached the same conclusion, but as our two lenses differed in certain respects, he was prepared to manufacture both styles.

Jim Little, of Oklahoma City, was one of the faculty members at the second phaco course that we gave at Charing Cross Hospital. One evening over dinner, I showed Jim my lens design, which he took away and spent most of that night modifying. It was this modified tripod design that was manufactured by Rayner in 1975 as the Little-Arnott lens mark 1 and became one of Rayner' most popular lens styles. The Pearce and Little-Arnott lenses paved the way for cataract surgery to be combined with an implant in the posterior chamber of the eye, but the credit for this innovation must be given to John Pearce.

Soon after the launch of the Little-Arnott lens mark 1, Veronica and I once again made our annual pilgrimage to the convention of the America Academy of Ophthalmology in Dallas, Texas. On our way, we stopped in New York to stay with the Kelmans, where we heard that my brother John and his wife Annie had had their first son, Alexander.

Charlie had sold his comparatively humble house in Roslyn and had moved into an extraordinarily modern house in Long Island, one side of which was totally panelled in glass. The difference in the two houses reflected the changed status that he had achieved in his career. Yet I knew of nobody who deserved his riches and wealth more than Charlie Kelman.

At this time, I gave Charlie one of my Little-Arnott mark 1 implant lenses. This lens had a central optical portion from which spread out three legs to help gain fixation in the posterior capsule of the eye. One leg was positioned at the 12 o'clock meridian and the other two inferior legs at four and eight o'clock. I might have known that Charlie, with his inventive mind, would have improved even further on what was already a good lens design.

Charlie's overriding interest in cataract surgery was to achieve an ever-smaller incision into the eye for removal of the cataract and the insertion of a lens implant. Looking at my lens, he noticed that the lateral splay of the two lower legs was wider than the diameter of the optics of the lens. He therefore produced a lens in which one of the two inferior legs was removed and the remaining leg was modified with a curved lateral expansion radiating from its end towards the position where the other removed leg had been. Thus the implant still had three-point fixation, but could be inserted through an incision that was no larger than the optical portion of the implant. This lens was affectionately nicknamed 'the saxophone lens'.

Charlie originally designed his lens, like my own, for the posterior chamber but subsequently changed its positioning into the anterior chamber of the eye, as he had difficulty placing the upper haptic behind the iris. This was a problem associated with all rigid posterior-chamber lenses. Charlie subsequently modified this rigid implant to one with flexible loops, which has remained one of the most popular anterior-chamber implants for the past two decades.

At around this time Hugh Dudley, professor of general surgery at St Mary's Hospital, London, invited me to write a chapter on ophthalmology for Hamilton Bailey's *Emergency Surgery*. I was among 23 other international contributors, all of whom were leading surgeons in their specialty, such as cardiac, abdominal, vascular, kidney, neurosurgery and ENT. As the list of contributors was given in alphabetical order, my name appeared above my other distinguished colleagues in medicine. Hamilton Bailey's has become one of the best-known sources of information for physicians who have to carry out emergency surgery in remote places with little or no access to sophisticated technical aids.

That Christmas, in 1975, Veronica's father Arvid lost his younger brother Werner, whom he had not seen or contacted for more than 50 years. Werner had escaped from communist Russia to Germany, where he lived through the Second World War on the side of the enemy. Arvid was passionately proud of Russia and his adopted new homeland, England, and felt that Werner's life was a betrayal of his own ideals. When Werner knew he was dying, he sent a letter to Arvid and said he hoped that they could depart this life as relatives and friends. Enclosed was a farewell present – a tin containing 20 German cigarettes. Arvid was very emotionally touched.

CHAPTER 21
Svyatoslav Fyodorov

1976 was to follow the same pattern as the previous few years, with courses being given by us at Charing Cross and in America. Our first course of the year was in March, and our American guests were Jared Emery from Odessa and Bill Harris from Dallas. We took Bill Harris and his girlfriend Bunny to our bungalow in Manorbier, South Wales, for the weekend. Being used to the open spaces of the plains around Dallas, they found it strange that farming was carried out in such small fields, but they loved our green and wooded countryside. It gave us huge pleasure to show them Oxford and the Brecon Beacons, and their excitement was tangible when we took them around the banqueting hall, towers and crumbling ramparts of the 1000-year-old Manorbier Castle.

Both Bill Harris and Jared Emery joined me on the course for surgery in the operating theatre and helped with the teaching. Also with us was Mosha Lazar, from Israel. Remembering how he had destroyed Charlie Kelman's Jaguar in New York, I did not volunteer to lend him our family car! Jared Emery and I had a constructive lunch, as together we designed a diamond instrument that could make a perfect 3-mm opening into the eye before the lens nucleus was removed with the phaco machine. The cutting edge was triangular and faceted. This 'diamond keratome', as it was called, went into production and is still on the market. During the early 1990s, an American ophthalmic surgeon, Howard Fine, leader of the second generation of phaco surgeons, wrote a textbook on phaco and illustrated the front cover with a picture of the diamond keratome knife, which he had just developed. I pointed out that we had developed the identical instrument some 15 years earlier. He subsequently acknowledged our design in his book and wrote to me quoting a saying of Abraham Lincoln: 'The only thing that is new in the world is what one has missed in the history books.'

Over the months leading up to this course, Veronica and I had had a number of meetings with Ernest Ford of Rayner Optical Company, to discuss the design of a new posterior-chamber lens. My original Little-Arnott lens mark 1 tripod design was giving excellent results, but I felt that having four-point fixation on the posterior lens capsule rather than three-point could make an improvement. The end product was a single-piece, rigid PMMA lens with a central optic from which four semi-circular flanges radiated symmetrically at the 10, two, four and eight o'clock meridians. Jim Little was not involved in the development of this rectangular lens, but, as I liked the name 'Little-Arnott' and as Jim was a good friend and a highly respected surgeon, I allowed Rayner to designate it as the Little-Arnott mark 3.

I gave a sterile sample of this lens to Bill Harris, who called to say that he had inserted the lens in one of his patients and was most impressed with its performance.

Over the next 10 years, Veronica and I continued to hold regular phaco courses of instruction at Charing Cross. As always, I would invite a top international surgeon as my guest: these included Dick Kratz, Bob Azar, John Sheets and Henry Clayman. One regular visitor at this time was Ulrich Dardenne who would come over from Bonn to enjoy a respite from the harassment of his German colleagues.

In May, after supporting our two great friends Charlie Kelman and Bob Sinskey on their respective phaco courses in New York and California, we booked a holiday in Sea Island, South Georgia. The flight from Atlanta to St Simond's airport in Sea Island was in an ancient twin-piston engine Douglas DC3 Dakota – a plane that had been the main form of military transport during the war. This flight was rather exhilarating. Mountainous storm clouds stretched up thousands of feet into the sky, and our elderly plane had to take a circuitous route, weaving and bumping its way to our destination through any available gaps in the clouds.

When not reading or writing by our hotel pool, we explored the underdeveloped countryside on a 'bicycle made for two'. Sea Island had remained locked in a time capsule for more than 100 years. Once famed for its cotton, it had fallen onto hard times with the abolition of slavery after the American Civil War. The plantations were mostly abandoned, as were the stone buildings in which the slaves had been housed. So preserved and undeveloped was the whole area that it was like living in the mid-1800s.

To coincide with my 47th birthday, Veronica and I flew to Aberdeen, Scotland, at the invitation of Mr Rae, the senior ophthalmic consultant at the Aberdeen Royal Infirmary. The hospital had acquired a phaco-emulsification machine from Cavitron and my task was to 'hold the hands of the surgeons', as they performed their first phaco operations. They had all attended one or more of my courses at Charing Cross and had become adept at practising the procedure on pig eyes. But today they would be in the theatre performing phaco surgery on real patients. They must all have felt the same apprehension as a trainee pilot on his first solo flight. By custom, we carefully examined the patients scheduled for surgery and the procedure was fully explained to them. The first patient elected me to do the operation – and so started phaco surgery in the second hospital in the United Kingdom. Having by now performed many hundreds of KPE procedures, the operation was almost second nature to me.

Sitting beside the surgeons who were just starting to embrace this field of surgery made me realize why it was taking so long for this technique to become established. Although they were all extremely experienced, they had to learn a totally new set of skills, which must have made them feel like medical students. After a very long day, I left the hospital feeling totally exhausted. It is very difficult supervising the progress of a new style of operation. At dinner that night, the atmosphere was charged with bravado – we were like a football team that had won a major match. Within months, patients were benefiting from their newly acquired and hard-earned skills.

The following day, Veronica and I left Aberdeen in our bright yellow rental car and drove up to the Highlands of Scotland to soak in the beauty and majesty of the glens, lakes and pine forests. Some years previously I had operated on the professor of medicine at Charing Cross Hospital, and, as a 'thank you', he had given me a bottle of Glenfiddich malt whisky, which from then on became our favourite evening tipple. Ever since then I had wanted to visit the distillery, which we did on our way down to stay the night with Hugh and Jane Blakeney in Granton-on-Spey. Jane had attended the beautician course with Veronica at Atkinsons and was now married to Hugh, the agent for the Seafield Estate. He was responsible for organizing fishing, shooting and deer-stalking parties. They lived in a Georgian house encompassed by the River Spey. Jane had become totally absorbed into this style of life, which was extremely social because of the number of guests that came to this part of the Highlands for its sport. They gave us a new taste for the country life.

Veronica took the children and an endless stream of their friends to Manorbier for the summer. Stephen was now a mature young teenager, relishing his time at Shiplake College and spending an increasing amount of time rowing on the Thames. Tania, our daughter, was making good progress at the Nesta Brooking School. Despite having twice been refused entry to the Royal Ballet School, she had not only been awarded a Checcetti scholarship but had also been highly commended at the Mabel Ryan awards held in the Barbican. Robert, as always, was quietly trying to catch up with his much older siblings. I would join them for weekends, taking the overnight sleeper train.

In the autumn we made another extended visit to the New World. After attending a microsurgical congress in Montreal, we flew to Los Angeles to stay with the Sinskeys in Malibu for the annual meeting of the American Society for Cataract and Implant Surgery. It was here I learned that an American pharmaceutical company was marketing a copy of the rectangular posterior-chamber lens that I had given Bill Harris in the spring – as the 'Harris-Arnott' lens. Bill was later credited as the first American surgeon to re-embrace the concept of implanting an intraocular lens in the posterior chamber after phaco removal of the cataractous lens. I did not make a fuss about the production and designation of this lens without my approval, but this was the first instance of a problem that would affect me for many years to come.

On the first day of the meeting, I gave a presentation to 5000 delegates, reading a paper entitled 'The Kelman phaco-emulsification cataract operation in combination with a posterior-chamber lens implant.' The address was well received, and I was particularly pleased to be congratulated by Cornelius Binkhorst, the inventor of the iris-clip lens, and Brad Straatsma, the chairman of the meeting. Charlie Kelman gave a paper on his posterior-chamber lens, which was the modification of my own.

Towards the end of the morning session, during one of the presentations, a man with cropped black hair entered the hall and started to walk, with a limp, down the side stairs towards a vacant seat. It was the Russian ophthalmic surgeon, Professor Svyatoslav Fyodorov. When he was recognized, the meeting came to a grinding halt, and the delegates got to their feet to give him a standing ovation. Professor Fyodorov and his colleague Professor Krasnov were the two foremost Russian surgeons and, with the cold war still in progress, only one was allowed out of the Soviet Union at any given time. This time it was Slava's turn to be out of Russia.

On the Sunday we had a quiet day at Malibu with the Sinskeys, who had invited a few of their friends for brunch. The Sinskey's house was on the edge of the beach, which steeply sloped down to the Pacific Ocean, and was pounded every half minute by the waves breaking onto the shore. The house had a ground-floor balcony, on which drinks had been laid out for the guests. Miles Galin, one of America's pioneer implant surgeons, arrived with the great Svyatoslav Fyodorov. After Svyatoslav had downed a couple of strong Bloody Marys, he asked if anybody would like to join him for a swim. Despite the fact that I was ravenous, having had no breakfast, I volunteered. When Svyatoslav was a student he had slipped and fallen under a tram, and one of his legs had been amputated below the knee. With this defect, I wondered how he would negotiate the steep slope down to the ocean.

I need not have worried. He vaulted over the balcony of the house and, half way down the precipitous beach, stopped to unstrap his artificial leg, which was salvaged by Veronica. He then proceeded to walk into the sea, standing vertically on his hands like a circus artist. Once afloat, he swam away from the beach at a fast pace, adopting the relaxed freestyle stroke of a champion swimmer. Following behind him, all I could see ahead of me was one waggling foot. Some 200 metres off the shore was a strip of kelp, a type of seaweed that floats on the surface, with roots that drop down to the bottom of the seabed. I warned him that it would be dangerous to swim through this weed, but he ploughed on out to sea. Some time later we passed the fishing boats and still he continued to swim. Finally exhausted, I managed to reach him and gripping onto his big toe, told him: 'Svyatoslav, I have had enough.' He stopped swimming immediately, and I realized that he had been simply determined to demonstrate his superiority over the 'Brit.'

We lay on our backs warmed by the sun and were so far out to sea that we could see the Californian coastline from Santa Barbara to Santa Catalina Island. We talked for more than an hour and immediately struck up a lifelong friendship. Relaxing with him, some miles out to sea in the Pacific Ocean, I learned about his background. His father had been a Russian general who had fallen foul of Stalin and had been sent to a labour camp in Siberia. Svyatoslav had hoped to become a fighter pilot, but his incident with the trolley car had put an end to that career. Medicine profited by his alternative choice. He qualified at the Rostov-on-Don State Medical Institute in 1952 and then took an appointment in Cheboksary. He had heard about the work that Harold Ridley was doing with artificial lens implants, and he began his own experimentation and made his own intraocular lens implants. There was an immediate outcry from the local medical establishment, which prompted Svyatoslav to move to the northerly city of Archangel on the White Sea. Here, despite many early failures, he continued trying to find a viable plastic prosthesis to substitute the opaque crystalline lens after cataract surgery. Svyatoslav told me that another reason for moving to Archangel was so that he could be near his elderly father. He rose rapidly to become head of the department of eye diseases at the Archangel Medical Institute, before taking a similar position in the Stomatological Institute in Moscow.

He was a relentless and politically astute worker and in a short time founded the Moscow Research Laboratory of Experimental and Clinical Problems of Eye Surgery, which later became the enormous, world-famous Research Institute of Eye Microsurgery. Among his many unique contributions to ophthalmology, he was responsible for pioneering refractive surgery, 'radial keratotomy', for the correction of myopia, astigmatism and hypermetropia, which became popularly known as the 'Russian operation'.

He was fond of saying that his research into the rectification of these conditions was prompted by a chance encounter with a highly myopic 16-year-old boy who had suffered multiple lacerations to his cornea. After the boy's eye had healed, Slava noticed that his myopia had improved. This led him to believe that strategically made surgical 'cuts' on the anterior surface of the cornea would have the same effect. He was also obsessed with the notion of providing predictive eye surgery to the greatest number of people at the most economical cost and pioneered 'assembly line' surgery.

Despite profiting from Communism and being awarded the highest Soviet honours, including the Order of the October Revolution, the Order of the Red Banner of Labour, the Order of Lenin Order and the title of Hero of Social Labour, he loathed Communism and distrusted its leaders.

During my first conversation with Slava, in the Pacific Ocean, his English was rather sparse, although even then, when referring to his surgery, his thoroughbred horses or the Californian coastline, he would punctuate every sentence with 'it's beautiful'.

We had a more leisurely swim back to the Sinskey's house, where brunch was almost finished. Veronica was anxious as we had been away for so long, but Bob Sinskey's only comment was: 'Weren't you guys worried about the sharks?' Ignorance can be bliss!

From Los Angeles, we took a Greyhound bus through the Mojave Desert to Las Vegas, where we checked into the Hilton Hotel for another small ophthalmic congress. Our bedroom was very dark and dingy and just as we were debating whether or not to change our room, Charlie Kelman rang: 'What are you two doing down there?' he said, 'I have booked the penthouse suites.' We took the lift to the top floor and entered a different world. The suites were the most palatial we'd ever seen. The sitting room could have hosted 100 guests at a cocktail party. On either side of this room were the bedrooms, both of which had extra large king-size beds, complete with rather disconcerting overhead mirrors!

The subject matter of the congress was intraocular lenses. I read a paper on the diamond keratome. This meeting was rather exclusive, and it was becoming apparent that the surgeons who had taken up the challenge of phaco were mostly the same ones to combine cataract surgery with lens implantation.

This small group of American pioneers in phaco surgery were now becoming our good friends: Bob and Annie Sinskey, Bill Harris and Bunny, Dick and Karen Kratz, Skip and Sheila Bechert, Jim and Maureen Little, Norman Jaffe and John and Rachel Sheets. Also present were John and Cherie Beale, Guy and Michele Knolle, Herb Gould, Bill Vallerton, Don Praeger, Jared Emery, Ron Barnet and Henry Hirschman. Ulrich Dardenne from Bonn, Germany, was the only other European surgeon at this meeting. Ulrich had started doing phaco two years after me and had the second Cavitron phaco machine in Europe. So incensed was the old guard in the establishment of German ophthalmology that they were trying to expel Ulrich from the German Ophthalmological Society. Much time was spent discussing his problem and our similar experiences. Such is the price one pays for success!

In the US, several other societies started, including the American Society of Contemporary Ophthalmology, which was founded by Randall and David Bellows, of which I was vice-president.

I always tried to split my working day into two – doing surgery in the morning and examining my patients in the afternoon. As I was the only surgeon performing small-incisional cataract surgery, the administrators of the various hospitals I worked in were sensitive about ensuring that my patients were kept separate from other cataract patients, as the phaco postoperative results were so much more impressive.

At lunch time I would try to snatch a 20-minute siesta before examining my full waiting room of patients. One afternoon I was interrupted by Veronica, who was accompanied by five-year-old Robert who had a large gash over his left eyebrow. He had hit his head on the sharp edge of the kitchen counter, and I gave him the choice of going to Charing Cross Hospital or having the wound stitched up by me on the spot. He settled for the latter. I injected each side of the wound with a local anaesthetic and sutured the wound. Robert did not utter a sound as my needle repeatedly pierced his skin. Throughout this operation I worried about the extended wait I was inflicting on my poor patients.

On an almost daily basis I would be joined in the operating theatre by a colleague from the UK or overseas, who would sit next to me and look down the assistant's eyepiece of the microscope to watch my surgery. One was a colleague from America who advised me that he was doing a research project on phaco. Delighted in his interest, I gladly welcomed him and allowed him to use my phaco machine to conduct his trials on rabbits' eyes. I was perhaps naïve in not checking the nature of his research but was shocked and saddened when I read the outcome of his unscientific research, which was published in a 1976 edition of the *British Journal of Ophthalmology*.

The phaco machine works by having a 1-mm wide hollow tip that oscillates at 65,000 cycles per second. Part of the skill of the surgeon who does the phaco operation is to ensure that this tip is activated only when in contact with the cataractous lens, so avoiding damage to the surrounding delicate tissues of the eye. This surgeon's perfidious research was to demonstrate that if the phaco tip was left activated in the anterior chamber of the eye the cells on the back of the cornea, which are vital for maintaining the integrity of the cornea, would be destroyed in one minute. It certainly wasn't necessary to sacrifice a few rabbits' eyes to prove this most obvious point.

Upon reading this nonsense, I immediately telephoned the editor, Sir Stephen Miller, to make my protestations about this untenable and ridiculous article, stating that it should never have been published. I reminded Steve that the conventional way of doing a cataract operation was to make a large incision into the eye and to use a probe that, at minus 175°C, adheres to the cataractous lens so that it can be removed from the eye. I suggested that, if this probe was inserted into the anterior chamber and activated, the ice ball at the end of the probe would destroy the corneal endothelial cells in considerably less than one minute.

Sir Stephen Miller totally agreed with my argument and suggested that I wrote an article in response. I pointed out to him that any article published in a 'peer' journal can never be retracted and could forever be used as a future reference. Sir Stephen was a fair and honest person and, on realizing what had occurred, immediately established an editorial committee that from then on scrutinized all articles before publication. The presentation was so ludicrous that it made no impact on surgery, but the American colleague unwittingly helped the journal's credibility by ensuring that in future only 'peer-reviewed' articles were published.

Sunday 12 December 1976 was an important day for British ophthalmology. Peter and Diana Choyce drove Veronica and me in their ancient Mulliner-bodied Rolls-Royce to John Pearce's house outside Bromsgrove. We were there to inaugurate the United Kingdom Intraocular Implant Society – ever after called the UKIIS. Unlike the American counterpart, the ASCRS, which had been inaugurated some years previously with hundreds of founder members, the UKIIS was started with only a handful of surgeons. The constitution of the society was drawn up and the officers appointed. There were so few founder members that everyone present was given an appointment. Neil Dallas was made chairman, Piers Percival treasurer, John Pearce secretary, Peter Choyce south-east and Midlands representative, Michael Roper-Hall north England representative, Walter Rich south-west England representative and Hung Cheng a committee member. I was made the representative for Ireland, but with all my other commitments, I was a dilatory contributor, and my appointment subsequently lapsed.

CHAPTER 22
Helping live surgery into the world

Our small ophthalmic cottage industry was soon to experience unprecedented growth. Other practitioners gradually began to join the pioneering group and this heralded a complete change in our profession. The advances in cataract surgery by a few of us had not only made it one of the most successful operations in the human body but also one of the most lucrative. The altruistic researches, such as those conducted by Sir Harold Ridley and Rayner, with the invention of the artificial lens implant and the later modifications made by Peter Choyce, John Pearce and myself, were about to change.

Before long, companies including Nestlé of Switzerland, 3M, Johnson and Johnson, Smith & Nephew and American Cyanamid would be operating strategic business units in this rapidly expanding sector. Spurred on by the profits from the sale of phaco machines, lens implants, instruments and pharmaceuticals, their research further hastened the advances in ophthalmology. From this time onwards, all ophthalmic meetings had large trade fairs displaying the new products available.

The evolving nature of the cataract operation is one of the most extraordinary stories in medicine. By the end of 1976 the stage was set for the large-scale introduction of modern cataract surgery in America, Europe and the UK. Alas, there were still relatively few 'actors' available to perform it. In Europe, only four hospitals possessed a phaco machine: Charing Cross Hospital in London, Aberdeen Royal Infirmary, Neil Manson's department in Newcastle and Ulrich Dardenne's in Bonn, Germany. The surgeons of Moorfields were still years away from acknowledging the merits of this operation, although for some time its Institute of Ophthalmology had invited me to give an annual lecture on cataract surgery to its students.

In January 1977, Veronica and I were invited, for the first time, to give a clinical demonstration of phaco in a European hospital. We flew to Frankfurt and joined Charlie Kelman in the Intercontinental Hotel. As always with Charlie, we enjoyed several days of really hard work and good relaxation.

Veronica was particularly pleased at this invitation, as she had made contact with Ursula, the daughter of her late Uncle Werner who had lived in Frankfurt. This was the first time in 60 years that a member of Veronica's family had met a member of her German side of the family. The meeting of these two first cousins was rather poignant and personified the troubles in Europe that had torn so many families apart. Werner had fled to Germany after the Bolshevik Revolution, where he had married and had five children. Ursula was the youngest daughter. During the Second World War, Werner supported the Third Reich, while his elder brother, Arvid, Veronica's father, was a commissioned officer in the British Intelligence Service.

For a number of years we kept in contact with Ursula, but just when we felt as if we had truly re-established a bond with this side of the Langué family, Ursula was sent to Poland by her company to explore future opportunities for tourism. She never returned and was one of the many innocent civilians who lost their lives during the violent protests against Russian martial law. With Ursula's disappearance we finally lost all connection with the German Langué family.

The Frankfurt course was a turning point in the evolution of German ophthalmology and paved the way for Ulrich Dardenne to have his rights restored in the German Ophthalmologic Society. At the phaco course were some 30 senior professors representing most of the major hospitals in the Federal Republic of Germany. Charlie Kelman and I shared the surgery and, as anticipated, our German hosts presented us with six patients with particularly complicated cataracts. Charlie and I had to really struggle through these difficult operations, which was made worse by the open scepticism of our audience. Fortunately, we completed the list without any complications, and even our hard-hearted hosts had to admit that they were impressed.

Many of my colleagues and many general practitioners were now aware of the benefits associated with phaco surgery, yet the cost of the phaco machine, the long and difficult process of mastering the procedure and the ongoing obstructions from the ophthalmic establishment were creating barriers for many ophthalmologists. Public demand far exceeded the profession's ability to deliver.

As a consequence, the demographics of my practice changed from being a general ophthalmic practice to one that dealt with the most difficult ophthalmic conditions in patients from all over the UK and Europe. In many instances these patients were referred when conventional cataract surgery posed too much of a risk – either because the patient had other pre-existing conditions or because they had lost the sight of their other functioning eye, usually as a result of failed surgery. Not only would an operation involve a great deal of responsibility, but it required the patients to be given a substantial amount of reassurance.

Many of them would enter my consulting room apprehensive and distrustful. I had to establish confidence in a few minutes. Despite envisaging great problems at surgery, it was important to make light of the situation. Unless the patient had a secondary condition, such as a malignancy or degeneration of the ocular tissues such as the retina, it was usually possible to guarantee some form of visual restoration – no matter how complicated the procedure. During the time span of surgery, the surgeon and patient walk together over a bridge above the troubled water. This unique relationship lasts for only a few short postoperative days before normality is restored to the patient and the surgeon's skills are again put into true perspective.

Two patients operated on during the early part of 1977 exemplified these relationships of fear, trust and loyalty. Jimmy Hudson, a senior member of the ophthalmic establishment who had always remained very loyal to my cause despite the concerns of his colleagues, referred one of these patients. He was a young Armenian barrister with advanced cataracts in both eyes. So petrified was he about his state that even giving an opinion about his eyes presented a problem. He would sit in the consulting room chair with his eyes clamped shut, which made examination virtually impossible. After considerable coaxing and reassurance, I was able to make an assessment of his condition, with the recommendation that he needed bilateral cataract extraction. With some reluctance he accepted the situation and agreed to have the phaco procedure without a lens implant, which he considered too risky. Both phaco operations were completed successfully, and he returned to his practice as a criminal lawyer. He cut a remarkable figure in the criminal courts, looking just like Ronnie Corbett with his short stature and thick pebble glasses. Despite being a brilliant advocate, he was somewhat of a loner and looked upon our practice as an extension of his family. On occasions he would ask my secretary, Joy, to be his escort to official functions.

The other unusual patient I operated upon at this time was Sir Anthony Blunt. He was at the peak of his career and, among other activities, was the curator of the Queen's picture galleries. So courteous and well mannered was he that I commented to Veronica about this most elegant person. He underwent a routine phaco and cataract extraction. We were mortified when, some weeks later, he was exposed, along with Kim Philby, Guy Burgess and Donald Maclean, as the fourth member of the infamous Cambridge spy ring who betrayed British secrets to the Soviet Union. Sadly we watched as he was disowned by the establishment and stripped of his title. We never knew whether or not he was responsible for the death of our own British agents, but my ignorant respect for Anthony Blunt and my Hippocratic Oath spurred me on to communicate with him. I wrote saying that he was still my patient and I would like to operate on his second eye, at his convenience. In reply he wrote a charming letter of acceptance, but died of a broken heart before I could be of any further assistance.

Veronica and I now embarked on another ophthalmic project that would once again inadvertently change our lives and the structure of British ophthalmology. We decided to host another live surgical symposium. With the total backing of our administrators Mr Barker and Mr Hart, we merged with

Bob Sinskey's society in Los Angeles and announced the second international congress of phaco and cataract methodology.

Aided by our friend Huw Thomas who, as one of the original ITV newscasters, had an in-depth knowledge of television and communication systems, we went into top gear. We decided to perform the live surgery on our patients in Charing Cross Hospital with a 'microwave' television relay beamed via the Post Office Tower to the congress hall of the Intercontinental Hotel in Park Lane. Some 350 delegates were able to watch real-time surgery on large screens placed around the hall in the hotel. We took over the large cardiac theatre suite for the week and installed a stage large enough to accommodate all the ophthalmic and anaesthetic equipment, as well as the television cameras and crew. We had one camera plugged into the microscope and another to film the moderator and staff in the theatre.

This was undoubtedly the most advanced ophthalmic congress ever held in England – and probably in Europe. Using a hospital like this would soon be a thing of the past. No other London hospital had the facilities of Charing Cross, and administrators such as ours were a rarity. All too soon our hospitals would be invaded by tiers of administrators and managers with 'protected learning time facilitators' rubbing shoulders with 'equality and diversity managers' and 'five-a-day coordinators'. In those days, there was not a bloated bureaucracy of managers clogging and making increasingly sclerotic the enterprises of our world-famous teaching hospitals. This congress once again demonstrated how the private and public sectors can work together with mutual trust. Added to this, some 30 of my NHS patients had surgery during this congress, which made a useful dent in my waiting list.

The congress started on Tuesday 3 May 1978. That morning, I ill-advisedly had 15 patients to examine in Harley Street before joining the opening of the congress in the hotel. All would have gone according to plan if my ancient Jensen CV8 car had not broken down in the middle of Piccadilly Circus. As always, Veronica came to the rescue, supervising the official opening. Most of the rest of that day was spent shepherding the members of the faculty to meet their prospective patients in the ward at Charing Cross Hospital.

That evening we joined 56 members of our faculty for a reception in the hotel. As usual, my few friends in the British establishment were there – as was Dr Charles De Voe, Charlie's supreme ally in America. Once again we had many leading surgeons from Great Britain, South Africa, Brazil, Argentina, France, Germany, the Netherlands, Canada and North America. Amazingly, the majority of these world leaders were still performing large-incision cataract surgery. Be that as it may, the 350 delegates sitting in the congress centre in the Intercontinental Hotel enjoyed witnessing superb surgery.

The operation I performed at that congress was phaco, with implantation of one of my Arnott lenses. Charlie Kelman was by my side in the theatre, giving the commentary with his usual wit. Halfway through the operation Charlie, speaking into the microphone said: 'It is wonderful seeing my phaco

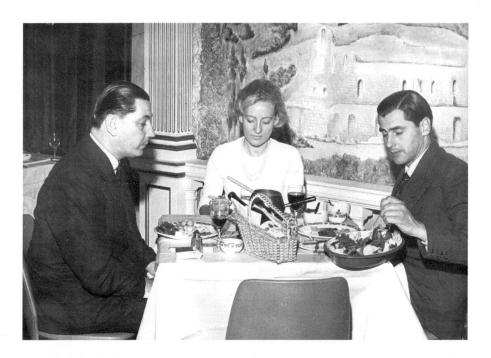

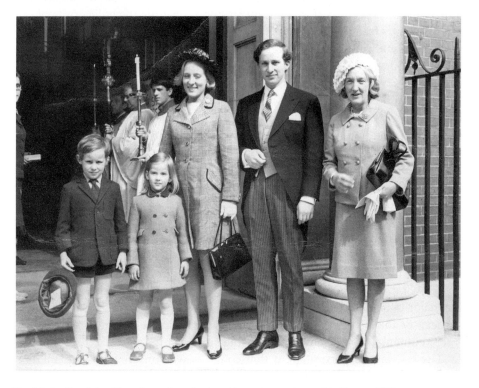

Top: My brother John, Veronica and me having dinner in a restaurant in Rome - 1966

Bottom: Veronica with Stephen and Tania, her brother Charles and her mother Joy -1976

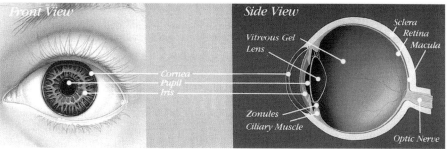

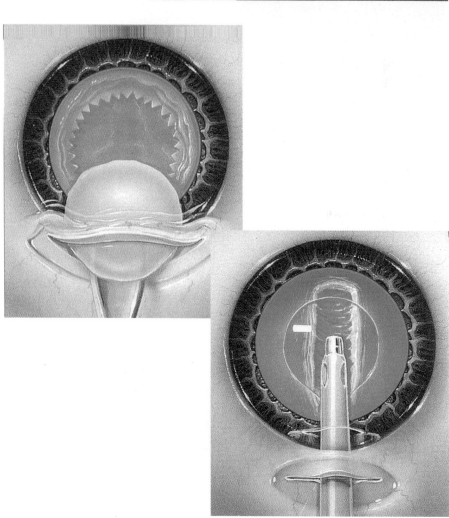

Top: The anatomy of the eye

Centre: Manual removal of the lens through a large incision

Bottom: Phaco removal of the lens through a microincision

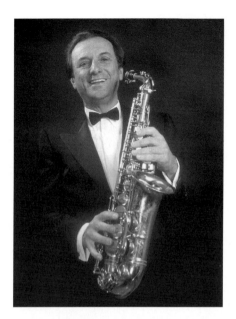

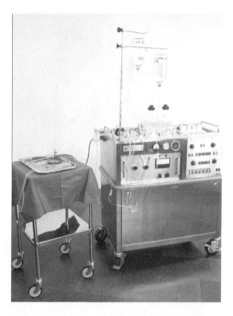

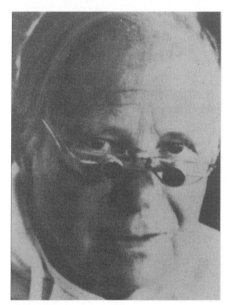

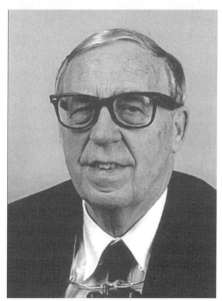

Top left: Professor Charles Kelman, MD, inventor of the phaco small-incision eye surgery and an early designer of lens implantation, playing his saxophone in New York

Top right: An early Cavitron phaco unit - c. 1971

Bottom left: Dr Cornelius D Binkhorst, pioneer of supported iris-clip lens implant

Bottom right: Dr Jan G F Worst, early pioneer of iris-clip lenses and the developer of the Worst lens for examining the rear of the eye

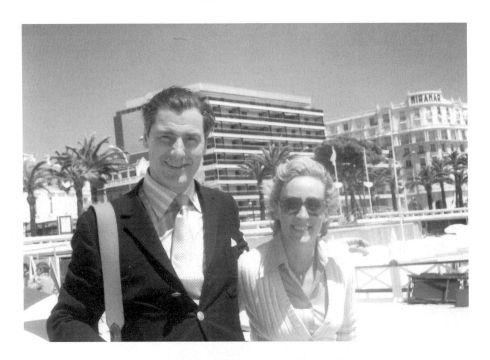

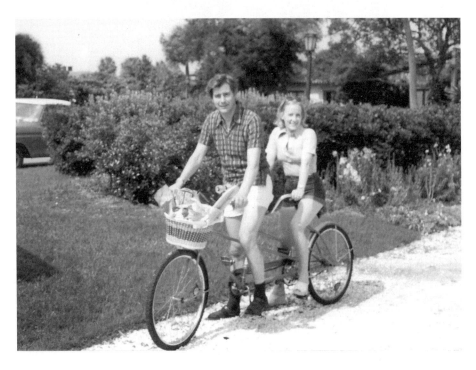

Top: Veronica and me on our first visit to the US to attend the American Academy of Ophthalmology meeting, Las Vegas, Nevada - 1970

Bottom: Holidaying in Sea Island, Georgia, USA - 1976

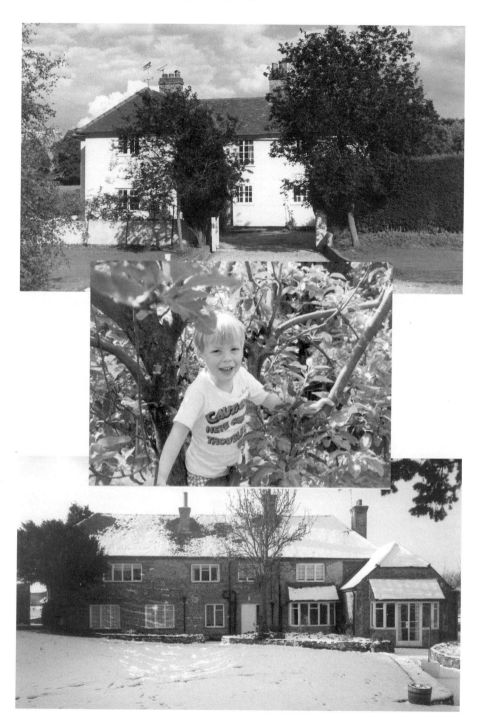

Top: The Langué's home at West Green Cottage, Hartley Wintney, Hampshire

Centre: Robert Arnott - 1974

Bottom: Trottsford Farm, Headley, Hampshire, in the snow

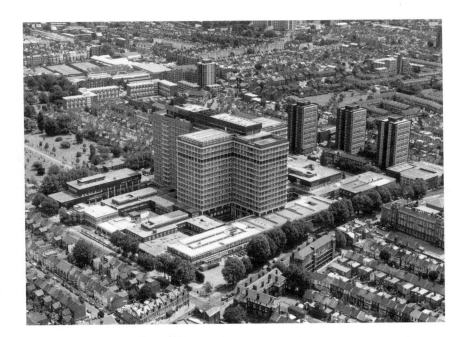

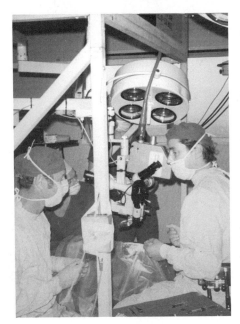

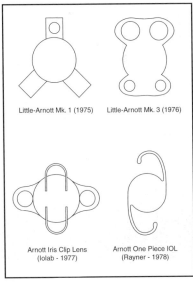

Top: An aerial view of the new Charing Cross Hospital, London, where I was ophthalmic consultant until 1994

Bottom left: Dr Robert Sinskey and Eric Arnott operating at the second international live microsurgical symposium at Charing Cross - 1978

Bottom right: My early posterior-chamber lenses (1975-8), including the world's first one-piece PMMA lens with totally encircling loops.

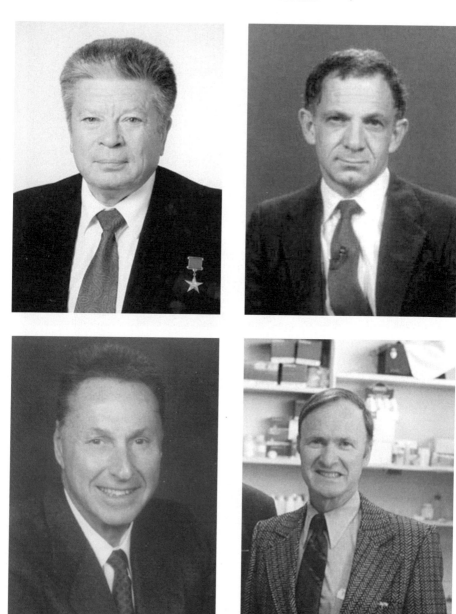

Top left: Professor Svyatoslav Fyodorov, designer of Sputnik lens implantation, who introduced assembly line surgery

Top right: Dr Stephen P Shearing, MD, inventor of the Shearing intra-ocular lens - the first flexible loop posterior-chamber implant

Bottom left: Dr Robert Sinskey MD, early pioneer of phaco and lens implantation and inventor of the Sinskey flexible three-piece posterior-chamber lens

Bottom right: Dr Richard P Kratz, early pioneer of phaco, developer of tunnel incision into the eye for surgery and designer of the Kratz flexible loop posterior-chamber lens implant

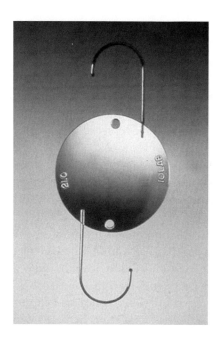

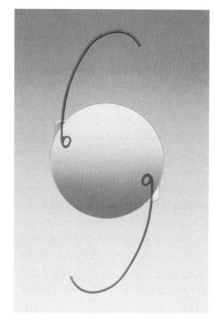

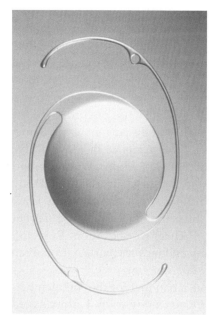

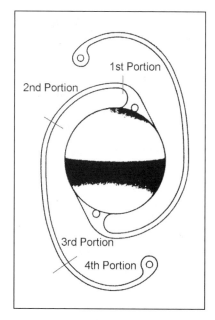

Top left: Shearing three-piece (one optic, two loops) J-loop posterior chamber intraocular lens - 1977

Top right: Sinskey three-piece (one optic, two loops) modified J-loop posterior-chamber intraocular lens - 1980

Bottom left: A later modification of my one-piece totally encircling loop-style lens - c. 1986

Bottom right: Arnott AR4 one-piece totally encircling loop (TELL) posterior-chamber lens, showing the position of the four portions of the loops - c. 1982 surgery being done so brilliantly. You are viewing an operation being performed by one of the world's...Eric – I am having difficulty reading your writing.'

One member of the audience was rather unique. Betty Kenwood, the writer of *Jennifer's Diary* for *Harpers and Queen* magazine, had known us for many years from our private stand in the Phoenix Park Racecourse. She sat in the last row of the hall making copious notes. It was bizarre later to see the news of our congress wedged between the other social events of the week.

As two years before, our patients much enjoyed being operated upon by the ophthalmic greats from around the world, and several struck up an ongoing relationship with their surgeon. Michael Krasnov from Moscow was one of the surgeons who kept in constant touch with his British patient.

On the third morning of the congress, after my usual morning one-mile swim, I was surprised to see news units from the BBC and ITV, as well as our normal crew. On this occasion, I assisted David Hiles from Toronto, who was operating on a 10-year-old boy with a dense cataract. A high court judge, having sentenced the boy's father to a short term in prison, was so concerned about the family's welfare that he had taken them under his wing, and he had referred this boy to me.

The following day we were the big story on the television news – second only to President Jimmy Carter's visit to his ancestral home in Washington, England. At a time when medical advances were not generally considered news items, half the country saw our meeting. Veronica, with her usual good taste and sense of the occasion, organized three excellent evenings of entertainment. On the first evening, after the reception, the faculty went to the House of Commons. Lord Morys Aberdare, the leader of the House of Lords, had asked Tory MP, Dr G Vaughan, to host our dinner. Most of the current world names in anterior-ocular segment surgery were there. From America there were Charlie Kelman, Bob Sinskey, Dick Kratz, Ron Barnet, Jim Little, Arnie Pearlstone, Frank Hurite, Dick Troutman, Don Praeger, Miles Galin, David Hiles and Jared Emery. Our old friend Gordon Krolman from Canada and Enrique Malbran from Argentina completed our faculty from the New World. Cornelius Binkhorst, with Jan Worst from Holland, Michael Krasnov from Russia, Jorg Draeger and Ulrich Dardenne from Germany and Jacque Charleau from France, represented Europe.

The second evening's entertainment was a banquet for the 350 members at the Café Royal. Dr Nigel Southwark, the Queen's physician, had managed to obtain the Duke and Duchess of Gloucester as our patrons. Dress was black tie. To avoid the evening traffic congestion, Veronica and I had decided to change in our nearby consulting rooms. I was mortified to find that I had forgotten to pack my evening black shoes and would have to attend the dinner wearing brown boots. We arrived to find that there was a power cut and the formal presentations were made by candlelight, so luckily no one noticed my brown shoes!

Royal protocol suggests that the opposite side of the dining table where royalty is seated should remain unoccupied so that those attending the function could have an unimpeded view of their distinguished patrons. Grace had just been said when two American late arrivals rushed into the hall and sat directly opposite the Duke and Duchess of Gloucester. With true royal courtesy, the young duke raised no comment. Matters were made slightly worse when this couple lit up, after the soup course, long before the royal toast with the permission to smoke had been given. When the Duke of Gloucester stood up to make his speech, he tore up his official script and made a most moving address on how, during that evening, he had come to realize what our small profession was achieving for the good of humanity.

For the final night's entertainment, the Mayfair Theatre had been booked for the evening. Huw Thomas was the compère of the show and Charlie Kelman, Laurie Holloway and Leon Goosens the performers. Charlie Kelman always travelled with his saxophone. Leon Goosens, my patient, who was by this time quite elderly, had been the world's foremost oboist until he had badly damaged his lips in a car accident. He had to totally relearn how to replay the oboe, before, once again, becoming the world's greatest.

After the congress, we gave a party in the theatre suite for the surgeons, the patients, our staff and the camera crew. Several bottles of Moët & Chandon were consumed in the superb ambience of the operating rooms on the 14th floor, with panoramic views over London. When it was time to say farewell, the BBC camera crew came to us and said that they had not realized that their work could be so worthwhile. The following day they returned to the daily routine of televising football matches.

To unwind, Veronica and I spent the weekend in a small country hotel near Monte Carlo with the Kelmans. We felt like guests joining a weekend house party in a home that boasted only a few bedrooms – none of which had a lock on the door. The pace of life in this remote retreat was far too slow for our American friends, but Veronica and I loved it. There was little to do apart from walking along the beach or languishing around the swimming pool.

It was while relaxing around the pool that Veronica made a casual comment that would greatly influence our future lives. 'I have been thinking,' she said, 'we have just completed a major international congress, leading surgeons from around the world demonstrated their techniques to several hundred delegates, but something was missing; there was not a single Indian or Asian surgeon there.'

I realized that she had raised a very pertinent issue. India had many outstanding surgeons who operated on hundreds of thousands of blind patients. Lens implantation was already available for a limited number of patients, and institutes were opening that would over the ensuing years develop and produce lens implants for the millions of patients requiring this treatment. A few surgeons from America and Europe were already assisting in programmes helping to resolve the major problem of preventable blindness. One of these was Jan Worst, from the Netherlands – my former teacher. He taught at many eye camps and introduced a lens implant that clipped onto the front surface of the iris called the 'lobster claw lens'. But no one was teaching phaco, which had a much faster healing time and so avoided the problems associated with postoperative infection.

By the time we had returned from our weekend, we were resolute to include India in our future teaching programme. We were determined to take teaching of small-incision surgery there.

Part Seven. Random Harvest

CHAPTER 23
A passage to India

Our dreams of going to India were helped by the arrival of my Indian house surgeon at Charing Cross Hospital. Major SK Upadhyay, whom we affectionately called 'the Major', was already fairly mature by the time he joined our team. He had served as a medical officer in the Indian Army and seen active service in the conflict against Pakistan. Seconded to the United Nations, he served with them for several years.

Shortly after our second international congress, the three of us went to India and embarked on a love affair that lasted many decades. I had for many years realized that the proud Indian ophthalmic surgeons did not want foreigners to do surgery on their patients but required only their teaching and technology. In India, lens implants were already being made, and in years production would reach millions per year. Two centres were in the forefront – the Aravind hospitals in Madurai under the directorship of G Venkataswamy and a hospital in Nepal run by Albert Henig. Without the availability of any funds to use automated phaco, alternative methods of surgery were developed for removing the lens nucleus, and in this they were influenced by the technique of Michael Blumenthal of Israel. Albert Galand of Belgium also had a specialized way of removing the lens nucleus – the so-called 'envelope technique.' Following the lead of two American surgeons, Richard Kratz and Paul Ernst, they adopted tunnelling incisions into the eye, which, having a valve-like action in the closure of the surgical wound, tended to be self-sealing. Their teaching spread to Africa, where British surgeons such as Andrew Richards attended teaching centres supported by Sight Savers International. Sometimes we would attend and even chair the meetings of the Indian Ophthalmological Society. I'd lecture and demonstrate advanced techniques at various hospitals around the country. During most of our visits to India we had the comforts of first-class Western hotels, but at times we had to share the sparse hospitality of our hosts in the remote eye camps of the country.

At first we were shocked to see the incredible poverty: shanty towns lay alongside the runway to the airport; thousands of open corrugated or bamboo shacks lined dirt tracks, which were often flooded by the monsoon rains; the inhabitants, with little to do, squatted in front of their scant homes; and the children, often naked, played in the mud or dust in the street outside their homes. Yet, with all this poverty and total inadequacy, their homes seemed well maintained and as clean as was possible.

From our chauffeur-driven car, courtesy of one of my patients, we would be surrounded by beggars, women with newborn babies cradled in their arms or men who had often purposely cut off their arms or legs to help their trade. Children with large luminous eyes would tap on the car window beseeching our help. Occasionally Veronica and I were able to open the car window and give a few rupees to one of them, but for the most part our driver would do his best to accelerate away. On our first trip we stayed at the magnificent Taj Mahal Hotel, overlooking the Indian Ocean.

We became acutely aware of the need for the young surgeons of India to learn the recently introduced world advances in cataract surgery. It was in no way a case that Indian eye surgery was lagging behind the rest of the world. Just as an Indian Susruta had, some 2500 years earlier, invented the couching operating for cataracts, so now had surgeons in the Western world invented lens implantation and small-incision cataract surgery.

The first charity we became involved with was the Seva Foundation. This had been largely responsible for the elimination of smallpox and was becoming increasingly involved in the treatment of preventable blindness. Seva invited us to Kathmandu to demonstrate in the local hospital, assuring us that my surgery would be only on poor Nepalese patients. Veronica, Stephen and I found Kathmandu one of the most romantic cities we had ever visited. Like every other town in Asia, the streets were bustling with bicycles, rickshaws, three-wheeler taxies, ancient Morris Ambassador cars, multicoloured trucks and buses. There seemed to be no rules of the road, and the right of way at crossroads was given to the driver who had the greatest nerve and the loudest horn. Priority was given only to the occasional elephant or the innumerable herds of 'sacred' cows, which took great pleasure in resting on the busiest thoroughfares.

From any part of the city could be seen the Himalayan Mountains, whose sides rose almost vertically to majestic snow-covered peaks. Every few yards there were ancient colourful Hindu or Buddhist temples, and posters of Buddha or Shiva were seen at every turn. During this visit to Nepal we were able to go to the countryside and visit the birthplace of Buddha.

Despite the noise and traffic pollution, Kathmandu had an overwhelming sense of peace and reverence. Our Oriental-style hotel had an outdoor swimming pool: a large steel tank filled with opalescent dark pea-green water. It was uncertain whether or not even the locals would be immune to the bacterial contamination within, but with my love of swimming and need for exercise, I did swim in its murky waters. Veronica confined her exercises to aerobic classes in our bedroom. Our visit took second place in media coverage to the activities of our fellow hotel guests, who were preparing for yet another ascent up Mount Everest. We much enjoyed their company and the youthful expectations they held for success in their climb to the summit.

Having examined my patients and prepared the staff, we returned to the hospital for the surgical session. Expecting to see one patient and one anaesthetist, we were surprised to find dozens of young ophthalmic surgeons waiting in the operating theatre. There was standing-room only, and I felt like I was trying to get onto a London Underground train during the rush hour.

Sitting at the head of the table, I realized there wasn't even space for me to move my arms while manipulating the instruments. Some of my visitors had their faces 10 inches away from me, and others were using the supports of the overhead-operating microscope as their viewing gallery, obscuring even the theatre ceiling. While operating in these claustrophobic conditions, I became conscious that my patients were not poor Nepalese but prominent members of the local society, including the minister of health. As I'd experienced elsewhere, the local surgeons were reluctant to operate on celebrities, fearing that a less than perfect result would tarnish their reputation. Stifled by lack of air, I managed to complete an otherwise normal surgical list, but, as never before, I required the close presence and tacit support of my wife Veronica. Later we were able to laugh about it. A few patients would hopefully have had their sight restored and more surgeons had viewed my surgery than ever before.

On another occasion, the directors of the Jaslok Hospital invited us to give a week's seminar, with live surgery, to 150 delegates from around India. The patients all seemed very pleased at the prospect of having a technique, not currently available, performed by an international eye surgeon. They had been carefully selected: one was a hospital director and another was the father of the theatre sister! But when we went into the operating theatre to discuss the arrangements for the next day's surgery, we found it totally deserted. The staff had all gone home for the night. I looked aghast at our host and said: 'How do you expect me to do a surgical list on 40 patients, in a strange operating theatre, with a staff totally ignorant of my technique?' In two hours, the whole theatre staff had returned to the hospital from their homes. We had a full dress rehearsal, which lacked only the patients! By the end of the day we knew that we had a good crew. The following morning it was a total joy, working with staff that could have been assisting us for years. The theatre sister was full of pride at being able to take part in the operation on her own father.

This surgical demonstration was the first of its kind in India, and it made a major impact. We had the most receptive audience possible, and the majority returned to their home towns determined to pursue this surgical path in the future. One year later, we found that the surgical procedures we had demonstrated were gaining great momentum with young surgeons from all over India desperate for modern teaching.

I had been invited as chief guest at the annual Indian Ophthalmologic Society meeting in Madras. This was to be held in a large congress hall in a wedding village. After my opening address, I visited some of the patients I'd operated on in London over the previous months. During the afternoon session I was to act as chairman, introducing the various speakers. On entering the wedding village with the Major, the younger members of the Indian Ophthalmic Society's committee confronted us. Their spokesman said: 'We humbly apologize, but the afternoon session of our congress has been postponed, as the government has taken over the hall in preparation for next week's general election.' I was genuinely disappointed to miss the afternoon's lectures. He went on: 'Perhaps we could benefit from your speaking to some of us in a small substitute lecture theatre.' With little else to do, we followed our guests down the street to the lecture theatre, which was not exactly small and was filled with more than 200 young ophthalmic surgeons. For some three hours we had a question and answer discussion covering most of the innovations of current cataract surgery. Leaving a very appreciative audience, I heard my name being called over the tannoy system. The president of the Indian Ophthalmic Society then rebuked me for not having acted as chairman for the afternoon session. Full of embarrassment, I suddenly realized that the younger members of the society had brazenly kidnapped me so that they could have my undivided attention for their teaching needs. There was subsequently quite a row at the next committee meeting. Common sense prevailed, and future congresses included symposia given exclusively by the overseas guest visitors.

Every year hundreds of patients would come to London from all parts of India, among them the elderly Mr Tata, a legend in his time and the equivalent of Henry Ford of the US. Many of these patients became good friends, and one, Bipin Ghandi, would insist on giving us the use of his chauffeur-driven car every time we were in his country.

Apart from being made aware of the need to help our Indian colleagues, our televised congress at Charing Cross Hospital had other repercussions. An erstwhile friend suggested that I should be brought before the disciplinary board of the Ophthalmologic Society of the UK and reprimanded for advertising medical skills on television. The fact that this had been merely part of the news bulletins of the day was not taken into account. Fortunately this threat did not materialize, but over the next few years I suffered a great deal of open hostility from my colleagues in the profession. Thanks to their jealousy, I lost forever my established place in the institutional hierarchy of British ophthalmology.

The congress had also the more important effect of bringing about a change of attitude towards small-incision phaco and lens-implant surgery. As a result of the television coverage, younger active surgeons were compelled, for their own professional survival, to learn these techniques.

I also had to modify the phaco operation in order to deal with certain eyes in which the removal of the hard nucleus was too difficult. By manually converting the small phaco incision into the much larger conventional one, it was possible to remove the hard intact lens nucleus. The operation could then continue using the automated irrigating/aspirating system of the Cavitron machine. This modified technique gave surgeons an escape route if the need arose, and the majority gradually became 'converted' to small-incision cataract surgery.

Due to the public exposure we received from this congress, the workload in our Harley Street practice, as well as at Charing Cross Hospital, was becoming impossible, and changes had to be made. Frederick Hoare once again came to my rescue. Just as he had insisted that I refurbish my consulting rooms three years ago, so he now suggested a move to bigger premises.

Finding a larger clinic in the golden square medical mile of Harley Street was no mean feat, but we did manage to acquire two adjacent apartments, numbers 11 and 12 Milford House in a new development just off Harley Street, which we customized for our needs. Three ophthalmic colleagues joined our unit.

John Grindle was an outstanding physician yet he had had great difficulty in obtaining his fellowship and sat the exam no fewer than eight times. A lesser mortal would have capitulated long before he finally acquired his FRCS. The other two colleagues were my previous interns at Charing Cross Hospital. Lyn Jenkins, as well as being an ophthalmologist, was a general practitioner with a practice near Bishop's Stortford. It was very convenient having his expertise as a physician. The third colleague to join us at Milford House was Major Upadhyay. To help with surgery of the retina, we enlisted Tony Chignell of St Thomas' Hospital and David McCloud and Bob Cooling of Moorfields.

Our ophthalmic technician Don Victor Franco De Baux was also a heraldry expert, who worked part-time for Sotheby's auctioneers. His main duty in our clinic was to establish the strength of the lens implant. This could be found by knowing the curvature of the front surface of the cornea and the length of the eye. As we were performing more than 20 operations a week, this involved considerable hours of examination. Despite his artistic background, Victor became expert at this and had a very important function in ensuring our patients achieved the best possible postoperative vision.

Don Victor introduced many Spanish and Portuguese patients to the clinic – he knew a very interesting cross-section of Spanish society, some of whom had served with General Franco during the Spanish Civil War in the 1930s. One of these patients was the Duque de Lerma, whose estate was in Algeciras, in the southerly part of Spain. After my surgery on his eyes he sent me a signed copy of his autobiography, which is now in my library of biographies written by my patients. The duke was an ace fighter pilot and in his book recounts the air strategy of the Spanish Civil War. When the duke sent me his book, he enclosed a letter in which he wrote: 'You also operated upon the widow of our greatest test pilot and later ace fighter pilot Garcia Morato. On page 75 of my book you will read how he was shot down in flames and lost his life.'

Another patient was the Marquis de Santa Cruz, whose ancestor should have been the Admiral in charge of the Spanish Armada but was unable to lead the invading flotilla because of illness. His replacement was the Duque de Medina Sidonia, a grandee and landowner, whose poor knowledge of the sea helped Drake to gain the victory. He came to my rooms while staying in London for the 400th anniversary of the armada.

During one of my consulting sessions I had two patients from Pakistan. One was President Bhutto's mother-in-law and the other was a relative of the former president, General Khan. Such was the hatred between these two families that they had to be kept separate, at the extreme ends of our unit.

Another two patients, who rather ill-advisedly were given appointments on the same day, were Lord Porchester and Dick Hearn. Lord Porchester was the Queen's racing manager and Dick Hearn the former trainer of the Queen's racehorses. Lord Porchester had relieved Dick Hearn of his duties to the Queen's racing stables. I had a great respect and admiration for both of these greats in the racing world, and it saddened me to consider that with all they had achieved in that sport, they could hold such bitterness towards each other. Dick was an example of how success can be achieved in the face of adversity. Despite having been crushed by his horse on one of his rides and becoming a paraplegic, he managed to hold his place as one of Britain's top racing trainers. His devoted wife was 'literally' his legs and guided him everywhere. On the day after his surgery he was 'flying' around the fields in his wheelchair, watching his horses do their morning sprints and gallops.

Another patient was David Gould, the prison officer in charge of Stoke Mandeville Prison. He became very interested in our hospital and wanted to donate a piece of equipment to support us. With the help of his fellow officers he organized a sponsored 100-mile relay run, from one end of the Ridgeway to the other. Veronica and I went to Aylesbury market, where he was attracting sponsors, and met the 12 officers who finished just over their target of 10 hours. Some weeks later David presented us with an ultrasound scanner which could accurately measure the length of the eye, a necessary prerequisite for determining the strength of a lens implant following cataract surgery. We struck up quite a friendship with the prison officers, which would have continued, but for the ophthalmologists at Stoke Mandeville, who were incensed that this charitable event had not been carried out for their own hospital.

That autumn I went with a group of fellow ophthalmologists to a meeting in Johannesburg. Dick Troutman, one of New York's most celebrated eye surgeons, and I were invited to perform surgery in the city hospital, which would be videoed to the ophthalmic congress. This demonstration turned out to be quite a surgical contest to test the skills of the Americans versus the Brits. I had as my partners Michael Roper-Hall, from Birmingham, Jimmy Hudson, from London, and Piers Percival from Scarborough.

At this congress in South Africa I met Ed Levin and his son David, who had interests in several medical companies. They gave me samples of poly hydroxyethyl methacrylate (poly-HEMA), a soft material that was suitable for lens implantation. Edward Epstein, a senior South African ophthalmic surgeon, had been using implants made from this material for some years.

Richard Packard had just become my senior registrar at Charing Cross Hospital and together we researched, using the material on anaesthetized rabbits. We discovered that a lens of this material could be rolled and inserted into the eye through a smaller incision than a rigid implant. After many months, we submitted our findings to the *American Journal of Ophthalmology*. Like many other great advances in medicine, the importance of our work was not appreciated, and the article was rejected. Our paper was finally accepted by the *British Journal of Ophthalmology*, but publication was delayed by more than a year, and it was not until 1981 that it appeared in volume 65. Despite this delay, our paper went to print some six months ahead of any other article on foldable lens implants. Without this delay in publication, our paper would have constituted 'prior art' and could have blocked many future patent applications for foldable lenses.

At this time, one of my most entertaining invitations was to Milan to help Lucio Buratto, then a very young and earnest surgeon, become initiated into modern cataract surgery. I was invited to attend for two days to operate and teach the phaco technique in his hospital, with the assistance of my theatre assistant from the Royal Masonic Hospital, Di Hardy. On the day scheduled for my flight to Milan, I was very delayed by having to do an emergency operation. Taking a later flight, I was met by Lucio who told me: 'Your theatre sister is happily settled into your suite at the five-star hotel.' I tried to explain that there was no way that my Russian wife would accept me staying in the same bedroom as another girl. With great difficulty I managed to make him understand my predicament, but nonetheless he felt that we English were very eccentric!

So my theatre sister had the penthouse suite in the Scala Hotel in Milan, while I had sleepless nights in a little motel under a motorway – some four miles out of the city. I used to creep in to beg breakfast from her in her palatial suite every morning. From then on all my colleagues in the Royal Masonic Hospital called my posh theatre sister 'Lady Di'.

The course was a success as far as Lucio was concerned, and he has since become one of the leading ocular anterior-segment surgeons in Italy. We did a number of operations together and it was obvious, even in those early days, that he had great talent. Towards the end of the operating list, he began to show signs of anxiety, as the last patient scheduled for surgery was the mayor of Milan, who had an only eye. I agreed to perform this operation on his behalf.

CHAPTER 24
Country lifestyle

In the summer of 1977, Veronica and I decided to introduce our children to the New World, where we had forged deep friendships with our American ophthalmic colleagues. Our first stop was the Kelman's house in Long Island. The children were fascinated by this large modern house. The staircase was a ramp, sided by a wall of glass facing the garden. In the hallway, on a patchwork multicoloured carpet, was a Steinway piano. The Kelmans did not return home that evening until 11 pm, which gave our family time to examine numerous household gadgets we'd never seen before. The children were sleeping when, creeping into their bedroom, Charlie said: 'Gee it's lovely having you to stay with us.' In a very sleepy voice Tania replied: 'Me too.' Charlie loved children and took them for a 'romp' in his Hughes jet helicopter. He flew over New York City, under the Hudson Bridge and encircled the Statue of Liberty. This was even better than Disneyland.

After two days we moved on to Westport, Connecticut, to stay with the Pearlstones and their children David, Nancy, Leslie and Martha. They lived in a typical home in a complex where racoons still roamed in the surrounding woodlands. The Pearlstones had a large swimming pool (much appreciated, as we had arrived in the middle of a heatwave), where we enjoyed many parties. Then we journeyed south to Miami, Florida and on to the Bahamas. We were staying on Bimini, an island shaped like a question mark, the most westerly in the Bahamian chain. Ernest Hemingway had his island retreat in one of the colonial, gaily painted homes in the village, and it was from here that he did his deep-sea fishing, immortalized in his classic book *The Old Man and the Sea*.

Driving north, we entered a tropical paradise, where palm trees lined the sides of the track, beyond which were sandy shores, faced by the Atlantic Ocean and, to the right, a blue lagoon. We were staying with the Littles in their substantial house built in the mid 1930s by a Detroit industrialist who had produced chromium plating for the enormous garish American cars of the time. Some of his millions of dollars had been invested in this part of the island of Bimini. Around the roof of this rectangular house was a parapet designed as a roller-skating track. The Littles had inherited from him a large glass dining-room table, with wrought-iron legs, which could seat 25 guests. The previous owner had enjoyed entertaining his dinner guests with nude ladies lying under the table, who could be fondled by the diners' bare feet. Despite this seemingly abnormal departure from a conventional dinner party, the owner of the house admirably fulfilled his duties as the senior citizen. Every Christmas he would go to church and distribute $5 bills to all the children on the island. And when the islanders were threatened by a hurricane, the barricaded big house became their refuge. Guests were accommodated in wooden chalets, joining the Little family during the day in the big house. Jim and Margaret Little took us to the Anchorage Club, with their children Jimmy, Cathy and Jan. Later that day we were joined by other friends: an oil driller who Jim had employed for his land in Oklahoma, and Miles Galin, an ophthalmic surgeon from New York who had just bought a Lear jet. This was a very different lifestyle indeed!

Jim took us by boat to the island of Cat Cay, which was like being on Treasure Island: it was almost deserted, having been devastated by a hurricane, but the clubhouse had been rebuilt and we had the golf course to ourselves. Returning from this lonely island we hit a severe storm. In minutes the sky darkened, visibility was reduced to almost zero and our little boat was lashed with torrential rain. Jim Little skilfully steered the buffeting boat through the frenzied sea, as our family clung for support to any available fixture. After some time the storm abated as rapidly as it had arisen, and once again, in clear sunshine, we saw the safety of the Bimini Lagoon ahead.

To the north of the island were some perfectly symmetrical sunken boulders known as the Stones of Atlantis, which the natives claimed were the remnants of the lost island of Atlanta. The house guests would swim out to these rocks teeming with fish, which included sharks and barracuda. I would normally do a prebreakfast swim along the shore. On my first day I was rather alarmed to note that I had a swimming companion, a large silver barracuda, who was pacing me some 10 yards to my right. Every time I turned he followed my manoeuvre. I tried to seem unconcerned but at the end of the swim, when level with the house, I ran in panic through the shallow water and onto the beach. Later I was told this fish was considered to be one of the island pets, who seemed to love the company of all their swimming guests. From then on I swam every day accompanied by my silent friend. Robert, aged six, learnt to drive a golf buggy, which he rode around the island for most of the day. Veronica and I loved walking, hand in hand, along the golden beach to the tip of the island. Stephen and Tania had a field day rallying in the Little's Ford Maverick car on the beach. They once became hopelessly bogged, but were fortunately rescued by a trespassing local who towed them out.

From Bimini we went to the Rio Grande. We had just left Denver City when we heard on the radio that 'The King of Rock', Elvis Presley, had died. Funny that throughout life one can instantly recall where one was, when one of our more outstanding citizens passes on to a better world. We drove via the Colorado Springs, Pueblo and Almarosa to the as yet unspoilt part of the Wild West in Colorado.

We were staying in a log cabin lent to us by a friend of Bill Harris, our great friend and colleague, high up in the Rio Grande. The house had not been lived in for some weeks, and there was a fair amount of garden rubbish that needed to be removed. Veronica and I were enjoying an evening tipple when we were alerted by screams from our children. Stephen had piled all the rubbish into a 44-gallon drum behind the house and tried to light it by pouring petrol from the first-floor balcony and throwing a lighted match onto it. This started a conflagration. We were panic stricken that the fire would spread through the tinder-dry scrub and start a forest fire, but fortunately we managed to put it out without any serious damage.

We could fish for trout in the Rio Grande River, which ran right alongside the cabin. We also drove up a mountain to fish in 'Beaver Pond'. This was real Western country and the locals still wore gun belts. Stephen was always looking for the two gun-toting cowboys coming out of the saloon swing doors he had seen in countless movies.

On the last day our guide, Butch Weaver, took us up the Elk Trail in a Suzuki 4x4. As we drove up the mountain, we felt as far away from civilization as we had ever been. The rough track, wending its way between the trees, suddenly opened onto a plain, with a surrounding vista totally untouched by man. We rode horses for some 16 miles through the mountain paths, with young Robert on horseback for the first time. This was a fantasy moment to imagine the time before white settlers, when indigent Native Americans and elk ruled the land.

The final leg was with the Sinskeys in Malibu and a trip to Disneyland. Stephen, Tania and Robert were made very aware during this holiday of the great warmth and hospitality of all our American friends and fully appreciated why we so loved returning.

During these years, when I was particularly busy, it was more economical for me to fly to the US in Concorde. It was possible to return in the early evening and do a normal day's list the following day. The economy of time more than justified the extra expense of flying by Concorde, especially as it was little more than that of first-class travel.

The journey itself was conducive to reducing jet lag. The flying time halved and the cabin pressure was lower, so body functions were less affected. On Concorde I found I could concentrate fully, and on one trip Emanuel Rosen and I composed the framework of a whole book on ocular surgery.

The first time I flew in Concorde I sat, with my seat-belt fastened, wondering how noisy it would be in the plane during the acceleration to Mach 2. Surprisingly, the noise of the engines was hardly apparent in the cabin. The initial take-off was little different until the afterburners were lit to give the plane further boost for lift-off, which was noisier but gave a pleasant feeling of acceleration and a sensation of being pushed in the back. Once airborne, the afterburners were switched off, to reduce the noise level for the residents living below. For the next half an hour, the journey was similar to that on any other jet, until the coastline was cleared and the supersonic flight could commence.

Even in subsonic flight the airspeed is some 100 km per hour faster than in other jets, so it takes little time before Mach 1 is passed and the aircraft has reached supersonic flight. In the cabin you can barely tell when you've reached Mach 2 and 55,000 feet: but there is an extraordinary sense of peace. Beyond the beautiful sweep of the Concorde wing you can see the curved horizon of the earth. In the cabin there is no sense of movement or turbulence as you travel a mile every two and a half seconds. We always left Concorde feeling very privileged at having been afforded this unique journey between the continents.

There was one further perk for the Concorde passenger. Luggage was guaranteed to be delivered within 12 minutes of landing. On one occasion my briefcase was left behind at Heathrow, and it was finally delivered to me some seven hours later in New York. For this inconvenience I was given £500 compensation!

Supersonic flying was not always straightforward. Problems did arise and there was a period when the timetable was very unreliable. Despite these delays there was always the certainty that we were flying in the safest of planes.

We also flew to visit Tania, who had gained a scholarship to the Julliard School of Ballet in New York. It was hard for Veronica, as she and Tania were very close. But this connection helped keep them together and Veronica never missed one of Tania's shows. Once when Tania had hurt her ankle and couldn't dance, Veronica flew over to be with her and they spent a week together in Florida to recuperate. On one trip John F Kennedy International Airport had been shut down by a blizzard. At touchdown the view from the aircraft window was obscured by high banks of snow. The plane could not reach the landing pod and we had to make the final journey to the terminus in a snowmobile. There was single-line traffic into the city and most of the roads were still closed. The normally bustling Park Avenue had been taken over by tobogganists. I joined Veronica and Tania in her West Side apartment and we dined in the twinkling fairyland grotto of the Inn on the Park.

Veronica and I always dressed for travel as if we were going to a party. This habit of a lifetime helped me on one occasion when Stephen and I went to America for a business meeting. Stephen booked economy tickets, but on our homeward journey at the British Airways desk, the manageress mistook us for first-class passengers and upgraded us to Concorde. The blue blazer, tie and grey flannel trousers we were wearing certainly improved that day!

Another flight on Concorde from Washington was particularly memorable. It was the Independence Day holiday, so Concorde could take a direct route towards Europe, flying over airspace belonging to the American Armed Forces. At the English Channel, I realized that we were flying supersonic further into it than was usual. I asked the stewardess if we were trying to break a record. She asked me to keep it quiet, but they hoped to break the previous record of two hours, 57 minutes by two minutes. If only air traffic control had been aware of the import of the moment – they stacked us over Heathrow for 10 minutes and the flight missed the record book by eight minutes!

Incidents did happen on these Concorde flights. On one we roared down the runway at Kennedy, but suddenly there was a screech of brakes and Concorde came to rest at the end of the runway. Over the intercom the captain said: 'Humble apologies for our aborted take off, but one of the afterburners has failed to ignite.' The plane was taken to the remotest part of the airport to be repaired, and then with full revs of the engine, there was a thunderous noise, which must have woken up all the residents of New York. After an even greater roar, the engine went into full function. Thereafter the flight was uneventful and we landed in Heathrow as dawn was breaking.

In another incident, we were making our final approach to Kennedy Airport when the landing had to be aborted, as a 747 jumbo jet had been too slow clearing the runway. Full power was applied to the engines and Concorde climbed like a rocket back into the sky.

There was an element of informality on that plane that is lacking on other flights. On boarding Concorde on my way back from America, I met Captain Black at the entrance door of the plane. 'I hope you will have a good flight,' he said.

'I wish it to be better than my last two,' I retorted, 'We had a failed take-off and the next an aborted landing.' Looking slightly embarrassed he admitted that he had been the captain on both of those flights and asked me to join him in the cockpit before landing at Heathrow to confirm that he did a good job this time. I sat next to the engineer and behind the two pilots, mesmerized by my situation. Looking forward it was dark, with a blank horizon until suddenly the lights of Heathrow came into view. This was our last flight on Concorde but a fantastic way to say farewell to such a wonderful ambassador for our country.

At this time Veronica and I started to change the style of our domestic life. In September 1977, we packed up the holiday home in Wales. This brought to an end our long relationship with that part of the country, and we would now have to look for pastures new. Our situation in Ireland was also becoming more fragile. The Phoenix Park Racecourse was struggling, and it was only a matter of time before the restrictions of the racing board forced its closure. Brother John and his wife Annie had by now two children Alexander and Andrew. Yet in John's seemingly idyllic family life, he was living in the shadow of failing health and the increasing debts of our racecourse.

During all these changes, we bought a smallholding in Hampshire after seeing it in *Country Life* magazine. It was semi-detached and lay alongside a sandpit; Trottsford Farm had half the farmhouse, the outbuildings and three acres of land. The owner of the house, Murray Cook, was a retired Canadian naval captain who had been rearing turkeys on the farm. The outbuildings were in a very dilapidated state. The medieval tithe barn had been rebuilt in 1815 and the wooden timbers of the roof had come from Nelson's warships. The barn had seen better days. One whole wall had collapsed and the roof was listing heavily into this vacant space. It seemed doubtful whether or not the roof could survive another storm. There was turkey litter some 12-feet deep on the floor. An old ice-cream van lay abandoned in the farmyard. The interior of the house was little better: a pub bar took up most of the hall, which, complete with stools, stocked a liberal supply of spirits. In one of the bedrooms was an old smoke hole in a chimney, which overlay a large inglenook fireplace in the study below. There was a cellar from which a priest's passage had formerly passed to the barn.

The house was in the upper reaches of the Churt Valley and the surrounding views were panoramic, with oak trees and pines spreading up the distant hills. The garden, lying along one side of the house, was semi-walled and contained four ancient yew trees and a gnarled walnut tree. Although in some state of disrepair the whole place felt warm and welcoming, and we knew it was our home for the future. Murray and Fiona Cook were the perfect sellers and we had great pleasure in dealing with them. They even organized a cocktail party for us to meet the locals, although I rather spoilt the gesture by leaving for an emergency operation. One's call to medicine is always lurking in the wings.

It was many months before we could move in. Like so many seventeenth-century farmhouses, maintenance was a problem: new water and electricity systems had to be installed and the interior was almost totally refurbished. With some reluctance I agreed with Veronica to have the pub removed from the hall. Our builders had some difficulty locating the sewage system and dug zigzagged six-foot-deep trenches all around the house, still without finding the sewer, which was eventually located under the rubbish heap.

Almost immediately after exchanging contracts, we watched a 20-foot high bank being built within yards of the garden. True to the agent's predictions, a sand-excavating pit was being prepared adjacent to our property. Amazing how one can adjust to these inconveniences. We lived next to this working pit for the next seven years, hardly realizing its existence.

Six months later, the builders were still very much in evidence. Veronica and I were determined to move in before another summer passed, so we spent our first night in sleeping bags on the floor of our bare bedroom. Despite the discomfort we were in our own little country home, which seemed like a palace.

We were foolish enough to entertain one of our American colleagues at Trottsford, long before it was really habitable. Buol Heslin, one of Charlie Kelman's assistants, was confronted by a scene of desolation. The builders had decided, without using coverings, to sand down the parquet floor in the hall, and all the contents of the house were covered with a copious layer of wood dust. Our guest immediately decided to do a six-mile jog around the beautiful surrounding countryside to get some fresh air. The following day he went from the sublime to the ridiculous, taking a tour around Blenheim Palace, the estate of Winston Churchill's family. He was most impressed with the imprint of an eye over the entrance portcullis. On returning to Trottsford, he found all five of us, 20-foot up in a tree house built in one of our oak trees. We are sure he returned to America totally convinced that the Brits were crazy.

Two years later we decided to build a tennis court on land bought from our neighbours David and Camilla Hadfield. We had lived in great harmony with John and Joan Beresford, who had owned the other half of the farmhouse for many years and they kindly gave us the first option on it when they retired in the 1990s. Thanks to the Hadfields and Beresfords, Trottsford became a single property.

Thus started our years at Trottsford, and our first impressions of warmth and welcome were fully justified. As in any property there were problems, particularly with difficult neighbours, but on the whole this small farmhouse gave all our family and friends a haven away from the outside world. Veronica's father, Arvid, had an idea that we should use the outbuildings to breed Californian white rabbits for fun and profit. Our seven bucks and 250 does had an idyllic existence, mating and raising their offspring in comfortable warm cages, under the supervision of a full-time farm manager. A van came from Buxteds every month to collect the rabbits that, at six months, were ready for the pot. As in so many other farming ventures the product sold for little and the mark-up went to the retailers. Almost from its inception we realized that it would be very difficult to make a profit.

One of my patients and a friend, Lord Victor De Rothschild, was at that time facing allegations from Chapman Pincher, accusing him of being the 'fifth' Soviet spy. At the height of his personal troubles Victor wrote us a letter, which simply read: 'Dear Arnott. How are the rabbits? Yours, Victor.'

Another patient, unwittingly associated with our rabbits, was Woodrow Wyatt. On one of our annual days in Woodrow and Verushka's box at Royal Ascot, Veronica had sat next to Tim Sainsbury at lunch. During the course of the conversation he warned Veronica that the bottom was about to fall out of the British rabbit industry because of much cheaper Chinese imports. We sold all our stock of rabbits and equipment just days before Buxteds wrote announcing that they would be making no more collections.

The other small business we ran at Trottsford was much more successful and gave Veronica many years of pleasure. She converted a garage and adjoining old stone building into a studio for aerobic classes. On one of our trips to San Francisco she had attended a step aerobics class, and later became one of the first teachers to introduce it into the UK. Tania joined Veronica in teaching these classes and they made a wonderful team, giving their clients very professional but fun classes. As mother and daughter, they were so in tune with each other that they'd turn up to give a class, saying 'Are you teaching or me?' and the classes were always greatly appreciated.

Veronica loved gardening and she spent endless hours building up the garden, with herbaceous borders and beds of roses. She transformed Trottsford from an ugly duckling to a beautiful swan. But Veronica did much more than that by creating a welcoming home, not only for our immediate family but also for our children's friends. Robert's numerous mates would invade our farm every weekend. They came to treat Veronica as Bob's sister, rather than his mother, and would spend the time with us totally without parental control. Such was Veronica's understanding of the young that the privileges she gave them were never abused.

Robert particularly enjoyed the riverbank and the fields of Trottsford for riding, first a 'Bat Boy' junior motorbike, followed by a clapped-out old Morris 1000 car. This, sporting a number plate, BOB 14, finally went out of circulation when it collided with one of our farm gates. But fortune was on his side: one of my patients was the Queen Mother of Oman. After the death of her husband, this lady had groomed her son to take over as the Sultan of Oman and he'd trained at Sandhurst. His mother was always a guiding influence and a great power in the running of the country. She was also an incredibly brave woman: once, at her summer palace in Salala, when the countryside was shrouded in mist, the local Yemeni tribesmen became restless and threatened to attack the palace. Realizing the gravity of the situation, the queen mother evacuated the palace and agreed to meet the tribesmen. At the appointed time, she opened the gates and said to them: 'I am totally alone, please come in.' The horsemen poured into the palace and left in peace some hours later.

Her operation was performed without incident. She later related to me that the drive home to Wargrave Manor was one of the most pleasurable in her life. She sat on the bed of her ambulance, alone, looking out of the window without her ubiquitous security officers. I drove out to Wargrave Manor several times and on one occasion found her in floods of tears. She had just heard that her best friend Mrs Ghandi, the Prime Minister of India, had been assassinated.

While making my proposed final visit to Wargrave Manor she asked if I could possibly return for tea the following Sunday.

'That is difficult,' I said, 'as it is our son's half-term from school.'

'Please bring him, with Veronica,' she replied.

We also took with us Veronica's mother, who was staying with us. After a lovely afternoon, with typical Arabic hospitality, Veronica and I were given gold Rolex watches, Joy a designer watch and Bob an envelope. Returning home in our car Bob opened his envelope and £50 notes flew everywhere. He was so thrilled he thought he'd never have to work!

'Oh yes you will,' replied Veronica, scooping up the notes and putting them into her handbag. Bob had been given £2000, half of which sum was put into his savings account and the other half used to buy a 22-year-old Land Rover. Bob had many years of fun driving this 4 × 4 around our small property. He even achieved the almost impossible by turning it over.

As chairman of the Blind Asian Association, I would attend their annual meeting on a midsummer's day, when the hall of the Royal National Institute for the Blind's building in Great Portland Street was filled with sweating members of our association. At Veronica's suggestion the meeting was transferred to Trottsford, where the members could enjoy a day in the country. We held open house one Sunday each May and the ancient red London double-decker bus hired for the occasion invariably caused mayhem on the route from London to Trottsford. It once broke down on the M3 motorway, and dozens of blind Asians wandered along the hard shoulder. In another incident its roof all but rammed the Railway Bridge in nearby Wrecclesham, causing a monumental traffic jam. One member of the association was a blind girl with congenital osteitis fibrosa who, being too frail to make the journey by bus, had the luxury of an ambulance. She had already suffered 64 bone fractures, and sadly suffered her 65th being lifted out of the ambulance at Trottsford. Despite her disabilities she was an inspiration to all and even eventually gained a university degree.

Our Blind Asian Association day at Trottsford was always one of the happiest in the year, with our guests loving the open spaces of our small estate. Escorted between two sighted people, each blind person would be taken around the garden and many enjoyed a swim in our pool. The proceedings of the day were carried out in the ancient tithe barn within which, by some extrasensory perception, our guests would become almost immediately aware of its interior structure. After lunch there was a variety show, which, while requiring sight for its full appreciation, was much enjoyed by all the members of the society. A regular contributor was Lyn Jenkins, one of our associates in the Harley Street Clinic, who would accompany his beautiful daughter on a 1772 Johannes Cuyper violin.

CHAPTER 25
Joining the inventors

On future trips to America, Veronica and I became more and more involved in lens implantation. Until late 1977, the implants used in America were mostly European designs. The Choyce Mk VIII had been modified by an American surgeon, Gerry Tennant, and had a large market share. John Pearce's tripod posterior-chamber lens had a limited American market, as did my Harris-Arnott posterior-chamber rectangular lens. The most popular lenses were the Binkhorst and Worst iris-clip lenses, which were designed by two Dutch surgeons.

Having already designed two single-plane posterior-chamber implants, in 1976 I had gone to see Ernest Ford of Rayner with the idea of producing a modified iris-clip lens. My idea was to suspend the optical portion behind the pupil, rather than in front of it, as in the designs of Binkhorst and Worst. This lens was marketed as the Little-Arnott lens mark 4. Jorg Boberg-Ans, an eminent Danish pioneer implant surgeon, produced a lens very similar to my own.

I prepared a major paper on phaco cataract surgery, associated with the insertion of my modified iris-clip lens, for the annual Los Angeles meeting of the American Society of Cataract and Refractive Surgery, the ASCRS. I was most excited at the prospect of giving my presentation to the 5000 delegates, fully expecting it to be a show-stopper.

Oh dear, I had been pipped to the post by Steve Shearing, who practised in Las Vegas. From the time his first slide was shown on the big screen I realized that my implant was totally obsolete. He had modified a 1950 vintage anterior-chamber lens with biodegradable nylon loops to a posterior-chamber lens with prolene non-biodegradable loops. This was the first posterior-chamber lens to have flexible loops, as opposed to the rigid loops of lenses such as John Pearce's and my own tripod lens. I read my paper with little enthusiasm. I would have to go back to the drawing board!

The whole implant market headed in this direction, with anterior-chamber and clip lenses taking very much a second place. It was the method rather than the design of the lens that gave Steve's concept such importance. His lens had a 5-mm optical portion to which were attached two diametrically opposed prolene loops shaped like the letter 'J'. Although this lens was a technological breakthrough in the advancement of cataract surgery, it was by no means the final solution to lens implantation.

Steve Shearing was also a member of the Sinskey-Kratz Californian phaco group which met in Los Angeles several times a year. During one of these lunchtime sessions, there was a discussion as to how improvements could be made to the Shearing lens. Jim Little held a Shearing lens in one hand and a pair of forceps in the other and started to manipulate the shape of the prolene loops. In his slow Oklahoma drawl he said: 'This loop needs an itsy-bitsy more bend here and a tiddly short curve there.' At that lunch we were unknowingly advancing the frontiers of lens implantation.

In months, the Sinskey, Sheets and Kratz styles of lenses had joined the international market. Among other American ophthalmologists, not proponents of phaco surgery, who produced new lens designs, were Jaswant Pannu, Aziz Anis and Bill Simcoe. Bill Simcoe also produced many instruments for extracapsular extraction. His lens had long loops that coiled into the posterior chamber of the eye. Bill was the first surgeon to appreciate that if the lens-implant loops came into contact with the posterior capsule, they could become adherent to it.

In April 1978, I attended an elite congress organized by Don and Helen Praeger in the NY Medical Centre, Valhalla, Valley of the Skulls. Only some 20 other top international surgeons, including Svyatoslav Fyodorov, Charlie Kelman, Bob Sinskey, Cornelius Binkhorst, Dick Kratz, Herve Byron, Dick Keats and Henry Clayman, had been invited. The meeting would have been unremarkable but for a paper by an ophthalmic pathologist on the structure of the human lens and the changes that occur in its remnants after phaco or extracapsular cataract extraction. He stated:

'In both the phaco and extracapsular cataract operation the clear posterior capsule is not removed at the time of surgery. In the postoperative period, clouding of this previously clear capsular membrane can compromise the restored vision. Within weeks it may be covered with grey scar tissue and within months by a substance resembling frogspawn, called Elschnig Pearls.'

'During the cataract operation the anterior capsule of the lens is opened and partially excised, before the contained opaque contents of the lens are removed, either with the phaco machine or manually. At the end of the operation there remains only the intact posterior capsule, a membrane a few microns thick, and the peripheral remnants of the anterior capsule. Under the anterior capsule is a single layer of cells which, if not removed at the time of cataract surgery, have the ability to form fibrotic tissue. These cells by migrating onto the posterior capsule are the cause of the fibrous scar, which so often develops on this membrane in the weeks following surgery.'

'There is another layer of cells lying within the retained recess of the capsular bag which, in the normal lens is responsible for the growth of new lens fibres. If not washed out at the time of the operation, these continue to produce fibres postoperatively. With the contents and structure of the lens having gone, these aberrant lens fibres will lie on the posterior capsule forming the Elschnig Pearls. Pushed from behind by other new cells they pass from the periphery towards the centre of the posterior capsule. After several months they reach its central point, producing a severe loss of vision.'

This lecture in Valhalla laid bare the secrets of our 'sick patient' – the cataractous lens. I realized this professor was bestowing 'pearls' of wisdom on us. Little consideration had been given to replacing the removed lens with an implant that would use the natural processes occurring in the retained portion of the lens. I came away realizing that the anterior subcapsular cells left behind could, being converted to fibrous tissue, be very instrumental in fixating and sealing a lens implant in the capsular bag.

This would require a totally new lens design, with loops shaped like a ring to line the recess of the capsular bag. The fibrotic process induced by the anterior subcapsular cells would cause adherence of this ring to the capsular bag and, with its wide arc of contact, give great stability. The adherence of the ring to the posterior capsule would also have the added advantage of acting as a barrier against the spread of the Elschnig Pearls.

In February 1979 I approached Peter La Haye, founder of Iolab, California, with these concepts and asked him to manufacture an iris-clip lens with totally encircling posterior loops. On 29 June 1979 I implanted the first Iolab 'totally encircling loop lens' in the presence of Joseph Stevens, their production manager, and Richard Packard, my senior registrar at Charing Cross Hospital. This lens proved to be too difficult to insert, and although the visual results were excellent, production of this implant was discontinued after only six had been made. Aziz Anis had also recognized the importance of having a lens with maximum contact in the walls of the capsular bag and his implant also had rigid totally encircling closed loops.

Once again I had to return to the drawing board chastened, but grateful to Peter La Haye for his help in a failed project, which must have cost Iolab a considerable amount. The results of six operations with this lens did confirm that this style of implant had real benefits for the patient. But changes needed to be made to facilitate its insertion into the eye. The modifications incorporated were the design of a lens with two diametrically opposed open-ended, totally encircling flexible loops, produced from a single piece of PMMA plastic.

By October 1979 I had been actively pioneering lenses for five years, and five styles had been manufactured for me by Rayner. When I first discussed with Ernest Ford the possibility of making a lens with flexible haptics out of a single piece of PMMA, it defied all known manufacturing techniques. Ernest was at all times most helpful and cooperative and it was a real joy working with him. Using my specifications, he produced the world's first one-piece PMMA lens. From the surgeon's view it looked perfect, but it could not be put into production as the long loops were too prone to break. After several prototypes, sadly the whole project was abandoned.

In 1981 we had a family tragedy when John, just two years older than me, suddenly died at the early age of 53, leaving a young widow and two small children aged five and three. John had a service in St Patrick's, Dublin, in which the vast cathedral was filled to capacity – such was his popularity in the country. For some years my brother had had troubles with the finances of the Phoenix

Park Racecourse, mainly because of the Irish Racing Board's restrictions on admission charges. It was almost impossible to make a profit with only 12 days of racing a year. After John's death, two great friends, John Wilson-Wright and Denny Wardell, took on the unenviable task of winding up the course. It was eventually sold to a syndicate that included Robert Sangster and the racing trainer Vincent O'Brien, but the staff, including the manager Teddy Tighe, was retained. The new management had no more success than the old, and eventually racing was discontinued. The racecourse, where in its day, royalty, heads of state and distinguished people from all over the world had been entertained, closed and became yet another derelict site.

Alone in Los Angeles, I had a sense of deep despondency and huge sadness at John's death like I had never felt before. I was desperately missing my brother but also realized how deeply I needed Veronica and her unstinting support. I returned with, if it were possible, an even greater love for her.

We went together shortly afterwards to the Loews Hotel in Monte Carlo, with Arnie and Marion Pearlstone and two of their friends. This hotel had been built out over rocks on the edge of the main centre of Monte Carlo. The Formula 1 motor-racing track passes under the hotel before entering the straight stretch along the sea front. The bedrooms were suspended over the sea, which gave the sensation of being on a ship. Although we were officially attending an ophthalmic congress in Nice, we very much looked on our stay as a holiday. Our friends loved playing Black Jack in the hotel's casino. On one of these occasions Connie was wiling away the time on the 'one-arm bandits', waiting for her husband to finish his game at the tables. All gambling stopped for a few moments as Connie hit the jackpot and thousands of coins tinkled out of the machine and rolled over the floor: she had won 3000 francs.

At the meeting, we visited the Cilco (Californian Implant Lens Company) stand and noticed a brochure advertising a new one-piece PMMA lens implant with open flexible 'J' loops. Could this company have the answer to our dreams? We met Randy Alexander, the vice president of Cilco Marketing, in the hospitality suite and saw a sample of his one-piece PMMA Sinskey-style lens.

I immediately told him: 'We have designed a revolutionary new lens, which we would be interested to know if your company could produce as a one-piece PMMA implant.' I went to work on a white table napkin, the only paper to hand, and drew a sketch of the lens I had envisaged.

This showed the round circular optical portion of the lens, with the two symmetrically opposed encircling open-ended loops, each of which had four portions. The first portion extending radially out some 2 mm from the 12 and six o'clock meridians of the optical portion of the lens would have enough width to give some added stability. The second portion starting from a sharp bend at the outward extremity of the first portion would extend circumferentially around the optics for some 2–3 hours before ending and merging into the third portion of the loop. This third portion had a lesser curvature, thus spreading it away from the optical portion. The fourth portion extending from the distal portion of the third would be more curved to equal the curvature of the recess of the capsular bag. The end of one loop would overlap some part of the opposite loop. The total diameter of the loops would be 12–14 mm but when inserted into the eye would compress down to 10.5 mm, the diameter of the capsular bag.

'This is exactly the lens we are looking for,' retorted Randy, as he folded up the paper napkin and put it in his pocket. Thus started a love–hate relationship that would last for many years. That folded table napkin, with its rough sketch, would become in the future a most important document in the Cilco files. We wanted our lens to be not only an optical but also an anatomical replacement for the lens removed at cataract surgery. The buttressing effect of the fragile and microscopically thin posterior capsule of the lens could be markedly enhanced by the totally encircling loop lens, with its rigid optical portion and loops sealed in the confines of the lens bag. Children and patients with an only eye could more safely be considered for lens implantation.

Over the following year Veronica and I continued on the ophthalmic circuit giving or attending conferences, and several meetings were of particular import. Sir Stephen Miller, the hospitalier of the St John Eye Hospital of Jerusalem, asked us to demonstrate modern cataract surgery to his staff. The Order of St John plays a unique role in the troubled lands of Israel and Palestine. The hospital is staffed almost entirely by British nurses, with surgeons from Canada, Australia, England, America and elsewhere. It looks after the ophthalmic needs of a very high percentage of the Palestinian population, who have to cross the Israeli–Palestinian border to attend the hospital. I did three days of operating and assisting at surgery on patients who had the most complicated ophthalmic problems.

In our off-duty periods we were given unique tours by the reception desk Palestinian guide, who had an in-depth knowledge of the country. We were shown the stables of the crusaders, which lay directly under the Golden Mosque. We descended to Jericho and had what is now forbidden, a dip in the Dead Sea. Veronica always took a personal interest in this hospital and for many years was on its ladies guild. In 1992 she was made a Serving Sister of the Order of St John of Jerusalem.

In May 1982, with Emmanuel Rosen, Bill Haining and Huw and Anne Thomas, we held our third international ophthalmic congress at the Gleneagles Hotel in Scotland. This was the most perfect venue, being surrounded by two 18-hole golf courses, the King's Course and the Queen's Course, as well as the Prince's Course. Reliving a round on the King's Course is a wonderful cure for insomnia – every hole has its own individual charm.

The interior is like a Victorian hunting lodge, with a superb sports centre and swimming pool. Veronica was very much the hostess of this congress. Like its predecessors it attracted most of the top international ophthalmic surgeons and was a serious scientific meeting. The new generation of posterior-chamber lenses of Shearing, Sinskey, Sheets, Simcoe, Kelman, Pannu, Anis and Harris had only recently come on the world market and most were presenting papers at this congress.

My one-piece PMMA lens was still a closely guarded secret, but we did have a serious discussion about its future with Jim Cooke, president of Cilco, and his representative Randy Alexander. Two of our American colleagues and friends, Skip Beckard and Barry Thrasher, were also at this meeting, which was held in the informal surroundings of the hotel drawing room. These American surgeons would have to do 'core' studies to verify that the implant was safe and suitable for the international and American markets. Our two surgical friends agreed to join the project, along with Norman Jaffe from Miami. Norman had for some years championed the use of implants, and his association with this new lens was considered to be of inestimable value.

Veronica had organized a social programme that was frivolous and fun. There was a golf tournament in which the delegates with the lowest handicap played on the King's Course and the rest on Queen's Course. We were relegated to the Queen's Course with Arnie and Marion Pearlstone and played by the 'Queensbury Rules'. On the first hole, Marion landed her ball in the drink, and a new ball was put on the green, with no penalty point. A ball lost in the rough would be replaced by another just lying on the fairway, again with no penalty point. The four of us had a wonderful afternoon of golf with 'irregularities' and much laughter and merriment.

The Gleneagles banquet was a Scottish event, with Bill Haining presiding at the top table. The haggis was ceremonially brought into the dining hall, preceded by a member of the Argyll and Sutherland Highland Regiment playing the bagpipes. Bill, wearing his 'hunting clan kilt', stabbed the 'sausage' with his dirk knife. The dinner continued in this Scottish vein, and Norman Ashton, our foremost British ophthalmic pathologist, gave a brilliant and witty speech, after which he presented the results of the golf tournament. Charlie Kelman had won the Golf Cup for his round on the King's Course Cup and Marion the Ladies' Trophy. Charlie left the next day, too early to hear that the marking had been inaccurate and he had actually come second. We had to produce another cup for the legitimate winner.

On a summer's day in August 1982, the UK's Cilco representative came to my consulting rooms clutching 20 of my new lenses. I knew from experience that these implants would be totally safe in the eyes of my patients. On Monday 14 August 1982, I had five patients scheduled for cataract surgery with lens implantation at the Royal Masonic. In the theatre were the anaesthetist Charles Foster, the theatre sister, Judy Moedy (or Lady Di, after our experience in Milan), and the UK representative of Cilco.

I performed the first operation that afternoon, with a mixture of excitement and anxiety. With the implant held by forceps in my right hand, I lifted the upper lip of the section into the eye with a fine spatula, held in my other hand. On passing through the incision into the eye, the lateral portion of the encircling loops compressed in towards the optical portion of the lens. Once the extremity of one loop had gained the recess of the capsular bag in the six o'clock meridian, the other loop was left extended outside the eye. Using a fine spatula with a bent end, I engaged one of the positioning holes in the lens and dialled this other loop into the eye. The lens glided beautifully into the capsular bag, with the loops lying semi-compressed in an almost perfect circular configuration. During the course of the morning the other four operations were carried out with the same simplicity. The following day I performed another five cataract and lens-implant operations. I had to be a little circumspect during this list, as I had the representative of a rival lens company in the theatre with some visiting guests from Rome. I implanted one of the rival company's lenses and four of my own. Having operated on nine patients over the course of two days, I broke off for the summer holiday recess, feeling elated with what our team had achieved.

CHAPTER 26
The calm before the storm

We decided to take our rapidly growing family on a boat holiday in the Mediterranean. Stephen, by now a young man of 20, had left behind him his years of studying. In his final year at Shiplake College he had been in the school's rowing eight. We had followed the 1st VIII's progress in the Princess Elizabeth Challenge Cup races at the Henley Royal Regatta. They beat the opposition, which included Sir William Borlase's School and Bedford Modern. What excitement we felt watching this small college take on the might of Eton College in the semi-final. We were filled with admiration as the Shiplake crew, which included Stephen and our future son-in-law Nick Whishaw, battled neck and neck throughout the length of the Henley course. Eton drew away in the final 500 metres. Under the caption 'The agony of defeat', the *Sunday Observer* showed the Shiplake crew slumped over their oars after crossing the finishing line.

Tania was at this time 19 and pursuing a ballet career. After some years at the Nester Brooking School of Ballet, she studied for two more years at the Rambert Academy in Twickenham. With her future still unresolved we had an incredible stroke of good fortune. Veronica's cousin Sheila Dunsany, while staying with us at Lansdowne Crescent, went to a dinner party at which she met a New York City Banker, Paul Arpen. Paul told Sheila that part of his trip to the UK was to find a suitable student for an arts scholarship to study theatre, music or ballet in the US. He was about to return without having found a suitable candidate. Sheila immediately expounded on the talents of her ballerina cousin Tania.

As a result of that chance meeting we took Tania for an audition to join the Julliard Ballet School in the Lincoln Centre, New York. Tania was accepted as a scholarship student and so started her career. After her first year, she joined us for our boat holiday in Turkey.

Robert was at this time only 11. He had been shown around Eaton House, a day school in central London, and offered a choice between that or boarding at Sunningdale. Without any hesitation Bob said 'Sunningdale'. We were surprised that such a young boy could be so decisive. Time proved him to be right with his decision. From the moment he entered the school, he made friends for life. The heads, Tim, Pru and Nick Dawson, became good friends and often came to Trottsford. On one occasion Stephen took Pru on the pillion seat of his motorbike, cross-country, around the farm. It was only later that we heard that she was three months pregnant at the time.

Bob was at school at the time that my brother John died. On returning from Ireland Veronica informed the Dawsons that she would like to attend the Sunday school service and break the news to Robert. Veronica was 10 minutes late, as she had been held up at the railway crossing in Sunningdale. They waited until she arrived before starting the service. Bob was having this holiday with us at the end of his third year in Sunningdale.

So gathered from four corners, we flew to Rhodes and joined our boat *Rupert Phillips*, skippered by John Yates and his girlfriend. We had a thoroughly enjoyable and relaxing two weeks cruising the totally unspoiled coast of Turkey.

After this holiday Veronica and I returned to the thrust of our ever-changing journey through life. I went with our accountant to file an application for a patent on my lens design. We spent three hours with the patent attorney, Mr Jennings, during which the principles, novelties and characteristics of the implant were described and he used the engineering drawings as a model for the patent. Within the year an application was also filed for an American patent.

Having our small farm in Hampshire and with Stephen and Tania having left the nest, it was time for us to move on from Lansdowne Crescent. We bought a small mock Georgian House in Abbotsbury Road, Holland Park. During our time there we suffered some of our worst experiences with successively the loss of Veronica's father, Arvid, and her brother Charles being diagnosed with terminal leukaemia.

There were also times of happiness. Our younger son Robert left Sunningdale to go to Harrow and on our visits to Harrow Hill, I thought how little everything had changed since my own time there 40 years earlier. We had wonderful picnics on the playing fields, when we would sit on rugs by our car watching the various sporting events. On these occasions we always joined Sonia Rogers, whose son Tony was, and still is, one of our son Robert's best friends.

In March 1983 Cilco allowed us to go public with our new lens. To a packed conference hall in Phoenix, Arizona, I demonstrated for 45 minutes, the features and capabilities of this new lens implant. Randy Alexander, the marketing director of Cilco, said his company would give their full support and produce a brochure.

It was so exciting to present this implant design and demonstrate how it should be used. Using this lens I performed many thousands of operations on patients from all around the world, including the composer Sir William Walton, who had this operation four days before his 70th birthday, when a concert was given for him at the Royal Albert Hall to celebrate his life's achievements.

I operated on many of our relatives, including both of my in-laws. Joy's operation was carried out under general anaesthesia, so she was unaware of my anxiety at operating on such a close relative. Arvid's operation was performed under local anaesthesia. With his characteristic Russian sense of humour, he banteringly kept asking for a large vodka. At the end of the operation he had a real emergency, desperately calling for a bed bottle; a request that, like the vodka, had to be refused.

I somehow felt very privileged at being asked to operate on relatives, who also included Pat Munro of Foulis and Desmond Murphy, who, following his operation and after retiring as a schoolmaster, became a very gifted water-colour painter. Our daughter Tania's mother-in-law, Geraldine Whishaw, also underwent surgery.

It always amazed me how many of my old school friends consulted me in my practice. Sir Francis Dashwood, a friend from prep school, took for granted the success of his operations and spent little time away from his busy schedules at West Wycombe Park and Lloyds of London.

Another patient, Hugo Southern, had been with me at Harrow. Having become reacquainted, he asked us to a cocktail party at which we met two former friends, Tom and Cline Kilner, who, it transpired, lived only two miles away from us at Trottsford Farm. I helped Tom with a severe ophthalmic problem, and, as a thank you, they gave us some Silky Bantam hens, which became part of our entourage at Trottsford for many years.

Having a large international practice, it was natural that one would meet people from all walks of life. Ian Kellam came to me as a young composer, requiring bilateral phaco and lens-implant operations. He was initially exam-ined by one of my assistants, John Grindle, who suggested that in lieu of a fee for his surgery he could write a piece of music dedicated to 'sight'. This he did and the result is *Fiat Lux*, which records many incidents that have occurred over the centuries involving vision. St Paul's loss of vision on the road to Damascus is portrayed in one of the movements. The score ends with 'Sunrise', a magnificent rendering requiring full choir and orchestra. This concert has been played at St Edmonsbury and St Alban's Cathedrals. The Ladies' Guild of Moorfields used it on one of their 'Fight for Sight' charity nights at St Martin's-in- the-Fields Church, London.

One of my most remarkable patients was Garfield Todd, the former prime minister of Zimbabwe. Following his surgery he sent out this circular:

'A letter from Garfield Todd – too late for Christmas 1981 and much too early for Christmas 1982. This letter is going to hundreds of friends – church groups, relatives, senators, MPs, children's groups – who have written to us over the past years. It is an attempt to say thank you for kindnesses shown, for messages of encouragement received, for prayers on our behalf, when as a family we went through difficult times of imprisonment, detention and rejection. Zimbabwe has its problems but for those of us who were caught up in the seven years of civil war the peace of today is a wonderful relief. Grace and I are now in our 70s and time is in top gear.

'What do you want for our 50th wedding anniversary,' asked Grace.

'To wake up with you for the 18,000th time,' I replied – and so it was. We are well, though age refuses to be entirely ignored. The blue in Grace's eyes has dimmed a little over the past few years.

'On April 10th we left London in search of a miracle. For several years my sight has been failing and in the past year it has so deteriorated that I could neither read nor write letters, nor could I recognize people. A very special friend arranged for me to meet ophthalmic surgeon Sir Stephen Miller. "I work with a young surgeon, Eric Arnott," said Sir Stephen. "He has perfected a technique which is the best and safest I know. We will open up the world for you again." On Wednesday afternoon I entered the Harley Street Clinic. On Thursday he removed the lens of my right eye, inserted a new acrylic one and on Friday I was discharged. Next week my left eye was done and a whole new world of light and colour came streaming in. Today I can actually read without spectacles but I do have them to correct a slight astigmatic error. I feel like bursting into poetry, but that is beyond my ability. I do, however, know something of the feeling of the man in the Bible who simply said: "I was blind and now I can see." And there was a second miracle for when I looked with my new eyes I found that the brilliance in Grace's eyes had been fully restored. There must be a moral in this story if I could see it.

'We had a wonderful month in London. Spring arrived as we did, and cherry trees and daffodils added their splendour to sunny days. To us it was a second honeymoon, all brought to a marvellous climax at Oriel College, Oxford, with a Church service and a choir, whose splendid singing voiced my own deep thankfulness. Then we dined at High Table. This letter is not one which needs an answer. It will not only express gratitude but also, for many friends, I hope it will explain why letters have not been answered.'

In early 1984 troubles over my inventorship arose, which would escalate over the ensuing years. Manuel Ferreira, a long-standing friend practising in Rio de Janeiro, spent one week every year socializing with us and observing my surgery. Before coming he had visited Norman Jaffe in Miami, where he had been shown a lens almost identical to mine that was to be marketed by Cilco.

In October of that year, Veronica and I attended the annual meeting of the American Academy of Ophthalmology in Atlanta. My presentation at that meeting was to be a billboard, some four feet high and six foot wide, on which were illustrations depicting the stages of the surgical cataract extraction and insertion of our totally encircling loop lens. One of my colleagues Dr George Chandra had elected to travel with us and be in charge of our 'rather large' contribution to the American academy. George is no taller than five foot five inches in height, and it was a sight seeing him walking out on the tarmac to our jumbo jet, holding, 'coolie-style,' the placard over his head. He had refused to let it out of his sight.

Excitedly we went to see the Cilco stand in the exhibition hall. Yet what we saw was a lens implant not totally identical to my design. It had been slightly modified by shortening the end of each of the two loops, so that they were not totally encircling. It bore the name of Jaffe. Veronica, George Chandra and I stood by the Cilco stand looking in dismay at this model, studying and discussing its features. In circumventing our patent by producing a lens with loops that were not quite totally encircling, the properties had been markedly diminished. Lens loops have the same characteristics as a swimming pool diving board, in that the length determines flexibility. By shortening the loops, a considerable amount of flexibility was lost, making the lens too rigid and more difficult to insert into the eye at the time of surgery.

That same day we rang our office manager to be told that our patent application had been granted. On returning to England, I once again commissioned Mike Duffy, our very experienced medical artist, to prepare further designs of my lens. At this time many thousands of my original encircling loop lenses had been implanted with excellent results, but it did have one fault. When inserting the lens into the patient's eye, it was just possible for the end of one loop to become jammed in the curvature of the other. I had experienced this problem during one operation, in which I had had to remove the implant from the eye, immediately after its insertion, and unravel the loops before its reinsertion. The patient suffered no harm, but I realized that it was imperative to modify the design of the lens. By widening the first portion of the loops the fault was rectified. These artists' drawings were sent to Cilco.

We were in the invidious position of having to improve the design of our lens, despite the fact that American surgeons were already implanting lenses of my original design under their own name. The defects of the original Jaffe lens had also been rectified by lengthening the loops to make them totally encircling, and the next generation of Jaffe lenses incorporating these changes became a good lens, but totally within the scope of my patent.

One of my lens designs had the optical portion narrowed, making it elliptical rather than circular, to narrow its width and facilitate its insertion through a smaller incision into the eye. This implant, named after an American surgeon called Ronald Coburn, proved to be very popular and I myself inserted many of them. Most of the other major intraocular lens companies started to produce my lens, some with and some without our permission. We were struggling in the web of international commercial wrongdoing and had no recourse but to seek legal advice from an American lawyer.

On 20 December 1984, Stephen, our accountant and I flew via Concorde to New York to meet Bradley Geist of Brumbaugh Graves Donohue and Raymond, an intellectual property firm. Bradley Geist pointed out that our patent was unnecessarily too restrictive. It stated: 'The end portion of one loop overlaps the second portion of the other' (the portion that lies just beyond the right angle bend in the first portion of the loop). That claim language should have read: 'The end portion of one loop overlies a portion of the other.' The careless insertion of the word 'second' markedly weakened our patent, which would now have to be reissued in what was called a protected reissue proceeding.

In the middle of the 1980s the senior executive of the Cromwell Hospital came to visit me. 'I would like to offer you the facilities of this hospital, if you would consider transferring some of your practice from Harley Street to here,' he said. This was too good an offer to refuse and under Stephen's direction we organized a satellite clinic. We were rather overstretched with our two separate practices, but it was very convenient being able to examine and operate on patients under the one roof in the Cromwell Hospital.

The reissue of our patent was finally granted and by the spring of 1986, Bradley Geist, as well as being our American lawyer, was becoming a firm family friend. It was his suggestion that resulted in our son Stephen coming to work full time as senior administrator in the Arnott Ophthalmic Clinic. I had neglected my finances for years, leaving everything to a newly qualified business manager. We benefited enormously by having Stephen on our team, and a new impetus was given to our practice and the quest to seek international justice for our lens-implant inventions. Stephen brought in an auditor who was so aghast at the state of our bank account that he assumed I must be keeping a mistress!

Stephen and I went to Huntington, West Virginia, to meet Cilco's senior representatives and to try and resolve the dispute over their infringement of our lens implant patent. It poured with rain throughout a rather dismal few days and nothing was achieved.

In September 1986 we had the wedding reception at Trottsford for our daughter and Nick Whishaw. The sand excavations next to our property had just been landscaped. What had previously been a hill by the side of our house was now a valley and, at the end of that wedding reception, the newly married couple drove from our garden along a lane by its side in their old yellow Morris Minor. By the light of a red autumnal setting sun, we witnessed, with the other 300 wedding guests, a romantic start to their honeymoon. Nick had been an old school friend of Stephen's who we had known and loved for many years. He endeared himself further to Veronica by discovering a distant relative in Russia who was vaguely related to Veronica's family, and if the line had continued, would have made Tania a baroness.

Early in the following year Veronica, Stephen and I attended a conference in Montreal. This was an ideal time to have another meeting with Cilco to try and resolve the dispute. Company directors were specially flown in from Huntington, Seattle and Washington, with their legal counsel, Sally Gray. My totally encircling loop lens, now sporting the names of Jaffe and Coburn, was becoming one of the most popular implants. We battled for more than five hours against the might of the large corporation.

Despite her rather foreboding appearance, with thick horn-rimmed spectacles and hair pinned back in a bun, Sally Gray was by far the most accommodating of all their representatives, and could have been mistaken for our own legal advisor. At the end of almost every discussion she would say: 'I agree with the Arnotts.' It was a case of the good cop/bad cop, and she masqueraded as the former. During that very lengthy meeting some progress was made.

For our return trip Stephen had booked us onto the Queen Elizabeth 2 (QE2). We had been given a penthouse cabin with its own balcony on the upper deck. We enjoyed a totally different perspective of travel. On board we made great friends with Alvah and Betty Chapman, newspaper tycoons from Miami, Vince Ostrom, a retired banker, and his wife, Dodie, plus Ambassador Del Rosario with his wife and Father Tom O'Brien, with a friend.

It is all too easy to slip into a ship's surreal routine. Every day we had to put our watches ahead by one hour. As early risers, Veronica and I did the mile walk around the empty promenade deck, seeing the previous day's refuse in the ship's wake. Swimming in the hold on a ship at sea is quite an experience and on one morning in a near gale, I had difficulty in preventing myself from being thrown out of the pool onto its surrounds. Every day was filled with activities, with courses on almost every conceivable subject, including computer studies. In the afternoons, there was a 12-bore clay pigeon shoot over the stern of the ship. After dinner and a cocktail party given by our friends, we would usually attend a floorshow before retiring to bed. All too soon we saw the white cliffs of the Isle of Wight and knew we were nearly home.

The following year in 1987, I attended the third congress of cataract and intraocular lenses in Rio de Janeiro as president elect. We were introducing a 'world first' to this meeting, with an address on the excimer laser.

Dr L'Esperance, a New York ophthalmic surgeon working in Columbia University, New York, with Professor Steve Trokel, Roger Steinert and Carmen Puliafito, alongside Professor John Marshall from London, had for some time been independently studying the use of ultraviolet light to produce a laser that could resculpt the tissues of the eye. LASER is the abbreviation of 'light amplitude stimulation of emitted radiation'. They had produced a laser machine, using the lethal ultraviolet light of the spectrum, that could totally destroy and ablate human tissue. The beauty of their invention was that each single pulse, when fired by the machine, would only 'ablate' a few microns of tissue. Thus the next stage in the future of ophthalmic refractive surgery was born, in which a patient with long or short sight could be treated by laser rather than spectacles or contact lenses. Some 60% of the focusing mechanism of the eye depends on the curvature of the front surface of the cornea. Increasing its curvature can reduce long sight, and flattening its curvature reduces short sight. With this laser the anterior surface of the cornea could be resculpted to serve the patient's needs.

Professor John Marshall had hoped to do the final research on this therapy at Charing Cross Hospital and had made me very aware of its potential. He had given me slides and details of this revolutionary advance in ophthalmology, which he allowed me to show to the delegates at the meeting in Rio. As a result of my addresses I had to attend television and press interviews. It was a truly memorable week of science and great sights to see.

Following the congress we went with Bob Sinskey to Manaus, a city in the middle of the Amazon jungle, which had previously been the rubber centre of

Brazil. It had been virtually abandoned some decades earlier when the rubber plantations had been transferred to Malaysia, and it was just starting to become a tourist attraction, with the town a mixture of ancient grace and modern concrete. The opera house was a replica of La Scala in Milan. Dr Miguel Padilha, the organizer of the Brazilian congress that we had just left, arranged for us to meet the local flying missionary doctor.

In this remote part of the Amazon jungle, the government was making efforts to preserve the habitats of the indigent native tribes, and each was granted 500 square miles of territory. Access to these areas was forbidden to all visitors, with the exception of the missionaries and medical doctors. Our flying doctor was a Pentecost missionary called Benny De Marchant, who flew a single-engine Cessna 206, fitted with water floats. Veronica, Stephen, Bob Sinskey and his girlfriend Betty Gold and I went with him on a unique missionary trip to the Kassuva Settlement. We flew for 180 miles with nothing but rivers and unspoilt Amazon jungle below us. We finally came in to land on the Nhamunba River. Benny taxied the Cessna to the landing stage where the chieftain, Pedro, met us with the itinerant missionaries, Orlando and his wife Jassava. Behind our hosts were the 300 other Indians of the settlement, all lined up in the order of seniority in their community.

Orlando and Jassava took us to their home, a circular wooden lodge with a reed roof set up on stilts to avoid the danger of snakes and other creatures entering their house. These two missionaries spoke the local dialect and were the first to compile a dictionary of the local Indian language. They had a very good relationship with the community and, at the time of our visit, were just recovering from the tragedy of the death of one of the children from dysentery the previous week.

We shared a rather indigestible lunch with them before being conducted around the settlement. All the houses, spotlessly clean, were made of timber and roofed with overhanging reed thatch. We went to the village bakery and watched the local papaya root being crushed before baking. In the church we experienced the wonder of listening to missionary music sung by a local choir. As guests, we were invited to contribute to this emotional impromptu service. Veronica, Stephen, Bob Sinskey, Betty Gold and I went onto the stage. The children sitting in the front two rows looked up at us in awe, waiting for an interpretation of Western-style religious lyrics. The five of us stood on stage, wondering what to contribute. Just about the only song we all knew how to sing was *Danny Boy*. This we sang to the 300 members of the congregation, who listened with due respect, until they realized we were indeed no rival choir. First of all the children in the front two rows started to giggle and then, with their elders, they all broke into thunderous laughter and rapturous applause. This small community showed us how an immediate bond can be developed between people of such different backgrounds. As we took off in the little Cessna, circumnavigating every bend of the river, the whole community turned out to wave farewell.

Following our stay in Manaus, and our unique visit to Kassuva, we travelled first by bus and then on a boat up the Rabu River to Lake Camaçari and the Pousadas Hotel, on an island many kilometres from any other habitation. The hotel was little more than a very luxurious log cabin and we were the only guests.

On Lake Camaçari we went fishing for piranha. These small fish, only 18 inches long, have razor-sharp teeth. They attack in a pack and will devour a body in minutes. A few days earlier a boat had turned over in the river at a tourist attraction. No trace of the occupants was ever found. The rivers are teeming with these fish, as their only natural predator, the alligator, is almost extinct from overhunting. Stephen and I landed one fish each!

Our guide took us across the lake and up a small tributary, deep into the Amazon jungle. The water level was fairly high and we could easily touch the overhead branches. At one point Veronica picked an orchid off one of the trees. After some time we entered a swamp and our river turned into a maze, with dozens of little tributaries. When we passed the same landmark several times we realized we were lost. After darkness descended we saw, with huge relief, a light ahead of us. We were lucky enough to have found a leopard hunter fishing in a small canoe. He asked for some fuel, as his tank was empty. We sat rigidly in our boat as he transferred petrol into his can, the whole time with a lit cigarette dangling from his lips. We pondered whether or not it would be preferable to be burned alive or eaten by the piranhas. As it turned out all went well and the hunter was able to guide us back to our island hotel.

Back in London we learned that John Marshall had visited the animal house at Charing Cross Hospital and was unimpressed with his reception and the facilities he would be given. He withdrew from our hospital, with the result that we lost our one prospect of having the first refractive excimer laser unit in the UK.

CHAPTER 27
Highs and lows

One of the outcomes of our meeting in Montreal was that Cilco agreed to produce a new lens of any design we wished. I duly submitted my idea, whereupon I was told that: 'This is too difficult to manufacture and further changes will have to be made before its production.'

In the autumn of 1987, Veronica, Stephen and I went to the annual meeting of the ASCRS in Dallas, Texas, where the Cilco marketing director presented us with a replica of my new lens – the AR12UO. What a disappointment: the modifications they had insisted on made it totally impractical to insert into a patient's eye. In fact I never did implant it. We left hardly able to thank our host for his feigned hospitality, totally unable to show any appreciation for the replica that we dubbed 'our lensis horribalis'.

The next day we visited the trade booths. It was déjà vu – as if we were back in Atlanta in 1984. Once again a model of a lens dominated the Cilco stand. It was the perfect replica of the lens I had designed and sent to Cilco some months previously. This new lens was the flagship of the new company formed by the merging of Cilco and Cooper Vision and was called the CVC1U. CV represented Cooper Vision, C1 Cilco and U for ultraviolet filter.

Stephen married Kathy Thompson in July 1989. They had an away match at Kathy's home, Midway Manor in Wiltshire, kindly hosted by her mother Rosemary, her father Colin Thompson and his wife Bridget. On that day happiness was mingled with sadness. Kathy's stepfather, Tim Walker, had died still only 46 years of age, one year earlier. On the evening of his death, he summoned Kathy and Stephen and give them his blessing for their future together.

This was the last major function that was held at Midway Manor in Wiltshire. The estate was for sale but, on this cloudless blazingly hot day, it still had the presence of all that Tim Walker upheld. Tim had been chairman of the WWF, and the grounds around his home were filled with many species of wild animals, which included llamas, tapirs, buffalo, ostriches and 17 species of owls, as well as a herd of zebras and Przwalski horses. Stephen and Bob gave speeches to the 450 guests. They had to compete with Derek Edwards, Kathy's uncle, who that year was alderman for the City of London. Veronica looked radiant and stood by my side throughout gazing proudly at her two boys. The bridal couple left for their honeymoon astride an elephant.

During that same year, Veronica and I decided that we were once again overhoused, when I noticed a new unoccupied block of flats on the riverbank at Hammersmith. It had a panoramic view of the Thames but Veronica described the three small rooms and spiral staircase as a 'matchbox'. A few days later we mutually decided that this small apartment would be perfect for the weekdays when I had to practice in London.

In 1990 Robert was studying architecture in Dundee. We went up to visit him and visit the home of our ancestors. After leaving Edinburgh behind us, we drove through Carlisle and joined up with our son Robert at Fiona Packard's parents' lovely country abode. After an evening with them we journeyed up the riverbank to Dundee. We stayed in the Holiday Inn and the next day visited the university and complex. I was amazed at the seeming quality of care that was being extended to our son. Veronica, I learned, took a different view and realized how unhappy our son was in this university. On returning to London, the first thing that Veronica did was to see that our son was educated in a different university. This turned out to be Oxford Brookes.

Following this, we went over the river at Dundee to our home country of Auchtermuchty in Fife. It was exciting surveying the lands that our ancestors had inhabited for hundreds of years. The Arnott Tower, the hallmark of our crest, was intact, but the original house had been demolished. We went to the Scottish Presbyterian Church and saw the tombs of our forebears, including Great Great Grandfather's grave, which showed he had been born in 1785. His eldest son Robert, born in 1805, had three brothers. One was responsible for the foundation of the Arnott Biscuit Company in Australia and another was my Great Grandfather. Robert had passed on the family home to his eldest son John, who died at the age of 32 while visiting his uncle in Australia, and so ended the Arnott lineage in Auchtermuchty. As we wandered through this remote but very beautiful cemetery, we were able to format a picture of our family that we had not previously appreciated.

It was during this same autumn that Saddam Hussein of Iraq invaded Kuwait, and we were preparing for the Gulf War. One of my patients, Lord Martin Charteris, the provost of Eton College, on whom I had performed bilateral cataract and lens-implant operations, had given us an open invitation to come to a service in the Eton College Chapel. Veronica's mother, Joy, whose brother Eric and many other members of the family had been educated at Eton, had much hoped to see the school one final time. Unwittingly I asked if we could come to the service on Sunday 11 November, which was Remembrance Day.

We were ushered up the steps to the raised provost's pew and were joined by Mary Rae, a very old friend of ours. The guest of honour was General Sir John Hackett, author of *The Third World War*. This venerable gentleman, standing very erect in the pulpit, said: 'Boys, take a good look at me, as I am as extinct as the dodo. I am the only man you will ever see who has drawn sword in battle.'

With that opening remark he continued his sermon by extolling the virtues of being a Christian and a soldier.

After a tour of the school, at lunch with some 20 guests, General Sir John Hackett rose to his feet and gave us an account of the tactics that would be used to win the forthcoming Gulf War. The Chaplain interrupted him in his discourse.

'General,' he said, 'the moment the body bags start entering the UK and America, public opinion will turn against the war.' Thus started one of the most fascinating discussions we ever witnessed. It transpired that the chaplain had been with the paratroopers during the Falklands War. He was present when some Argentinean prisoners of war were removing live ammunition from a warehouse when one shell exploded, causing excruciating suffering to the trapped prisoners. With no chance of their being saved, the chaplain had taken a fellow officer's revolver and put them out of their misery. He knew only too well the horrors of war.

Thanks to Martin Charteris's hospitality, Veronica's mother, Joy, had a most memorable last visit to Eton College. A few weeks later in January 1991, Joy suffered a severe stroke, which proved to be fatal. She had outlived her husband, Arvid, by only six years. Some 18 months later we also tragically lost Veronica's brother Charles, bringing to an end our side of the Langué family.

By 1991, at over 60, I had reduced my NHS sessions to just four a week so I could concentrate on our charity commitments and the development of lens implantation. One morning in February I was called to Charing Cross Hospital to cope with the victims of an IRA bomb that had exploded at Victoria station during the rush hour. I walked between the rows of injured to choose the patient I could most help. I found a young man covered in blood, whose face had been almost cut in two. He had been making a phone call with his head bent forward when the bomb had exploded in an aluminium wastebasket 20 feet away. A five-inch piece of shrapnel was still deeply impaled in his face.

I ordered my theatre to be immediately available and I stared at the devastated face, considering where best to start. The piece of shrapnel was removed without any difficulty. One eye was a mass of pulp and had to be excised. The other eye, although lying very exposed, had suffered little damage and was easily repaired. Having carried out my duties as an ophthalmic surgeon, which was second nature to me, I now had the responsibilities of being a neuro-, ENT and plastic surgeon. But I was not alone, having my very dedicated nursing staff and the ophthalmic and ENT surgical registrars. Working as a close-knit team, we isolated and closed off the exposed brain tissue, realigned the nose and repaired the surrounding sinuses. Finally we sutured the severely lacerated tissues of the face. The operation took four and a half hours, and during that time not a single member of our team left the theatre.

The patient made a very good recovery and, when fitted with one artificial eye, seemed hardly to have been injured. When recovering in the ward he set an example of fortitude to all our other patients. Some two weeks later I received a letter of complaint from one of the patients I had abandoned earlier in the morning: 'Private patients should be given priority over national health ones, no matter what the circumstances. The cancellation of my Monday afternoon appointment caused me a great inconvenience.'

CHAPTER 28
The Virginian Trial

By the early 1990s, most of the intraocular lens companies, such as Storz, Allergan, Rayner and Iolab, had entered into licensing agreements for the right to manufacture one-piece totally encircling loop, intraocular lenses of our designs. Others such as Intraoptics and Ioptex were still unwilling to acknowledge the validity of our various patents. Stephen and Bradley Geist decided to sue Ioptex as a prelude to taking on another major international ophthalmic company, Alcon, which by now had acquired Cooper-Vision Cilco. The reason for litigating Ioptex, a relatively small company, was to gain a war chest for fighting the next company. Also, under American law, discovery rules would permit us to examine file records of third-party companies, if relevant. Ioptex settled before the case came to trial. Bradley Geist's firm agreed to continue our case on a contingency fee base. If we lost the next case we would only have to pay disbursements, and if we won they would receive 40% of the awarded damages.

The trial of *Arnott v Alcon* took place in Alexandria, Virginia, in the beginning of January 1992. The court in Alexandria was chosen because it had jurisdiction but, more importantly, was known as 'rocket docket.' Cases tried in this court proceeded promptly.

Veronica and Stephen stayed up half of the first night with attorney Bradley Geist. It was wonderful having Bradley with us. A brilliant attorney, he had devoted most of the previous five years entirely to this case. Added to his sincerity and belief in our cause was his compulsiveness for detail and a deep knowledge. He had read David Apple's *Atlas of Lens Implantation*, more than 1000 pages long, from cover to cover, and he, like Stephen, knew more about lens implantation than most eye surgeons.

Two of his paralegals, Bill Placky and Tom Pease, drove through the night with all the legal files relevant to the case. Another attorney who Bradley brought with him was Marina Larson. Marina was the modern example of the blonde intelligent American female lawyer and working mother. She had been most diligent in assisting in the preparation of our case. Normally unkempt, she surprisingly appeared on the first day of the trial chic and looking like a model. After Bradley Geist, the most important member of our legal team was Bob Neuner, a senior partner who had been recruited for his jury trial experience. Irish in mentality and attitude, he was unflappable and a supreme optimist. During the difficult periods of the trial he was a consoling figure to whom we could always consult about the meanings of the legal tirades we had to suffer. Bradley Geist had very carefully picked the best from his firm.

Every morning Veronica and I would begin the day with a reading from Rabbi Bloom's book *Blue Angel*, which set a light religious mood for the day. We were fortunate in having a swimming pool in the hotel, and most mornings, at 6.30 am, the three of us did a leisurely one-mile swim. As the days stretched into weeks, the swimming pool attendant expressed amazement at how long our trial was taking.

On our first morning we walked to the office of John Anderson, a lawyer with the firm of McGuire, Woods, Battle and Booth. He looked like Anthony Perkins, from *Psycho,* but was a marvellous host and always full of optimism. His adversary on the opposing firm had been at law school with him. It was the start of a long weekend of preparation for the case lying ahead of us. A considerable amount of time was spent discussing the Park lens, which Alcon claimed was important prior art to our lens, as well as each of Alcon's 23 infringing lens designs.

John Park, an eye surgeon from Buffalo, had designed his lens at about the same time as me in 1981. Park received 100 lenses from Cilco, but abandoned the project after using only 85, as insertion proved too difficult and the lens was never put into production. Although having nearly totally encircling loops, his lens lacked virtually all the characteristics that I had achieved with mine. Despite the differences between these two lenses, much of the trial would depend on whether or not the Park lens would be found to be an experimental design that was never publicly available.

Over the previous months, most of the motions had been in our favour, including one preventing Alcon from taking the case away from Alexandria. Nevertheless, serious problems loomed on Friday 13 December 1991, when we nearly lost a summary motion, which would have prevented the case going to trial at all. Judge Ellis, who had been entrusted with our trial, could, at that time, see little difference between our lens and that of Park's. On 3 January, the lawyers spent all afternoon with Judge Ellis and the opposing attorney, at which time it was obvious that the judge was having difficulty understanding our position. He stated that he could possibly stop the trial at any stage and, moreover, he ruled out contractual damages.

Although I have a prodigious memory, it was my detailed diary notes from 1984 that saved the day.

On Tuesday 7 January, we were seated in the courtroom with 60 potential jurors. At precisely 9.30 am, the attorneys took up their positions and Judge Ellis strode into the courtroom, behind his marshal, and lowered himself into his chair. He was the very antithesis of our impression of a judge.

A former torpedo boat commander in the American Navy, now in his mid-40s, he had black hair cleverly arranged to conceal a bald spot, and the overall picture was of a man who, while having a great ambition, was totally honest and a strict disciplinarian. Despite any reservations he may have had concerning the validity of our patent, we realized on first seeing him that we were happy to place our ophthalmic future in his hands. He would be very instrumental in determining whether or not we left the trial as bankrupt 'has beens' or still in the centre stage of world ophthalmology.

Judge Ellis lectured the potential jurors on the importance of the American judicial system and the whole democratic process. Having been warned that the jury selection could take up the best part of the morning, we watched as eight potential jurors at a time were interrogated by both sides. After one and a half hours, three men and five women were selected, and at 11 am the case finally started.

Bradley Geist opened for the plaintiff and, after asking to be excused if his throat sounded hoarse (a ploy he used to gain a level of familiarity with the jury), summarized our case and the wrongs that had been done to us. Brian Medlock, whom thereafter we called 'Madlock', opened for the defence. He was the opposite of any of our team. He had thin bristly greying hair, chubby red cheeks and a pear neck above a stocky body. He was a Texan and a good advocate who could hold the attention of both judge and jury. His failure lay in his coarse bullying tactics and his presentation of material, which had been shoddily and inaccurately produced by his own support team. He totally incensed Veronica and me with his opening remarks by saying that: 'Pigs get fat and hogs get slaughtered and that it is Dr Arnott who is the hog.' Little did he know that in that part of the country 'hogs' was a revered term for some of the Washington Redskins' football players.

After this insult, he then claimed that some fine American surgeons had all produced prior art lens designs, namely Bill Simcoe with the barrier-protection concept and John Park with a version of a totally encircling loop lens. Bradley Geist's opening was far superior to that of Brian Medlock, who had the ability to tell only half-truths.

After the lunch recess I took the witness stand to be examined by Bob Neuner. Bradley had beautifully prepared our case with abundant illus-trations, many of which were also used by the defence. I got off to a creaky start by referring to the Judge as 'My lord' instead of 'Your honour'. This faux pas was rather appreciated by the judge, a closet Anglophile. Bob Neuner took me through the afternoon, allowing me in effect to give a series of lectures to the judge and jury. The judge continuously reminded me to just answer the questions briefly and succinctly. Nevertheless I was given my head and I started with a talk on the anatomy of the eye followed by a dissertation of lens styles of 1981. I then introduced the concept of my totally encircling loop lens (TELL). I went through my relationship with Cilco and the production of my invention from 1982–4. At the end of the afternoon I stated that Dr Jaffe had been given my lens design. We finished day one at 6 pm. After the jury had left, Judge Ellis turned to us and said he hoped a settlement would be reached. He quoted Voltaire saying that: 'He had lost one case, won the next but lost everything.' Looking at Bob Neuner, he carried on: 'I cannot yet see the story emerging.'

We started the morning at church before another examination by Bob Neuner. Ted Ciccone's litigation company had drawn on a large billboard a diagram with the precise measurement of each of the lenses that infringed either the original or reissue patent. Whereas on the previous day, Bob Neuner had acted rather like 'Colombo' the detective, with hesitations and constant fumbling of documents, on this occasion he was the true assured advocate.

A large billboard depicting my original AR4 totally encircling loop lens was placed in the centre of the courtroom only a few feet away from the jury, and I was asked to elaborate on the features of this lens in relationship to the claims of the reissue patent. Judge Ellis had given me permission to stand in the centre of the room. Having been briefed for so many hours by Bradley Geist, I was able to cover every segment of my invention, word by word and sentence by sentence, without even having to think. Each part of the lens was described in the scope and extent of the invention.

Following this, all the infringing lenses were placed on the easel and their configurations in relationship to the claims of the reissue patent were demonstrated. With some 23 lenses to present, this process became somewhat tedious but a very clear and definite message was emerging. Finally the board depicting the Park lens was produced. Bob Neuner urged me to go over the claims of my reissue patent in relationship to the Park lens. Apart from being a PMMA lens with encircling loops, the differences were quite fundamental. The Park lens had a diameter of only 10.5 mm and would simply lie on the capsular bag of the removed human lens, whereas each of the infringing lenses were at least 12 mm, thus allowing the loops to compress within the capsular bag. One loop had a first portion, which ran into a second with a fixed curvature, before extending into a third portion having two humps that faced outwards. This loop having no fourth portion was totally asymmetrical to the other and would give the lens a rather unstable three-point fixation when placed in the eye. Everyone in the courtroom must have by now been made aware that this lens did not have the same features as mine. Besides, even if there had been public knowledge of it before the introduction of my own invention, it was purely experimental and hence not available as prior art.

We recessed to a private room in a local hotel for lunch with the team 'in business' at one table and those 'resting' at another. I had lost my appetite and spent most of this time, lying on the floor of the dining room, being given a back massage by my Veronica. On returning to court I sat waiting apprehensively for the cross-examination. While only issues brought up in examination can be reviewed in cross-examination, there was concern about what the opposition might be brewing up, as they had been seen preparing slides and numerous pages of diagrams. After the opening of the afternoon session, Brian Medlock was given permission to have an overhead projector for screening pictures onto the courtroom wall. It was so large that I was totally hidden from my adversary, to which Bob Neuner raised an objection but was overruled by the judge. I thus missed Brian Medlock's flirtation with the jury. After every question he would turn to face them, nodding his head and grinning like a Cheshire cat.

Brian Medlock gave me, via the marshal, a mock-up of the empty capsular bag of the human lens. This model was a clear plastic disc some 10 inches in diameter, which had on one of its sides a clean-cut circular hole, some half the width of its surface. This was meant to represent the opening in the anterior capsule, which is made at the time of the surgical cataract procedure. From my previous deposition with Brian Medlock, I had learned how he considered the Park lens could be fixed on the posterior capsule. He thought that the capsular bag and lens could be compared to a sandwich, with the capsular bag as the outer bread covering and the lens the contained contents. His idea was that the anterior capsular flap coming down to press on the posterior capsule would keep the lens wrapped in the capsular bag. Inadvertently Brian Medlock had made a big mistake in giving me this model exhibit. In extracapsular cataract extraction, a hole is made into the anterior capsule of the lens before removing its contents. Up until 1986, in all forms of anterior capsulotomy, a needle would be used to make little nicks in the capsule, which would leave a serrated edge in its opening. In 1986, two surgeons Neumann, of Germany, and Gimbel, of Canada, independently thought out a new technique, in which the opening was formed by making a tear in it rather than nicks. This could create a circular hole with a clear edge, as in the model I was holding. I looked perplexed, wondering why I should be given a model pertaining to 1986 rather than the surgery of 1982, which was relevant to this case. After some little time Brian Medlock, realizing he had made a major faux pas, withdrew the model. Stephen sitting in the audience was equally aware of the mistake.

Medlock next went into the issue of joint ownership, suggesting that part of the design was Cilco's. Bradley Geist had fully prepared me on this point, advising me that Cilco were empowered to engineer and produce my concept within their capabilities. The actual construction of the lens, such as the use of fine rectangular loops, employed techniques embodied in many other surgeons' lens styles and was subsidiary to our patent.

The next round of the cross-examination did much to change the course of the trial and convince the jury that our case was valid and true. The image of the Jaffe JF1 lens illuminated one wall of the courtroom and onto this was superimposed a transparency overlay of the Jaffe JF3 lens. Brian Medlock suggested that there was little difference in the appearance of the two lens designs. A lens implant needs to vary from another by only a millimetre in its design to transform a 'useless pup' into a 'gracious ballerina'. He had exposed the weakness of the one lens and the supremacy of the other.

The JF1 lens, purposely designed not to have totally encircling loops was the 'pup', as it was almost impossible to insert into the human eye because of its shortened rather inflexible loops. The JF3 lens, with its slightly longer totally encircling loops, while coming within our patent, was a fundamentally better lens implant. With its flexibility and ease of insertion into the eye, it could be used by all surgeons of average ability. Confronting Brian Medlock from the other side of the large projector, it was not too difficult to make the judge and jury aware of these deliberations.

Medlock next produced the sketch I had drawn for Randy Alexander in the Cilco hospitality suite of the Towers Hotel way back in 1981. With great panache, he looked at the jury and claimed that there was no gusset or first portion of the loops. I had made only a very rough thumbnail sketch for Randy Alexander, but there was a definite gusset in the upper loop. The first portion of the loop could be seen coming vertically away from the optic at 12 o'clock, before the right-angle bend towards the second part. Brian Medlock looked horror-struck when it was pointed out to him, and rapidly withdrew this exhibit.

During a recess our local counsel, John Anderson, warned me to be more circumspect and deferential towards Brian Medlock, as I could well lose the sympathy of the jury. He need not have worried, as the closing session of the day dealt with the legal rather than the surgical implications of the lens design, which I had always found a difficult subject to master. The effort of trying to concentrate on these legal issues was beginning to make me feel rather insecure – being a surgeon not a lawyer. He next asked a very simple question: 'Does your lens give barrier protection to the posterior capsule?'

'Not only does it give barrier protection but the lens also has a high arc of contact and stability,' I replied, having avoided his trap. If I had affirmed my lens had barrier protection without further elaboration, the Simcoe lens would have been considered as prior art.

He next asked: 'Is 'essentially similar' the same as 'identical'?'

Not knowing the purpose of the question and wishing to avoid another trap, I said rather limply: 'Essentially similar means essentially similar.'

Feeling like a schoolboy after a very hard exam, I returned to the gallery and a big hug from Veronica.

The following morning our patent expert Tom Arnold went into the witness box. Judge Ellis cut his evidence very short, but he was able to emphasize that, although the Jaffe 1 lens did not infringe our patent, all the others did. Then it was Stephen's turn to sit in the witness box. Bob Neuner took Stephen slowly through the seven major American companies that had agreed to a royalty licence. The same repetitive question about each of these seven companies was listed, so as to emphasize that Cilco and Intraoptics were the only two firms out of line. Bob Neuner concentrated on the meetings that Stephen had had with the Cooper-Vision Cilco representatives in Huntington and Montreal. Stephen related how, in Montreal, we had concentrated on being allowed to design a lens totally as we wished, but that even this design, when given to Alcon, had been renamed. He was utterly convincing throughout.

At the start of the afternoon session, our opposing advocate asked if Stephen's cross-examination could be adjourned, so that their expert medical witness could give his evidence. A small dark-haired man wearing round brown spectacles went into the witness box with a rather arrogant expression on his face. Despite stating that he had been implanting lenses since 1978 and had tried more than 75 lens styles, he seemed to have only a cursory knowledge of both the Simcoe and Jaffe lenses. The first real excitement in the defence came when Bob Neuner cross-examined him on the similarity of the Park and Arnott lenses. The witness stated that the different configuration of the loops made little difference to a lens's performance and anyway the flexibility of loops could differ from one identical lens to the next. Bob Neuner paused in the proceedings to allow those in the courtroom time to digest this totally muddled and confusing piece of testimony.

The Park lens with asymmetrical loops has one with no fourth portion. Bob Neuner closed his cross-examination by asking the witness to mark, with a crayon, the extent of the fourth portion of the offending loop. The witness was, by this time, no doubt longing to get out of this court and take the next plane home. He stood in the centre of the court speechless, with his mouth opening and closing. After great hesitation he went to the board and, using the green crayon, traced over the whole end portion of the loop, which included the two bumps. His marking ended at the second portion of the loop, which had a continuous curve right up to the gusseted first portion. Unwittingly he had demonstrated that there were only three portions on this one loop.

Before adjourning for the weekend, Judge Ellis again recommended that the two parties should get together to attempt a settlement. So ended the first week of the trial. Despite the constant nagging anxiety, we were fortunate to enjoy some respite at a weekend organized by Bradley in the Farmington Country Club near Charlottesville. Our pent-up tension at the humiliations we had had to endure from our adversaries in the trial started to evaporate. We had a very special weekend, touring some of the most picturesque and historically important parts of America. The three of us later took a moonlight walk around the golf course to discuss with Bradley the possible terms for a settlement.

The following morning Bradley returned to Alexandria to have a council of war with his fellow attorneys. It was very generous of him to have given up so much time to us, when his mind must have been in constant turmoil over the vicissitudes of the case. Releasing the week's stress, I must have driven Stephen and Veronica mad with my imitation of 'Madlock' firing off questions. Worn down by my constant mimicking of Medlock, they made me promise not to mention his name again for the rest of the weekend.

On the Monday, Brian Medlock started Stephen's cross-examination. He dwelt at length on the varied royalties the other companies were giving us. Stephen emphasized very strongly that his father had little interest in finances and stated that our primary interest was to maintain accountability for our various lens styles. With these arrangements it was possible to know what each company was marketing and the teaching that was required for the surgeons starting this form of lens implantation. Stephen knew all about the design and production of lens implants and his case could not be flawed. Both the judge and jury must have been aware of his youthful integrity and honesty. Even so, it was music to Stephen's ears when he was finally told that there was only five minutes more of cross-examination. This friendly remark made by Brian Medlock showed that under his rather cold exterior there glowed an element of human warmth, and even he may have been impressed by Stephen's exemplary evidence in the witness box.

John Ostendorf, an elderly gentleman who was the acknowledged damages expert, was the next and last of our witnesses to enter the box. With the assistance of Marina Larson, it had been calculated that our rights and damages, if we won the case, should amount to $3.5 million. Brian Medlock metaphorically put on his boxing gloves for his cross-examination of John Ostendorf. It was very long and gruelling, and John had to listen to long extracts about totally irrelevant patent laws. John 'stuck to his guns' and left the jury very cognisant of our rights. As he finished, Veronica turned to me and said: 'I am very worried about John. He looks totally exhausted and is walking very slumped.'

The case for the plaintiff now rested, and it was the turn for the defendants to present their side. At the end of the previous week's session, their first witness, an expert ophthalmic surgeon, had markedly flawed their case. But Alcon, as a subsidiary of Nestlé, one of the world's largest corporations, still had much ammunition left and all the finances required to call on any witness. Despite this enormous backing, act two of the defence had, if possible, less panache than their first. For two hours, everyone in the courtroom suffered by having to listen to yet more totally irrelevant depositions about the Park lens.

At the end of the afternoon we heard depressing news. After leaving the court John Ostendorf had returned to his hotel. Soaking in the heat of a hot bath, John was disturbed by the phone and clambering out of the bath he had slipped on the marble and heard an ominous crack as his left hip fractured. He lay writhing in agony on the bathroom floor, the call unanswered. In considerable pain he eventually managed to crawl onto the bed, where he waited for us to return. He did not want to seek help until I had first seen and examined him. We found poor John in great pain, with his left leg splayed across the bed at a totally abnormal angle.

Having experienced, over the previous two weeks, the workings of the American judicial system, Veronica and I were now witnessing their medical services. How suddenly things can change – here we were rushing to hospital with one of our witnesses, who had paid such a high price in trying to help us.

Within minutes John had been X-rayed and taken to the operating theatre for the pinning of his fractured hip. His wife arrived by plane from New York, so we felt able to leave the hospital.

The next day produced some extraordinary evidence. The first witness was someone whom we had known for 12 years. Short and thick set, he had a firm protruding jaw – a seemingly confident and successful man. A biophysicist, he had been responsible for developing one-piece PMMA lens-implant technology for Cilco. He often consulted ophthalmic surgeons in the preparation of lens styles, which he would then market. The artist drawings of my original totally encircling loop lens had been sent to him. In the fall of 1983, I had attended a Cilco meeting at Hilton Head, South Carolina, during which he and I had discussed at length the refinements and changes to my next lens design.

On direct examination by Brian Medlock he was quite brilliant. He gave the court a 40-minute lecture on the various stages of the manufacturing process of the one-piece PMMA lens, supplemented with prototype diagrams and sketches. He elaborated on various styles of lenses he had made in late 1981 and 1982. Included was a lens identical to mine.

'Who invented the Arnott lens?' asked Brian Medlock.

'I did,' retorted the witness. So ended his examination.

Bob Neuner cross-examined him: 'Are you a paid expert of Nestlé's?'

'Yes.'

'Are you paid $1080 a day?'

'Yes.'

'Have you been working on this case for many weeks?'

'Yes.'

'Then you must have received a considerable amount of money to act as an expert witness?'

'Yes.'

'Having left Alcon some years ago, were you re-employed so that you could work on the Arnott case?'

'Yes.'

'Do you wish to change your testimony?'

'No.'

'Do you wish to change your testimony?'

'No.'

Bob Neuner now put on his best 'Colombo' expression and said, 'Did you design the Arnott lens?'

'Yes.'

An exhibit was produced showing the text of the 1985 *Simcoe v Alcon* trial. In this the witness had said under oath that he had not designed the Arnott lens. Standing very erect, Bob Neuner said: 'Your memory seems to be better in 1992 than it was in 1985.'

Judge Ellis, leaning forward towards the witness, said: 'You have not yet reached the stage of impeachment, but you are not far off.'

By this time, the top of his head was only just visible above the level of the witness box.

In the afternoon, one of the senior vice-presidents of Alcon was examined. He entered the witness box with head held high, wearing shoes so highly polished you could see your reflection in them. Brian Medlock introduced him as 'one of our heroic Vietnam veterans'. His direct examination was unremarkable. Despite the fact that, at the meeting in 1986, we had been promised royalties on all the Coburn lenses, the witness, in his testimony, claimed he always denied us the Coburn CP4LU lens, which was later renamed the JF3. He also claimed that Alcon, in their dealings with the Arnotts, had never sought legal advice.

In the cross-examination, Bob Neuner produced as an exhibit a letter from their patent solicitor to this executive. In this he stated that the Arnott patent was strong and should be taken seriously. The witness claimed not to have seen this letter, although it had been produced from his own files. With the disclaimer of the letter, it was very difficult for Bob Neuner to draw him into the relationship with his legal advisers, as only exhibits known to the witness can be used as substance for interrogation. After several abortive attempts at questioning the witness, the judge, who had sat for several minutes with his head in his hands, intervened. Looking at Bob Neuner, he said to him: 'I so sympathize with you. It reminds me of the time that I was at your stage in my own career.' Then turning to the witness, he asked him: 'Have you had any dealings about the Arnott lens with your legal representative?'

'No,' was the reply. Both judge and jury knew he was not telling the truth and he left the witness box with little credibility.

One of the company's artists was the last witness of the trial. He had previously, in a deposition, told Marina Larson that there was no similarity between the Arnott and Park-style lenses. He had to repeat the evidence in court, and these final remarks, from a witness for the defence, were of considerable help to our case.

At the end of the proceedings, Judge Ellis stated that all the issues would have to be decided by the jury. That evening we went to the hospital to visit John Ostendorf, who was making a good recovery. The only duties of the next day were to be the summing up by the two chief trial attorneys and the judge's directive to the jury.

Bob Neuner presented our case beautifully in his closing statements. He summarized the history of my lens designs. He closed by producing the large sketch of the Park lens on which their medical expert had, with a green crayon, traced in the hypothetical fourth portion of the asymmetrical loop.

By contrast, Brian Medlock summed up with statements that were totally at variance with the testimony given during the trial. He stated that I had used the Park lens design in the spring of 1984 as a springboard for my advanced lens and had myself pinched the Jaffe lens design.

After lunch, members of the jury were released to form their verdict. All our team adjourned to the local Irish pub and returned at 5 pm, hoping to hear the verdict. It was not until Friday evening, some two days later, that this was reached. The jury had 12 points to answer, split up into series of four. The judge said that all the first two series of four must be answered, but the last four only if the first eight were in the plaintiff's favour. The first four required the answer 'no' for the case to be favourable to the plaintiff.

The jury filed into the courtroom and sat in their leather-bound chairs, except for their foreman, who remained standing while being questioned by Judge Ellis.

1. Was the Arnott lens anticipated?

'No.'

2. Was the Park lens anticipated?

'No.'

3. Did the Park lens constitute prior art.

'No.'

4. Was the Park lens prior art.

'No.'

The next four questions dealt with contractual and infringement issues, such as whether or not the Jaffe lenses should have been in the contract, all of which we won. The only issue we lost was on the question of whether or not Alcon's infringement had been wilful and wanton. All in all we had received a very fair trial.

Whereas in criminal cases the jury's verdict is final, in civil cases the verdict has to be approved by the judge, which takes a matter of months. Despite these limitations we considered the case closed. We thanked God for the hospitality that had been shown to us and the judicial rights that had been extended to us foreigners. Even if we had lost the case, we would have respected the honesty and integrity of our trial. We spent the time on the flight to New York almost in a state of suspended animation.

In one day our credibility in ophthalmology had been re-established, with an American court judging that my one-piece totally encircling loop lens, the most popular on the market at that time, was my invention. We had not wished for acclaim but only our due rights.

During the following weeks, the opposition filed various motions to get the verdict overturned – all without success.

In May 1992, Judge Ellis upheld the jury verdict. As Alcon was dithering about whether or not to go to an appeal, which would have delayed a final settlement for many more months, Bradley Geist sought an injunctive relief against the production of all the infringing lenses. The judge gave a stay of four weeks, after which it came into effect. The result was immediate. A director of Alcon rang up Bradley Geist after four days, saying: 'Mr Geist, your injunction is causing great difficulties. The production of our lens implants is being severely affected.'

Bradley replied: 'You have only to pay what the jury awarded my client.'

Alcon put in two appeals to have the injunction lifted, without success.

On 12 June, they finally agreed to settle the case. This was almost the first time that a single family had stood up for its rights against the might of an international corporation and won. For this much of the credit must go to Stephen and Bradley Geist. All our team played such a major role, and Bob Neuner brought in expertise and excitement to the trial. As a thank you, we sent both Bradley and Bob cut-glass Baccarat 'hogs' with our implant lens crested on their flanks. Probably their grandchildren will one day be perplexed as to why they have such funny objects on their desks.

Despite our victory, we realized we were in no way millionaires. Our attorneys took 40% of the damages, and the residue was taxed at 40%. Stephen was able, with his proportion of the reward, to move from London into a more suitable family home in Hampshire. For us, our share would reprieve us from almost certain bankruptcy. All our debts from the previous Ioptex litigation were paid off, and we had enough reserves to make a modest gift to our children. Veronica and I decided to splash out and buy a new Porsche 911, which by complete coincidence had a number plate K12 JUN, the day of my birthday and ironically the day that the case finally came to an end.

Collecting our car, Veronica and I drove down the King's Road like two young lovers without a care in the world. Thus was completed one of the most interesting stages in our career together.

CHAPTER 29
No specs

There were many changes in our profession during the early 1990s. The NHS had gradually become burdened by tiers of management bureaucracy, and I was no longer in complete charge of my own ophthalmic department. My pioneering work in cataract extraction and lens implantation had been completed just in time, as it would have been almost impossible to introduce new concepts with the numerous committee meetings that were now the norm for any project.

With the introduction of computer technology, the lens implant companies were beginning to develop new instruments and lens designs without being so reliant on ophthalmologists. The third generation of my lens implant, such as Alcon's CVC1U, made of rigid PMMA, was among the most popular lenses made up until this time, with worldwide sales in excess of five million, but the emphasis was shifting to implants of soft materials that could be folded and put into the eye through a smaller incision. Physicists rather than surgeons were required for the development of the new forms of ophthalmic lasers that were entering the market. The surgeon's expertise was still required, but not to the same extent his inventiveness. It was rather as if, as in the aircraft industry, ophthalmology had progressed from the piston engine to the jet era.

Small-incision phaco cataract extraction and lens implantation, thanks to the work of the few, was now the standard operation in most hospitals throughout the world, and ophthalmologists were looking towards new horizons, with the treatment of refractive errors of the eye, such as long and short sight.

For years, surgeons such as William Jory in the UK, had been treating short sight surgically, with a procedure known as refractive keratotomy. In this operation, which had been developed in Russia by our long-time friend Svyatoslav Fyodorov, cuts were made in the cornea to flatten its surface and reduce its focusing power. His operation followed the concepts of a Japanese ophthalmologist called Sato, who had developed a similar form of refractive surgery many decades earlier. Sato's operation was doomed to failure, as he had made his cuts on the inner surface of the cornea, thus destroying the vital layer of endothelial cells that line its posterior surface.

On our first visit to Slava's clinic in Moscow in 1978, Veronica, Tania, and I had joined Svyatoslav in his office. He was watching on CCTV the performance of his junior surgeons, who had started the long day's surgical list. In true Russian style, he downed a large neat glass of vodka before joining them in the operating theatre. He invited us to join him, and Tania witnessed live eye surgery for the first time. His refractive surgery was most impressive, and he accentuated his results by having beautiful nurses on his staff, who had discarded their spectacles after being treated by him. Few surgeons from the West visited him at this time, and he entrusted to us his paper on refractive keratotomy and asked us to forward it to the American journals for publication.

With the introduction of the excimer laser, an alternative treatment for refractive errors of the eye became available. The excimer, with its ability to vaporize a few microns of tissue with each pulse, was the ideal instrument to sculpt and reshape the anterior surface of the cornea. Stephen leased one of these instruments from Summit Technology for the princely rental of $100,000 a year for four years, allowing the Arnott Eye Centre to enter this new branch of ophthalmology at the Cromwell. This was the first private excimer refractive unit in the south of England, and Professor John Marshall, carrying out research with a similar unit in St Thomas' Hospital, was very helpful in advising us about this new project.

The operation performed by this laser was uncomplicated, being almost entirely computer-orientated and completed in fewer than five minutes. Using the microscope, the surgeon initially sweeps away the delicate layer of cells that cover the anterior surface of the cornea. After programming the amount of refractive error into the computer, the surgeon adjusts the laser beam over the exposed surface of the cornea. Pressing a button simply fires the laser which, with each pulse, vaporizes and reshapes a few microns of the surface corneal tissue. Automated robotic surgery had truly arrived! Research over the previous 10 years had proved that this form of laser treatment was safe for the patient, as long as it was used within the prescribed limits. So initially we treated only patients with a modest amount of short sight.

In the months after its installation in the Cromwell Hospital, in 1992, hundreds of patients were treated with almost uniformly good results. The efficacy of this treatment was exemplified by the experience of our own son-in-law, Nick Whishaw. Within a week of his treatment, he surprised a burglar in the kitchen of his Hampshire home. The burglar fled up the drive and escaped in his car, hotly pursued by Nick, who was able to record its registration number. Police were alerted and in minutes the culprit was arrested. Tania was impressed – it was the first time in his life he had been able to read the number plate of a car without contact lenses or spectacles!

During this period we were able to help many patients whose career depended on normal unaided vision. One air test pilot was able to regain his job after our treatment. At the medical interview it was almost impossible for the examiner to see the results of our treatment. Despite these good results, the treatment was limited to patients with six or fewer units of short sight. A modified surgical procedure had been developed in America for the treatment of patients who might have up to 30 units of short sight.

The solution lay in ablating the deeper substance of the stroma of the cornea, which would indirectly change its anterior curvature. Access into the deeper layers of the cornea was gained with the use of a 'microkeratome', a machine that simulated a mini bacon-slicer.

After this machine had been clamped onto the eye, a revolving blade sliced off a disc of the cornea. The excimer laser could then be used to sculpt either the back surface of the corneal disc or the exposed flat surface of the remaining cornea. Following the treatment with the laser, the corneal disc was repositioned onto the eye.

We decided to be the first clinic in Britain to demonstrate this form of operation, which became known as LASIK. Several patients volunteered to improve their sight by having this procedure, including the daughter of one of my surgical colleagues. As, at this time, neither my partner Keith Williams nor I had been taught how to perform the operation, we enlisted the help of an Italian surgeon to undertake the surgery. A microkeratome was loaned from a German company. We organized quite an international set-up, with an American operation being performed by an Italian surgeon using German equipment in a British operating theatre.

The BBC's medical correspondent, James Wilkinson, joined us to film the occasion. Not being actively involved in the surgery, I stood in the wings of the theatre, with my surgical colleague whose daughter was to be treated. The first three operations went without a hitch, and we were all made very aware of the potential of this revolutionary form of surgery. The fourth patient was the daughter of my surgical colleague.

The operation started routinely. The microkeratome was fixated onto the cornea and started to make its slice through the substance of the cornea. We watched in horror as it jammed halfway through and the superficial disc of tissue was ripped off the surface of the eye. Our guest surgeon was left holding the microkeratome, in which was the slice of the patient's cornea, severely damaged by the machine failure.

I hurriedly scrubbed up and surveyed the remnants of the damaged cornea. I replaced the traumatized corneal disc and started to suture it back into place. With every stitch the cornea began to regain its normal appearance, and we realized that the patient would suffer no long-term ill effect. James Wilkinson could have had a field day reporting on the dangers of this eye operation, but instead presented a very fair documentary that featured in every BBC news bulletin over the following 24 hours.

During 1993 we seemed to be forever travelling. As a Serving Sister of the Order of St John of Jerusalem, Veronica was invited to visit the Holy Land. It was a change for me to be Veronica's guest. All the participants were members of the order and many were our friends. The hospitalier of the hospital, Sir Godfrey Milton-Thompson, and the secretary of the order,

Richard Duffield, were accompanied by their wives, Noreen and Rosemary. Reverend Michael Barklett and Sylvia Holmes were with us, and our tour guide was Michael Hodgson. He was very well read and had a great knowledge of the historical sights that we would be visiting. We spent a lot of time with other members of the group: Tara Elliot, her husband Alan, and their friends Mark and Nicola Cannon-Brookes. It was on account of meeting Mark Cannon-Brookes, who was a director of NCL Investments, that our son Robert got his first job in the London Stock Exchange.

Our tour started in Aqaba and on our coach trip along the Kings Highway to Petra we passed the desolate dunes of Wadi Rum, where Lawrence of Arabia's great triumph over the Turks took place. In the afternoon, we rode on ponies down a narrow steeply sloping gorge that entered a valley of extraordinary beauty. The vertical walls were dark red sandstone, onto which had been sculpted and architected the ancient City of Petra. Vast chambers had been hewn out of the rock.

Walking down the valley we passed the tombs of ancient Roman warriors and a Roman amphitheatre. The mysticism of this ancient world was mercifully lifted by the presence of a modern café, situated at the end of the valley, where we climbed some 800 steps to a sacrificial altar.

On the Sunday, Michael Barklett had organized a temporary church without walls in the unfinished part of the hotel. The early morning sun blazed into our makeshift chapel and, as a backdrop, there was the distant view of the bare Jordanian mountains.

On our drive to Amman we stopped to visit several crusader fortresses, including Shobak and Karak, circa 1140 AD, and Mount Nebo, which Moses climbed to survey the Promised Land.

Here we took some time to meet with HRH Prince Raad bin Zeid, the Lord Chamberlain of Jordan, a cousin of King Hussein and the rightful King of Iraq, on behalf of Lions Eye International. Despite showing some interest, the prince felt that ophthalmology was quite well funded in Jordan and no extra foreign finances were required. We did, however, go to the university, where I gave an address to some 50 members of the Jordanian Ophthalmic Society.

Having had a very enlightening time, Veronica and I returned to find that the other members of our group had not had a happy day. It had been planned for them to have an audience with King Hussein and Princess Muna. But the tour bus was refused permission to enter, and the very irritable party sat for some hours outside in the road. They never did gain entry to the palace, as the Women's Institute had pipped them to the post! Party spirits improved when the Order of St John had their function dinner in the Kashmere Restaurant. By coincidence, Prince Raad bin Zeid was the guest of honour.

The following morning we embarked on the main purpose of our trip, a visit to the Holy Land, and in our mini-bus followed the trails that Christ had walked some 2000 years earlier. We entered Israel by going over the Allenby Bridge onto the West Bank of the River Jordan, and then went via Jericho to Tiberius, a coastal town by the Sea of Galilee.

The tour around Galilee was truly biblical. First visited was the Mount of Beatitudes, where Mussolini had donated money for a church built of black marble with a golden dome, inlaid with caricatures of fishes. The sense of occasion was enhanced by the beautiful chanting of a choir. We went to a balcony overlooking the mount, and Michael Barklett read the Beatitudes, just as Jesus had to thousands on the hill below. It was a magical spiritual moment.

Our pilgrimage continued with a visit to the home of St Peter in Capernaum. This had been carefully excavated, and the rooms of his house could be seen through a glass floor of the museum. Only 100 metres away was the synagogue in which Christ had preached.

We hired a wooden 'Jesus boat' to explore the Sea of Galilee. It was probably very similar to those used at the time of Christ, except it had a diesel engine. Once at sea we dropped anchor, and Michael read the extract from *St Mark* chapter 6 about Jesus walking on the water. We listened to this sitting in a dead calm under a very hot sun, appreciating the peace and tranquillity while enjoying a picnic lunch. Afterwards, remaining by the coast, we visited the church that represented the miracle of the two fishes and the five loaves. Along the shore was the church where Christ appeared to Peter after the resurrection and had told him to 'Feed my flock'. At Nazareth, we saw the cave where Christ grew up.

Our last few days in the Holy Land were to be spent in Jerusalem, visiting most of the other major biblical scenes and attending an investiture in the Hospital of St John. The Lord Prior of the Hospital, Lord Vestey, supervised the inauguration of new officers and handed out prizes. I did not escape without giving yet another lecture.

At dinner in the Intercontinental Hotel with our friends, a rather distinguished-looking American entered the restaurant. As he was unaccompanied, we invited him to join our table. Dr James H Charlesworth was a theologian studying the Dead Sea Scrolls, a subject on which he subsequently gave a lecture to our entire group. He surmised that Essenes had hidden the scrolls in AD 68 before they were expelled by the Romans on their scourge of the holy lands. The Essenes attached importance to the effects of light and darkness and the interpretation of dreams. Some members of this order joined the early Christians and one was probably responsible for the editing of the *Gospel of St John*, reflecting Essene thinking that included references to the Holy Ghost.

I had to miss our planned trip to Bethlehem in order to look after Sylvia Holmes, who had been taken ill in Tiberius and whose condition had become grave. We had expected to be able to collect Sylvia and immediately escort her back to Jerusalem. We found her semi-comatose, dehydrated and running a high temperature. She had developed severe blood poisoning with early signs of meningitis. Luckily, I always carried an adequate medical kit stuffed with antibiotics. Few medical skills were required to treat Sylvia's infection, but it was essential to give her a massive dose of these antibiotics. Instructions were also given to force water down her, and I anticipated that, in seven hours, we would be able to stretcher her back to Jerusalem.

Using that time, Michael and I went to the Israeli border and entered a no-man's land between Israel and the Golan Heights. There were no customs barriers, no guards and nothing moved on the road. We drove for several miles through an abandoned countryside, littered with military debris, to reach Bethsaida. Where the headwaters of the River Jordan enter the Sea of Galilee there was a tranquil rather narrow waterway surrounded by trees, in which the only signs of life were some Arab children swimming in the river. We walked along a track through the scrub towards the now non-existent town of Bethsaida, when Michael said: 'This is the spot where Christ restored sight to the blind man.' It was a very special moment, and Michael gave me a stone from the path to remember it by. I would so loved to have been able to share this moment with Veronica.

Sylvia had to some extent recovered, and we were able to escort her back to Jerusalem, but it was weeks before she regained her full health.

Our colleague, Ulrich Dardenne, who in 1973 had introduced phaco into Germany, decided to give a 20th-anniversary congress in his home city of Bonn. Ulrich had not forgotten the support that we had given him during his early days when his own German Ophthalmologic Society had been so hostile, and we were his honoured guests. The Kelmans, Sinskeys and Kratzes had flown in from America, along with some of the younger generation of international ophthalmic surgeons who were quietly replacing us as the seniors in our profession, including Hans Koch and Jack Dodick, with their wives Helen and Lyn. Howard Fine was one who epitomized the changes in our profession. Although not directly inventing his own phaco machines or lens implants, he was most influential in promoting new ideas into our profession. He wore a different brightly coloured jacket at each congress we met. David Macintyre, an inventor of ophthalmic equipment and also many household gadgets, was also present.

Other European surgeons included Karl Jacobi from Germany, Fabio Dossi and Lucio Buratto from Italy, Philippe Sordille, Patrice De Large and Philippe Crozafon from France, Paddy Condon from Ireland and Richard Packard from England. Michael Blumenthal was Israel's foremost surgeon and over the years had been very supportive to the hospital of St John of Jerusalem. On one evening, by chance on my 64th birthday, this very mixed assembly was entertained on a boating excursion up the Rhine. As usual Charlie Kelman, playing his saxophone, gave the cabaret.

Later that month we attended a very different international congress, as guests of Howard and Judy Gimbel in Calgary, Canada. Howard was a very inventive phaco surgeon who owned his own hospital and was the pinnacle of a pyramid that employed dozens of staff. Like some other eminent surgeons, such as Jim Gills, he was deeply religious and would say a prayer before operating. Being a Seventh-day Adventist, Howard and Judy would not leave their home on a Saturday. Gimbel was a household name in Canada and even had his own advertising space on Air Canada planes. Along with Howard Stein, Marvin Kwitko and Gordon Krolman, he was among the greats in Canadian ophthalmology.

At this meeting Howard demonstrated live surgery to the delegates in his hospital, while the congress was held at the Banff Springs Hotel, some miles away in the Rocky Mountains. Bradley Geist, our American attorney, joined us on this trip, and we had an exhilarating boat ride on the white rapids of the Kicking Horse River in Columbia Yoko Park. The waters of the river are freezing and survival in them is only a matter of minutes. We were to use one hand for the paddle and the other to grip the railing of our dinghy. The surrounding mountain landscape was extraordinary and peaceful, until rounding a bend in the river, we saw ahead of us foaming white water. The boat took on a peculiar pitch: it came to a grinding halt, with its bow first rising vertically out of the water before dipping, the prelude for its plunge. Just when it seemed that we had reached the extreme capability of remaining in the boat, we would arrive in the calmer waters of the river below. There was little time to regain our equilibrium before we were hurled into the next series of rapids.

To add to our misery the skies descended on us, and through the latter part of our trip we were soaked with torrential rain. One of the boats went headlong into a rock, spilling three of its occupants into the torrent. Fortunately they were able to swim and clutch onto rocks before being rescued. Two hours later, we were home safe – very cold, bedraggled and totally exhausted. It was an experience we relished but would not want to repeat.

This congress was so typical of the many we attended over the years. While enjoying the splendours of the world and the company of our good friends, we were able to share our knowledge. These international congresses were very instrumental in formulating many of the advances in our profession.

CHAPTER 30
The Arnott Eye Centre

During the first years of using the excimer laser, the many hundreds of patients treated for short sight had almost uniformly excellent results and a marked improvement in the quality of their sight. The total success of this project was indirectly the cause of a severe problem in our unit at the Cromwell Hospital. To enhance the high-profile image of our unit, we decided to paint and redecorate our clinic. But overnight, our patients started to suffer unacceptable results from their refractive surgery. It transpired that our once-perfect excimer laser had suffered irreparable damage from the fumes of the paint used in the redecorating.

The laser beam is transmitted in the excimer machine by a series of very delicate mirrors, which are coated with a substance to enhance their reflective potential. The paint fumes had destroyed the coating of the mirrors, and ruined our wonderful laser, costing nearly half a million dollars. It proved impossible to repair these defects, and our machine had to be closed down. To continue doing refractive surgery we were forced to use the facilities of a rival hospital, so causing serious financial losses. Radical changes were needed if we were to remain financially solvent. Our thriving cataract practice was supporting the ailing refractive. We needed to construct a surgical clinic to encompass both. Stephen found the ideal site on the ground floor of Harley Street's only modern building. Dr Norman Ramsbottom, a foremost physician, took over a portion of this floor with his secretary Diane Dawood, and we rented the remaining 5000 square feet. In this building we developed a rather novel clinic. One end of the facility was an outpatient department for treatment with the excimer laser, and at the other end was our clinic for all the other ophthalmic patients. In the middle were two operating theatres.

Laser Vision Inc, which already had 20 excimer lasers in various hospitals around the country, was looking for a flagship clinic in London. Our custom-built new unit in Harley Street was totally suitable for their needs and they entered into a joint venture with us.

After the usual construction difficulties, our clinic looked superb, and the two operating theatres were 'state of the art'. This new clinic, which was an immediate success, was well received by our patients and the physicians and embassies that referred them. If surgery was required, all the pre-operative ancillary tests were carried out on site. With Keith Williams, who had joined us from America, we had a large workload of laser refractive surgery.

Once it was up and running, Veronica felt at a loose end. For years she had supported Stephen and me in every aspect of my career. Looking for pastures new, she decided to give an even greater commitment to charity events.

Working on the staff at Charing Cross Hospital was a hugely overqualified young man called Victor Marks. Stephen and he conceived the concept of the 'Great London Treasure Hunt'. This turned into a hugely ambitious project, which took on a life of its own.

The idea was that an unlimited number of sponsored teams of four would travel all around London on one day, looking for the answers to clues set by the A–Z Map Company. The first team back to the finishing station with all the answers would win. Every participant would be recognizable by having a 'Long John Silver' parrot emblem on their tunic, and the winner would be presented with a large golden parrot.

We required massive sponsorship for our Arnott Trust, which was the kernel of this function. Our first support came from Sir Richard Branson, who, with his usual appreciation for a challenge and the need for charity events, donated £125,000 towards his sponsored 'Virgin' teams. We also linked up with two major charities, the Wooden Spoon Society and Lions International, which in 1993 had decided to distribute all its donations to ophthalmic charities. Philip Daubigminy was the chairman of the British Division of Lions, and he, with his wife Minna, played a major part in the event.

Adjacent to our maisonette in Hammersmith, was a large area of land that had been given by Henry VIII to the Worshipful Company of Girdlers in honour of this vestment. For centuries it had been valueless until, in the latter part of the twentieth century, London spread out to encompass this area. The charity committee of this company, now well-endowed, generously donated £8000 for our cause.

The Royal Mail entered several teams, as did many dozens of companies, such as IBM, and several London teaching hospitals, including Guys and Charing Cross. All the monies raised by these teams would be given to the charity of their choice. Unfortunately, the Wooden Spoon Society and Arnott Trust bore the brunt of the considerable financial responsibilities of the event without ensuring that the teams allocated a small proportion of their sponsorship, and we both ended up well in the red.

Some 200 teams started the treasure hunt at 9 am on 11 September 1993. Stephen, Kathy, Tania and Nick formed one team, and Robert, with three friends, Al Hill, Steve Norton and John Castleman, another. Many of our friends, such as Tony Spooner, organized their own teams.

The clues were enormous fun to put together: the first clue was 'What lies by the altar of St Mary's, the Wren Church in the Strand?' (Answer, the internment of Nell Gwyn, King Charles II's mistress). Another was 'Where in Hyde Park does time stay still?' (Answer, the old clock by the Elf tree near the Bayswater Road).

Most of the clues were impossible to answer without going to the location, and Londoners watched as hundreds of teams, sporting the parrot emblem, rushed around London using various forms of transport, many in their own cars. The winning team got lucky and found a taxi driver who became enthused with the cause and drove without charge all over London, using all known shortcuts, so they finished an hour before anyone else. Veronica and I spent the morning with Philip and Minna Daubigminy in the control centre at the top of the BT Tower, where Simon Evens and volunteers saved our teams from getting lost. The whole event was televised on BBC and ITV news.

The official dinner and presentation was held at the Cat & Canary and presided over by Radio 2 presenter Ed Stewart. All teams had completed the course and the Inn was packed with more than a thousand people in party mood. Tonight there were no losers, and many tens of thousands of pounds had been raised for charity.

As the main catalyst for this event, Veronica had been invited to present the six-foot high 'golden parrot' to the winning team. Just before the presentation, as I was heading for the Gents to freshen up, I heard a commotion on the balcony above. A lady was cradling in her arms a man, who was naked above his trousers, unconscious, pallid and bathed in sweat. There were no signs of breathing and I could find no trace of a pulse.

Apparently he had inadvertently eaten a morsel of shellfish to which he was acutely allergic. I considered that my unwitting patient was suffering an attack of status asthmaticus and had almost reached the point of no return. I laid him flat on the floor and started external cardiac massage – not easy, as his chest was rigid with the muscular spasm. I sat astride him and pushed down onto his chest as hard as I could, 60 times a minute. Luckily another colleague appeared in time to give the kiss of life. Incredibly, a glimmer of a pulse returned and, after an eternity, the paramedics arrived with adrenaline and oxygen, and the patient started to breathe normally.

I was nearly late for the presentation, but had a powerful sense of pride at the organization of such a fun event that raised so much money.

CHAPTER 31
Operation eyeball

On my 65th birthday in 1994, Veronica held a party at Trottsford and we had a double celebration to also mark Robert's fundraising bike trip around the world. Each of the 16 tables in the marquee was decorated to represent one of the countries through which Bob and his friend Steve Norton were travelling: France, Italy, Zimbabwe, Botswana, South Africa, Pakistan, India, Nepal, Thailand, Malaysia, Singapore, Australia, New Zealand, Japan, USA, Scotland and England. On the day of our party, Bob and Steve were in Capetown, South Africa. A very old friend Judge Hubert Dunn, with his wife Quetta, gave a toast to the continued success of the two cyclists.

The bicycle trip had taken months to organize and we received hundreds of letters and donations, which totalled more than £83,000, from patients. The money raised was to go to various ophthalmic charities, which included buying an operating microscope for the King Edward VII Hospital, Midhurst. Many of my ophthalmic friends and patients became involved in hosting the boys on their route around the world. Lions International was also supportive and held various fundraising events where the two young men would 'sing for their supper'.

From the Royal Automobile Club, the boys were flagged on their way by hundreds of friends. A gang of us, including Ranulph Fiennes and David Essex, accompanied them on bikes down Pall Mall to Trafalgar Square, where we left them to fight with the London traffic on their own. We headed home before setting off for Dover in the early afternoon but caught up with them along the A2, already exhausted and beginning to wonder if it was all a great mistake. We trailed them into Dover and had a rather emotional dinner along with Steve's parents John and Sue. And so they started a journey of some 12,500 miles. With just their bikes and pannier bags, they seemed so vulnerable. Veronica and I plotted their progress on a large map, which took up a whole wall of our hall at Trottsford. After an easy and pleasurable ride across Europe, the second leg took them across Africa. They were well looked after in Harare, Zimbabwe, by a patient of mine, Mrs Bouzanis, on whom I had operated. She in turn put them in touch with a chief of police, who acted as their host during the visit and organized a police helicopter to take them over Victoria Falls.

As they crossed the border into South Africa, they entered the State of Bophutswana at a politically volatile time. Luckily, any fears for their safety were unfounded, and they experienced as much hospitality as anywhere else. Often they would cycle through a township accompanied by crowds of welcoming schoolchildren and local television crews.

Flying on to Islamabad, Robert found himself being taken for me, as he was met by an ophthalmic professor who said: 'We are so privileged to be able to welcome such a distinguished international ophthalmic surgeon who will demonstrate his surgery and lecture to our staff.'

Robert and Steve, sitting in the limousine, were overcome with embarrassment realizing that there was a problem of mistaken identity.

'I think you have mistaken me for my father. I have just finished my degree at Oxford Brookes University in Architecture,' replied Robert. At the hospital they were met by a reception committee of the staff lined up in the forecourt of the hospital. Without turning a hair, the head of the hospital introduced Robert: 'We are honoured to have as our guest Robert Arnott, who will talk to us about his ideas for our new hospital wing.' Robert did his best to offer some ideas!

They struggled with heat exhaustion through Pakistan and were stopped by customs officers at the Indian border, who wanted to saw their bike frames in two to ensure that they were not carrying cocaine. After many hours of confrontation, the differences were sorted out over cans of Coca-Cola.

Veronica and I flew to Mumbai, India, to meet up with them, and of course we contacted our old friend and patient Bipin and added in a few lectures to colleagues who had set up their own phaco clinics. This was probably the first time that well-used bikes had been seen in the lobby of the Taj Mahal! Major Upadhyay, my long-time colleague, had arranged an audience for Bob and Steve to meet Mother Teresa in her clinic in Calcutta. From Nepal they flew on to Bangkok, where they were relieved to find that the temperature was only a mere 37°C! The next leg to Singapore was a tough ride, on narrow roads filled with fast traffic and dangerous black mambas. One night they found an unoccupied house with a suspended wooden plinth in its hall. The two weary travellers jettisoned their tent and climbed up to this balcony for the most comfortable night's sleep of many weeks. They were woken the next morning by the incantations of the local Moslems, who were taking early morning prayer in their mosque below them!

In Perth, Australia, they stayed with Veronica's second cousin, Angela Duke, and met a man who held the world record for the fastest crossing of Australia by bicycle. He put to rest their fears of crossing the Nullarbor Plain, a desert that extends 1200 miles with only seven roadhouses (essentially large petrol stations) across the whole length of it.

With a tail wind and blue skies, they clocked up 120 miles a day, despite wasting one day searching for their tent, which had been blown half a mile away. Breakfast was a Mars bar, crisps and a can of Coca-Cola. They were gallantly watched over by truckers, who drove this most lonesome road every five days.

After 27 days and some 3000 miles later, they arrived in Sydney, where they stayed with an old friend Emma Hawkins. By this time both Robert and Steve had become quite professional at being interviewed on television.

In New Zealand they battled constant freezing rain and very hilly landscapes but found the countryside spell-bindingly beautiful. Their Japanese leg from Osaka to Tokyo was particularly difficult, made fraught by language barriers, indecipherable road signs, thick fog and extremely expensive Mars bars. They slept rough on the streets most nights, as even the most basic room was unaffordable!

In October Veronica and I flew to San Francisco for the annual meeting of the American Society of Cataract and Refractive Surgery. With impeccable timing, Robert and Steve joined us in the Prescott Hotel only minutes after we had checked into it. Having arrived in Los Angeles with time to spare, they had decided to bicycle up the 500 miles from Los Angeles to San Francisco on the spectacular Highway 1. After 465 miles, the back wheel of Bob's bike finally collapsed and the last 35 miles to our hotel was made in a Cadillac stretch-limousine.

What a celebration we had that night in our hotel! Much else was achieved that week. Stephen joined us to finalize our contract with the Laser Vision Inc of Missouri, agreeing that the joint venture should be 51% Laser Vision and 49% Arnott. As minority shareholders, we were taking a calculated risk but felt that this honourable American company would not take advantage of our vulnerability.

While in San Francisco, Bob and Loraine Sinskey took us up the Napa Valley to see their winery. The Sinskey wine was now becoming popular in America and other countries. His son Rob, with wife Marie, was running the company.

In San Francisco, we organized a press reception in honour of our two bicyclists and many of our ophthalmic friends. The owner of the Press Club, Izzy Stewart, immediately adopted us as friends and was with us throughout the whole of 'the Operation Eye Ball' evening. The current edition of *Ocular Surgery News*, which featured a whole page on Bob and Steve Norton's charitable event for ophthalmology, had arrived just in time to be on display.

The Sinskeys had supplied the wine for the evening free of charge. Jack Dodick was the opening speaker and was followed by Bob and Steve, who gave their differing accounts of their journey around the globe. As always, Charlie Kelman played sax and paid for the band. It was a truly marvellous event. The 140 guests included Emanuel Rosen, Hugh Williams and Ian Mackey from the UK, Philippe Crozafon and Danielle Aron-Rosa from France, Michael Blumenthal from Israel and Harold Stein from Canada. We also entertained in their own country Gerry Freeman, Herve Gould, Ron Barnet, Irv Kalb, Arnie and Marion Pearlstone, Henry Clayman, Howard Fine, Howard Gimbel, Samuel Masket, Steve Obstbaum and John Beale, along with many others.

We flew home, leaving Robert and Steve to cycle across America before making their flight back. Their trip took them over the foothills of the Rockies, before going through all the southern states. Despite being in one of the most civilized countries in the world, they met with more adversity than in any of the others through which they travelled. They had a very unfortunate experience with six kids hanging out the back of a pick-up truck wielding baseball bats. Armed with only their bicycle pumps, Bob and Steve bravely fought them off! Climbing over the Rocky Mountains they encountered logging truckers who threatened to run them off the road with their trucks, claiming that the cyclists were slowing down their daily schedule. On another occasion, a logger came at them with a hammer: fortunately they made it out unscathed!

Finally they reached Charleston and could almost smell home. On 9 December 1994, relatives and a gang of friends that included Ollie Vigors and Emma Hawkins met them at Heathrow. We had a great welcome home breakfast, before Stephen Arnott and Nick Whishaw joined them for the final leg from Edinburgh to London.

When they reached London a week later, we celebrated their safe return with a ball at the Riverside Club, Chiswick.

Around my 65th birthday I retired from the National Health Service and my appointment in Charing Cross Hospital was terminated. While saddened at leaving a hospital that had played such an important part in my career, I looked forward to the challenges of the future. There was our family responsibility in the new Arnott Eye Centre in Harley Street and still a surgical workload in my private practice. We also had to maintain our charitable commitment to the poorer countries of the world.

Part Eight. The Final Stretch

CHAPTER 32
Surgical demands

I realized that in a very few years I would have reached my 'sell-by date', but at the moment there was no tremor in my hands, and internationally my services were still being sought. In these mature years of my career several incidents particularly stood out.

One of my patients at the Cromwell Hospital was a relative of Mrs Bhutto, the president of Pakistan, and I was invited to go to Karachi to examine Mrs Bhutto's mother-in-law, on whom I had operated some two years previously. As I was due to lecture in Mumbai in several days' time, I agreed to go from India to Pakistan, with Veronica, for 24 hours, as long as the Bhuttos made all the arrangements for our trip to coincide with a meeting in Mumbai.

We were given VIP status all the way. The diagnosis of the patient was very easy. The posterior capsule of the lens, which had been left intact after the cataract surgery, had become opaque. By simply making an opening in this membrane with the yttrium aluminium garnet (YAG) laser, vision was immediately restored and we once again had a grateful patient. All accounts were settled and a generous $1500 expenses payment was also made! Shortly after this event, the chief executive of the Cromwell Hospital asked if I would undertake a trip to Europe in total secrecy. Veronica and I arrived in Geneva a few days later, with no idea where we were staying or why. A chauffeur-driven Mercedes took us to the Intercontinental Hotel, where we were told of our mission. His Highness Sheikh Zayed bin Sultan Al Nahyan, the ruler of the Federation of the United Arab Emirates, was taking his annual holiday in Geneva to avoid the midsummer heat of his own country. We had been summoned to give a consultation concerning the prince's failing sight.

I examined him and saw that he had developed a cataract. The diagnosis and its treatment could not have been simpler. As I had been extended the hospitality of using a Swiss ophthalmic colleague's equipment, I considered that it would be courteous to involve him in the examination. Turning to him, I said: 'I would be most grateful if you would confirm my diagnosis and the treatment that is required to restore his sight.' It took little time for him to agree with my opinion and we left his clinic.

The prince's personal physician Dr Sofara then told us that they had sought numerous opinions about the prince's eye problems, including the Wills Eye

Hospital and the Johns Hopkins Hospital. But they decided to ask me to perform the operation, which was a great honour.

Veronica and I were a little concerned that our schedules for the summer might be disrupted and agreed to drop any appointment except for one week in July, when we had plans to be on holiday with Patrick and June Hodson. After weeks of hearing nothing, we were finally summoned exactly in the middle of that holiday. After some wrangling, we reluctantly decided to leave our friends in the middle of the weekend and make our way to Geneva. We took the other members of our team: John Salt, the anaesthetist, Pam Austin, the theatre sister, and Joy Andrews, our private practice manageress. John Salt was very unhappy that we had been too deferential to the needs of the prince and felt that he should have fitted in to our schedules.

As it happened, the stay was rather more prolonged than we had anticipated. Before operating on Sheikh Zayed I was asked to do surgery on the head housekeeper, who also had a dense cataract, in order to reassure the prince that he had nothing to fear. After a further 24-hour delay we were scheduled to operate the following day. That night a cavalcade of 22 Mercedes limousines left the hotel with all the royal staff to drive to the hospital in the foothills of the Alps.

Operating on a person of importance can certainly prove dramatic. As we entered the building, the tension mounted, and we were greeted by the hospital administrators with due deference to our position, mixed with sympathy for our responsibility. This small clinic had been fully equipped with a Zeiss operating microscope and the most advanced phaco machine, along with one of the Alcon managers to service it during the operation. I used my set of gold-plated instruments and my Arnott lens implants. Along with John Salt and Pam Austin, there was, of most importance, Veronica by my side.

The patient had been perfectly prepared for the operation. The only problem was the opacification of the upper half of the cornea, the result of a previous trachomatous infection of the eye that made the viewing of the operating field rather poor. If I had been an airline pilot, the flight would have been cancelled because of poor visibility. I had no option but to make the most of a difficult situation. I concentrated on doing as much as possible of the operation viewing through the lower clear portion of the cornea. As the operation proceeded, I would nudge the parts of the cataract hidden from view down to lie below the area of clear cornea, where I could remove these remnants with the phaco machine. Little by little I managed to remove the cataractous lens. The insertion of the implant was also somewhat impeded by the paucity of visibility with the semi-opaque cornea but was achieved.

After a relaxing few hours seeing Geneva we visited our patient early in the morning to attend to the first dressing. Expecting to find him lying in bed with his eye covered, we were surprised to see him sitting by the side of his bed fully dressed, impatiently awaiting our arrival. All was well and he had excellent vision. On leaving the clinic, John Salt extended his hand to say goodbye to Dr Sofara. Wagging his finger at John, Dr Sofara said: 'What do you mean goodbye? You are expected to be here to give the Sheikh his official discharge tomorrow.'

Poor John was not pleased, but he had to stay the extra day. Veronica and I could hardly suppress our amusement at this turn of events.

Over the years I performed hundreds of cataract operations on young patients with congenital or developmental cataracts. What would have previously been very hazardous or risky surgery was rendered relatively simple with the use of Charlie Kelman's machine. One in particular made a great impression. Anton Ereira had been born with healthy eyes and normal vision, until, at school, his problems started. He gradually lost his sight, and when I first saw him at the age of six his vision was seriously compromised with the development of 'Lamella cataracts'. I performed his surgery with lens implants, first on one eye and then on the other, at the Edward VII Hospital, Midhurst. His mother was a model in coping with the needs of a child in distress. Anton was able to resume life as a normal schoolboy. What was remarkable about him was the amazing grasp he had of appreciating what had been achieved. Most patients are grateful, but Anton did much more than that. Every time we met over the ensuing years he would thank me for his sight. Shortly before I retired he said: 'I am going to become an eye surgeon so that I can give to others the same sight that was restored to me.' With dedication such as this, what worries have we for the future care of our patients?

During the last 10 years of my active career in ophthalmology, Veronica and I continued to enjoy a blissful life together. On our 30th wedding anniversary she presented me with a plaque that depicted some of the highlights of our career together: paintings of a pale yellow rose and a blue Agapanthus, her two favourite flowers, a replica of the eye, within which was our totally encircling lens implant, and a badge of the Phoenix Park Racecourse. Inscribed was a quotation of Victor Hugo:

'The greatest happiness in life is the conviction that we are loved,
  Loved for ourselves,
  or rather,
  Loved in spite of ourselves.'

Over the years I can honestly say that our love for each other had not diminished – in some subtle way it just matured. I hated travelling abroad alone, but with Veronica it was pure delight. We would hold hands on the flights and be thankful that we had the next few days together. Her company enhanced everything I did. It was a feeling of mutual total completeness. We so enjoyed sharing our holidays with friends, and once went to see Francis and Marcella Dashwood in their new apartment at the Anchorage, just outside Palma in Majorca. Despite living most of the year in West Wycombe Park, one of the most beautiful National Trust Palladian houses in Britain, Francis had an inordinate pride in his new property in Majorca. He and Marcella met us at the airport and drove us through what seemed like a concrete jungle. Veronica and I were incredulous that they had chosen this part of the world for their overseas retreat until, on rounding a bend, we entered an oasis. Built around a bay, overlooking a craggy island with its own Martello tower, was a development that resembled a miniature Venice. Three tiers of mock-Venetian buildings had been built on a hill, surrounded by pine trees. Each apartment had shutters painted in a different pastel colour. In between were gardens with artistically shaped swimming pools and palm trees.

In the centre of this complex was the amenity club, which resembled a miniature Arabian sheik's palace. The Dashwoods' apartment, in an octagonal tower perched on the edge of a cliff, had a panoramic view over the sea with Magaluf and Palma Nova on the distant horizon. It wasn't hard to be enthusiastic about the place, and pretty soon we had met the local estate agent, who as it happened owned the only apartment available in this 'unique' condominium. Unwittingly, Veronica and I had become members of the community of the Anchorage.

For 10 years we enjoyed this haven of peace, which we shared with the Dashwoods, other friends and all our growing family. We even combined it with work, acting as advisors for a Palma Group of Surgeons setting up their refractive clinic.

Our apartment was a maisonette with green and blue shutters. The interior was typically Spanish with marble floors throughout, and we added Majorcan curtains and fittings. Bay doors opened directly onto the gardens, beyond which was Contessa Beach, which, early in the morning, was our own private bay. Walking along the shore and up the hill in the dawn sunshine, we would sometimes have the nearby golf course to ourselves, which meant we didn't have to worry about hindering any players behind us. With the dew still on the turf, glittering with the reflection of the early morning sun, we would make our leisurely way around the course, probably playing, in this totally relaxed atmosphere, better golf than ever before.

I would often sit on the patio writing my papers for the next international congress. I could understand why Byron and other celebrated artists found inspiration to write in these islands of the Mediterranean.

Veronica and I would try to break away to this retreat every few weeks. We managed to adopt a Continental style of living, staying up till all hours of the night listening to music, playing Scrabble or backgammon. This was an idyllic peaceful time in our lives and it seemed that we were living in an endless summer. We would return to London on Monday to resume the next week's activities.

The rest of our family had different types of holiday in our apartment. Stephen and Tania, both happily married, found the Anchorage ideal for taking their young children on a non-expensive holiday in the sun. Robert, however, was still very much a bachelor, and his wild weekends were legendary. There were never enough beds for his mass of friends and most of the guests slept on the sofas or patio. Thankfully, the majority of their entertainment took place in the local ports, but on one occasion the security guard at the club ended up fully clothed in the pool at 2 am! Fortunately, he had a sense of humour.

On another riotous evening, Bob's friends were pushing him along the jetty in a shopping trolley when they 'lost control' and the wagon with its occupant ended up in the polluted waters of the harbour. Two days later, when we joined them, the apartment had been well scrubbed and looked immaculate, but a very sick Robert was confined to bed, suffering from the ill effects of his plunge. If I had not treated him, he would have been admitted to hospital.

The normally calm Mediterranean Sea, its virtual absence of tides and the warm climate, makes Majorca one of the most idyllic islands in the world for boating. Having flirted with sailing for most of our lives, Veronica and I decided to invest in a boat, a 10-metre Sea Ray Sundancer fitted with twin diesel engines. Our new Acushla, the fourth boat we would have in our family with this name, was brought overland from Sweden to Barcelona causing numerous traffic jams along its route. When it finally arrived, Veronica skipped with joy, saying: 'It's Acushla. It's Acushla!' I had rarely seen her look happier or more radiant. The following day with Tania and Nick, we sailed the 120 miles across to Porto Cristo, Majorca. Despite being very exposed to the elements, we had an exhilarating trip, and we then spent many hours at this little harbour practising our nautical skills – turning, reversing and berthing our boat.

Every year in the harbour of Porto Cristo is the Festival of the Virgin Mary, when all the locals who own a boat go to sea with a stature of the Virgin Mary raised in the bow. The estuary is so packed with boats that you could walk over them from one jetty to the other. At an allotted time all the boats set out to sea and the statues of the Virgin are cast into the Mediterranean, thus ensuring her blessing for yet another year. That night we witnessed a glorious firework display from the comfort of our boat.

Our favourite anchoring spot was by a lighthouse on the south-east tip, where we'd swim in blue opalescent waters as we island-hopped with friends. We also joined the congregation of the Anglican church in Palma. The local incumbent the Reverend Jim Hawthorn was a very untypical priest. Having been the chaplain on the QE2 and with his Irish upbringing, he brought a very cosmopolitan atmosphere to this very parochial, but international, parish.

Jim Hawthorn became an abiding friend. After the Sunday communion service, the three of us would often make our way to a Majorcan restaurant for a lunch of sea bass wrapped in salt and baked. Jim enjoyed abandoning the cleric's habit, preferring Bermuda shorts and a T-shirt. He was a constant support, particularly comforting Veronica when her brother Charles was dying from leukaemia. He rang her every week, giving her love and consolation at this difficult time.

Lord and Lady Romsey's daughter, aged eight, also died from leukaemia on the island of Majorca while on holiday. Jim Hawthorn gave the parents the support and succour they needed over this most traumatizing period. Some two years later, Prince Andrew visited Palma in a naval minesweeper. At a function given by the British consul, the prince approached Jim Hawthorn, who for once in his life was wearing his clerical uniform, and said: 'The Romseys insisted I met you, to say how grateful they are for the support you gave them at the time of their daughter's fatal illness.' Jim Hawthorn thanked the prince for his kind words and offered to entertain him while he was in Palma.

'I have no official commitments for next Sunday but sadly will not be able to come to your church, as my presence would cause too much disruption,' replied Andrew.

So the following Sunday Jim Hawthorn went in his ancient Ford Fiesta to the Palma dockyard and drove between the mass of press photographers, who took no notice of him. He collected Prince Andrew from his ship and had passed through security before the press realized they had lost their quarry. Like baying hounds, the press leapt into their cars to chase the battered Fiesta. Jim knew all the short cuts through the city of Palma and was easily able to shake off his pursuers, heading for our apartment, where they enjoyed a quiet Chinese takeaway and bottle of wine on our patio.

Jim also introduced us to his locum, Mike Brotherton, who also shared wonderful times with us and he became a great friend. He would later become instrumental in helping Veronica with her charitable commitment to India.

CHAPTER 33
Anglo–Russian–American cooperation

By 1996 ophthalmology had entered the twenty-first century. In Charing Cross Hospital, small-incisional phaco cataract extraction had been routinely performed since late 1971, and all the residents and surgeons associated with the hospital were taught the procedure. Charlie Kelman taught Vivian Highman at the same time as me in 1970. Richard Packard, Tim Leonard, David Spalton and Paul Kinnear all learnt phaco as members of the staff.

The take-up for this advanced surgery is well demonstrated by the Wellington Hospital in London. From its opening in 1973, thousands of cataract operations were performed, but my patients were the only ones having the benefit of phaco for the next 12 years. The second surgeon to do phaco in this hospital was Arthur Steele, who started to perform it in the mid-80s. From that time onwards other surgeons rapidly started to adapt. A Moorfields Foundation was set up in the hospital, in which Alison Shutt, the matron, worked with Pam Austin, the theatre superintendent, and Mohammad Dustagheer to organize a day unit. This attracted many of the younger surgeons, which included Julian Stevens, John Dart, Paul Rosen, Mike Falcon (who had operated on Harold Ridley's cataracts), John Brazier and David Gartry. Reg Daniel, Bruce Mathalone and Calvin Townsend had been long-term users of the hospital facilities.

Our superb clinic in 22 Harley Street was expanding and treating more and more patients, and we planned to use the two operating theatres and obviate the need for an outside hospital, which would cut down the overheads.

With this in mind, on a spring day in May 1996, I drove to the Midlands for a Laser Vision board meeting. Expecting routine business only, I attended it without Stephen or Veronica. It turned out to be anything but a normal session. The acting chairman told me: 'Our American company has formulated a new strategic direction. In future we will not work in partnership with any of the satellite units spaced around the world.'

'Where does that leave us?' I asked.

'Quite simply,' he replied. 'We have decided to suspend all marketing or advertising in the Arnott Laser Vision Centre until we have gained full control and the Arnott family have resigned.'

I looked at my erstwhile friends and colleagues sitting around the table and marvelled at their duplicity. I couldn't believe that our refractive unit, developed with such care, was about to be taken over so easily by newly acquired partners, whose only input had been financial. There was nothing I could do about it, but my sadness was later alleviated by the news of our new granddaughter Isabella's birth.

As usual, Veronica knew just what to do to cheer me after the setback. We drove with our bicycles to the New Forest, and in-between finalizing the settlement with our solicitor, we forgot our cares in the sunshine of the forest, lunching at the Marina on the Hamble. Again I was reminded that true happiness is merely about being with the person you love.

In November, Veronica and I attended one of the last of 'the old school' international congresses entitled 'Phaco on the Nile' in Luxor. Even the taxi drive from the airport was a journey through history, passing an old Egyptian temple and ex-King Farouk's Winter Palace before arriving at the Sheridan Hotel.

We had a wonderful tour of some of the world's most treasured antiquities including the Valley of the Kings, where we were allowed to enter, without an escort, Tutankhamen's tomb. The following day we joined the rest of the party on the Nile river boat that would be our congress centre for the next few days. We were again surrounded by friends: David and Ann Apple, who would soon become much involved in our next ophthalmic project, the Kelman family and our German hosts Hans and Helen Koch.

That evening we crossed the river to the West Bank and went to a small village. From there we could see in the distance the Temple of Hatshepsut, which was brilliantly floodlit. Like a scene from *Aida*, we walked under a starlit desert sky towards this temple with, on either side of us, camels carrying warriors who held blazing braziers. All of this was accompanied by the sound of *The triumphal entry*. The reception was held in a large tent in front of the temple hosted by the mayor of Luxor. With a harpist and ballet dancers, it was as if we were in some bygone age. The whole of this setting was on Holy Land and the nearest conveniences were in the village more than half a mile away!

The congress was a mixture of long scientific sessions and times of escape to this different civilization. On our 36th wedding anniversary, during dinner, Veronica and I were presented with an anniversary cake, after which all the members of the congress did a conga around the tables. We were all in Egyptian dress and Veronica chose stunning red robes topped with a royal fez.

The scientific sessions were held while the ship made her way towards Aswan. Most of the surgeons' wives would spend this time lounging around the decks, but Veronica was much in demand for her exercise classes. The last night of our stay in Egypt was spent in the Old Cataract Hotel. From this hotel we visited the Low Dam, built in 1902 by the British, and the High Dam, built by President Nasser and Russia in 1962. That evening we mounted camels for the trek up the mountainside to a site where we pitched tent for dinner. It seemed strange squatting in the middle of the desert, surrounded by camels and their handlers, in the company of all our ophthalmic friends!

Richard Packard sat next to Veronica on the flight home and for the first time intimated that he might be interested in taking over the Arnott Eye Centre when I retired.

Stephen and I spent many hours organizing a symposium to celebrate 25 years of phaco surgery in the UK and Europe. This was to take place in Chester, in the autumn of 1997, during the annual UK Implant and Refractive meeting. This symposium was actually taking place one year too late, as the first phaco operation in Europe was performed by me in the Fulham branch of Charing Cross Hospital on 27 October 1971. A silver plaque recording this event is one of the most treasured possessions I have from Veronica.

We were very privileged to have so many of our family with us, alongside our treasured staff of Joy Andrews and Pam Austin. Our greatest ophthalmic friends, Charles Kelman, Bob Sinskey, David Apple and Svyatoslav Fyodorov, with their wives, flew in from America and Russia. We also shared this occasion with the next generation of surgeons: Paddy Condon, Richard Packard and Helen Seward.

After this congress, Svyatoslav Fyodorov came to stay with us at Trottsford. By this time in 1997 he was recognized as the foremost Russian ophthalmic surgeon. He had recently opened a large ophthalmic hospital in Moscow, which was best known for conveyor-belt surgery, in which each surgeon performed only one stage of the operation. Patients on trollies laid out in a circle would pass from one surgeon to the next as the cataract operation progressed. If a surgeon overran his time, a bell would be rung and the conveyor belt would stop.

He established his own political party 'The People's Party for Self-Governing,' and in 1996 stood for election as a candidate for the president of the Russian Federation and received more than six million votes. Although his profile was high, it was not enough to get him elected, but he was elevated to the State Duma of the Federal Assembly of the Russian Federation. Svyatoslav had a very simple philosophy. He felt that the Russian people would work harder, live longer and be better motivated if they were rewarded according to the amount and quality of their work. He believed that the land and factories should be given back to the workers of Russia, who would organize their own management. In this way productivity and prosperity could be restored to their country. He partly adopted this system in his own vast hospital complex. Each member of staff, from Fyodorov to the most junior hospital porter, didn't take a salary, but shared a percentage of the net profits, according to their seniority. The number of patients treated and the anticipated resulting profit was illuminated on a large electronic notice board in the reception.

Svyatoslav introduced many other innovations into ophthalmology and had some 16 satellite eye units around Russia. For some years he had a small converted cruise ship, based in Gibraltar, which was essentially a floating ophthalmic hospital. His Western colleagues were both envious and sceptical

of this unit. After running very profitably for years under the total control of
Svyatoslav, the administrators, crew and some of the medical staff organized
a management buy-out. Svyatoslav in Russia was powerless to preserve his
interest in this ship. Without his support, the unit soon got into financial difficulties and bankruptcy followed within the year. This once graceful hospital is
now a rusting hulk in some Greek harbour.

Fyodorov had always been keen to restart another international eye centre,
and he invited Veronica, Stephen and me to join him in developing a new land-
based Gibraltar International Eye Institute, as a joint partnership born out of
our 25 years of friendship. Slava was fascinated by Veronica, partly because she
was half-Russian, but also by how her family had been so totally integrated
into the British way of life. Svyatoslav had been seriously defrauded by some
of his international ophthalmic colleagues and he often told Veronica that ours
was one of the few families he totally trusted. He put this into practice and
very much used Veronica as his overseas agent. He would call weekly with oft-
times impossible requests. The phone would ring and my wife would hear:
'V-e r-o-n-i-c-a. Could you please find a racehorse for me?' Or on another
occasion: '. . . a new back axle for my 1994 Mercedes Model S motorcar.' His
most difficult request was when he asked Stephen to find him a helicopter. We
put him in contact with George, Marquis of Milford-Haven, who was himself
a helicopter pilot. With arrangements having been made, the Fyodorovs came
to stay with us at Trottsford. A friend, Tony Spooner, drew a large white circle
on our lawn as a temporary helicopter pad. George took us all on a memorable
run to London – an hour's drive away but flown in only 12 minutes. Air traffic
control stacked our helicopter exactly over the Houses of Parliament to allow
a plane to take off from the City airport. There we were, hovering over the
most security-sensitive building in the country, in a craft piloted by a cousin
of the Queen, with one of the passengers being number six in the Russian
Politburo!

Slava immediately 'hit it off' with George Milford-Haven, and they became
good friends. As a result of this flight, a second-hand French helicopter,
ex-Yugoslavian Army, was delivered to Russia some months later.

We went many times to Moscow to plan arrangements for Gibraltar and
were always given VIP status. The Fyodorovs loved entertaining us in their
Dacha in Slavino, a substantial estate on the Volga River, 60 km from Moscow.
Nobody was allowed to own land in Russia and this estate was, in fact, an
extension of the world-famous Moscow Eye Microsurgical Complex.

Svyatoslav was a great philanthropist: he built dozens of chalets, all
with their own plot of land for his hospital employees and sold to them
to them at a discounted price. There was a health and recreational resort,
complete with a sports centre, gymnasium and swimming pool. The barren
wilderness of land was restocked with pedigree cattle and sheep. Milk, cream,
cheese and mushrooms were produced for the local community and the pure
spring water of the estate was bottled and sold throughout Russia. There

was also a Fyodorov hotel, restaurant, congress centre and an ophthalmic hospital.

Nearby was a derelict church, the Nativity of Our Lady, which had been stripped of all its ancient treasures after the Bolshevik Revolution. When the Fyodorovs started to restore this church, the ancient relics started to reappear. One by one the descendants of the local inhabitants returned the long-lost altar cross, icons, paintings and chalice. The golden dome of the church once again became the most prominent landmark, and an Orthodox priest was employed to administer to the community.

On our visits to Slavino we would spend hours with Svyatoslav and Irine – Slava in his chair by the fire, playing with his worry beads – swapping stories and discussing our very variant lives. But we had much in common too: Slava and Irine were as close as is possible for two human beings to be. They adored their children and doted on the other Slava, who was their grandchild. Young Slava with his mother Elina would often visit us in England. In all, we spent some considerable time in Russia, permitted to live as the Russians did then, and felt very honoured to have done so.

Everything in Svyatoslav's conversation was prefixed with the word 'beautiful', almost as if this was an expression of his own appreciation of life. Rather like my own Great Grandfather, the first Sir John Arnott, he felt that much of what he had acquired, during his successful career, should be given to the community. His worker's Self-Government Party, of which he was the leader with some 6,000,000 members, upheld the policy that the land and assets of Russia should be returned to the people, thus giving them an incentive to work and earn their own profits.

The proposed Eye Institute of Gibraltar would uphold many of these ideals: it would be international and serve the needs of NHS, charitable and private patients. We hoped many patients would bring their families and combine their treatment with a holiday in the warm Mediterranean sun.

Surgeons, doctors, nurses, technicians and administrators would also be employed from the 'market of the world'. Situated at the gateway between Europe and Africa, in the Mediterranean, it would have the benefit of being under British jurisdiction.

One of the venture capitalists raising the finance for this project was Mark Klabin, Svyatoslav's financial advisor and president of the Rosh Group. His family had a security-guarded property in Ascot, just two miles from Windsor Castle. Mark would be financing the clinic along with the Cambridge Research and Advisory Group (CRAG), another Anglo–Russian company chaired by Lord Whaddon. The most charismatic member of this company was Professor Vladimir Krislov, a scientist who had previously been involved in the Russian Space Programme supervising the surface coating of the satellite rockets and ensuring that they were smooth to within a few nanometres. With the end of the cold war, he was offered an appointment as a professor at Cambridge University, England. Another major investor would be Gary Tcherepakhor, whose agency made a fortune by selling cigarettes to Russia after the collapse of the Berlin wall. Such was the shortage and demand that cigarettes became an unofficial currency for barter.

Veronica seemed to be regaining her former Russian roots. She adored attending ballet performances at the Bolshoi in Moscow or the Kirov in St Petersburg. We once spoiled ourselves with a holiday on the Orient Express, a train that, twice a year, makes the longest rail trip in the world from Moscow to Beijing. A Swiss company had bought a number of pre-war Pullman railway carriages, one of which had been converted to shower rooms and two to dining cars, which served both French and conventional cuisine. All the wooden carriages were brightly painted green, yellow or red, and outside each was an attendant in red livery uniform. Our cabin was all Edwardian grace: it had walnut walls, chintz curtains, a writing desk and a spacious sofa. We were summoned to dinner and told to leave our room unlocked. Returning later, we found it converted into a bedroom. Our main companions on this trip were Peter Walter, a professional traveller in his 80s, and Ronald and Ginette Smallwood, a couple from Yorkshire.

For the first 24 hours our train was non-stop as it passed through Yaroslav, across the Volga River and over the Ural Mountains. Our first stop was at Tobol, the City of Tears, and the farewell point for those who once were sent into exile in Siberia. At Novosibirsk, 'the Chicago of Siberia', we walked around the cathedral and into the market. Our preconception that the Russians were poor and starving was totally altered: there were counters colourfully laden with vegetables, spices, fish, meat and all other types of food produce. This was not a show put on for visitors, as we were the only tourists within some hundreds of miles.

We travelled on through the Taiga Forest, which accounts for about 40% of Russia's landmass. At Irkutsk we learned how Russian aristocrats, exiled here after a failed coup against Tsar Nicholas I in the 1820s, had brought architecture, culture and efficient farming methods to this remote spot. The town, with its hall, market, shops and houses, could have been a colonial outpost in any corner of the world. The stone church, with leaded window panes, was typically mid-nineteenth century, and in yards of the porch was the tomb of a Russian princess, who had made the long journey from Moscow single-handed on a horse-drawn sledge to join her husband.

Stopping to paddle in Lake Baikal, we found it hard to remember that we were in the so-called barren arctic land of Siberia, as all around us were fruit trees, chickens, geese and ducks and evidence of the smallholder's efficient farming methods. Like children, we played with our friends the Smallwoods in the cabin of an abandoned steam engine, pretending we were the drivers and firemen.

It took 24 hours to circumnavigate the shore of Lake Baikal, the largest clear-water lake in the world, before we climbed over the Steppes and Plains to enter

Mongolia. We stopped at Ulan Bator, the capital city, from where Genghis Khan had set out to conquer the world. We were driven to the Mongolian Plains and spent the best part of the day with a nomadic tribe. Since time immemorial these people had been roaming these vast spaces with their horses, goats and cattle. During our visit, most of the men were racing their ponies around the wide open plain in preparation for the annual Mongolian Horse Show, the highlight of their year.

These nomads lived in large round tents built around an open central fire, which was fuelled by dried dung. Over tea one of the families told us their story: 'We were relieved to have been freed from occupation by the Russians, who pilfered most of our food and substituted it with a ration of tomatoes and potatoes. Our staple diet is goat's milk and meat, so we found this unpalatable. We are very concerned that, with the introduction of compulsory education for the children, our nomadic independence will come to an end.' We found these people, so far away from modern civilization, very erudite and interested at having this rare talk with friends from another existence.

That night our train went over the Gobi Desert, the highest in the world, before descending to the Chinese border, to the end of our epic journey. It says something about the hygiene of our Swiss hosts that, on this long rail journey, there was not a single case of food poisoning. From China we flew back to London.

On a cold autumn morning, in 1997, Veronica, Stephen and I went with Svyatoslav Fyodorov and Vladimir Kislov, the Russian agent of CRAG, to Gibraltar to see the home of our new unit. We met Gerry Nash, a genial Irish businessman, who would become a very integral part of our team. On this short visit we had meetings with Albert Isola, our legal advisor, and drew up plans for the marketing structure and financing of the company. We met the tourist minister, the Honorable Joseph Holliday, who was very aware of the boost that this project would give to their economy.

CHAPTER 34
Sai Baba and the Indian dream

Shortly after returning from Gibraltar, and some 20 years after our first visit to India, we received an invitation from Sai Baba to teach phaco and lens implantation in a hospital in Puttaparthy, which had recently been built for the treatment of ophthalmic and renal conditions. Bhagavan Sri Sathya Sai Baba was an Indian Swami who lived in an Ashram that was the focus for millions of devotees from around the world. He had built a community founded on principles of love, truth and peace and had an international reputation as a guru, miracle worker and healer.

Many international surgeons were always asking to help with the surgery at the Sai Baba Hospital in Puttaparthy, but none was welcomed without the express permission of Sai Baba himself. Veronica and I never knew why, from surgeons available from all around the world, we had been chosen. It may have had something to do with Major Upadhyay, who was also invited along with Pam Austin. Accompanying us on the flight were 15 tea chests containing medical equipment for Sai Baba's Hospital, the Sri Sathya Sai General, brought by Drs Bishwanathan and Kirin, which passed through customs without a single one being opened. We felt honoured to have been chosen to work in his hospital, although we little knew how life changing this trip would be.

After travelling for some 20 hours we arrived in Bangalore and the next day made the drive to Puttaparthy through uninhabited but beautiful countryside of high stone hills and vast areas of prairie. Then suddenly we could see well-tended farms and the road became smooth. We went through several arches proclaiming our entrance to Puttaparthy. The town had tree-lined streets, modern well-designed buildings and even a cricket field, which had a pavilion like the one at Lord's.

We finally arrived at a block of flats, to be met by our rather agitated host, Jit Aggarwal, who said: 'Why are you so late? We will almost certainly miss the meeting.' Like the Mad Hatter running to the tea party, Veronica and I had no idea where we were going as we were rushed into the street. We finally arrived at a stadium, little smaller than our own Wembley, where Veronica was taken to a separate part.

I entered the hall and, shoeless, followed my host across the vast crowded arena towards 'the veranda', which was reserved for important visitors, the academic professors of the schools and the senior members of the hospital. I picked my way through the guests, who were all wearing white trousers and tunics. They were sitting cross-legged in rows, facing a large carved Indian teak door, which was closed. I was ushered up to the front row and joined my companions in the same sitting position, feeling rather exposed in my grey trousers and blue blazer.

The ceremony had not as yet started and I had time to take in my surroundings. Some two yards in front of me was this ornate closed door. To my left was an opening into an atrium that could seat 100 people. In the front of this smaller hall was a raised red throne, and to either side and behind me were the rows of elders, squatting in the veranda. To my right was the vast expanse of the main hall, filled with thousands of devotees, with the ladies segregated from the gentlemen. Far across the hall I could just make out Veronica, who was sitting in the front row with Mrs Aggarwal and Pam Austin. During holy weeks, up to one quarter of a million devotees would be in or around the Ashram. The interior of the building was beautifully appointed. The glass roof was supported by light pink colonnades embossed in gold. The side walls did not extend to the ceiling, and birds flew in and out of the hall through this gap, as monkeys scampered along the top of the wall. There was a red carpet leading to the steps of the veranda. The thousands of people talking to each other in a whisper produced the effect of a low-pitched murmur, which was accentuated by the acoustics of the hall.

Suddenly there was a hush, as a diminutive person entered the Ashram through the far entrance. It was Sai Baba himself. The swami was wearing a plain plum-coloured robe, and he had a thick thatch of black hair that stood up and outwards, like a coronet around his head. His tanned face was creased with the experience of his 70 years in this world. He glided rather than walked up the red carpet in the centre of the hall, stopping to collect letters from devotees. The entire congregation, sitting cross-legged, held their hands together, as if in prayer, and followed his progress with their gaze. Having reached the veranda, he turned to the crowd and raised his hands in salutation, before mounting the steps.

When on the veranda he turned to me and in a gentle voice, with impeccable English said: 'Are you alone?'

'No,' I replied. 'My wife is in the hall.'

'I will see your wife with you tomorrow, in the meantime come with me.' Having thus spoken, he gestured to two students, two Russian ladies, a Dr Taylor, the major and me to go with him. He opened the big door and we followed him into a small room, in the corner of which was an ornate throne of ebony wood and red leather upholstery, on which he sat. The men squatted, with crossed legs, on the left and the ladies against the wall on the right. He wanted to know about my wife.

'She is Russian?' said the Major.

'No, she is not Russian,' replied Swami. 'Veronica is only half Russian.'

He seemed to know our thoughts, and his questions were only asked out of courtesy. He then turned to the two students and exhorted them to maintain the virtues of morality and truth. After this audience we all returned to our places in the main hall. Swami joined us later, as prayers and singing continued for the next hour. The incantations started with 'om', the creation, and then continued to bless all the other main religions. Despite my lack of knowledge of the language, I could make out references to Jesus Christ and Christianity. Sitting in the front row of the veranda I was the only person in the main hall who had a full view of Sai Baba. He faced his choir but seemed to be in deep meditation throughout. After the service we were introduced to Dr Sufaya, the principal of the hospital, and Dr Deepak Khosla, the senior ophthalmic surgeon. Outside the Ashram, joining up with Veronica and the other ladies, we walked through the town to the canteen. The bustling town had been built almost entirely by the SAI Foundation. In an inner area were the Ashram, houses and apartments for the staff, the canteen and hostels for invited guests such as us. The crowded streets were essentially filled with the devotees of Sai Baba, who had arrived from all the corners of the world to be in his presence. Some had come to spend time in Puttaparthy during their holiday in India, while others had spent months or years in the complex hoping to finally have an audience. It is recorded that one lady waited 20 years before personally meeting Swami.

On arriving at the canteen, Veronica and I were once again segregated. The food was vegetarian, mostly coming from the well-irrigated local fertile land. Apart from the segregation of the sexes, eating was communal, and we piled our trays with food, just as we had done at school. After supper, once again united with Veronica, our party wandered around the streets. The Aggarwals finally showed us to our accommodation in one of the hostels. Everyone working here was a volunteer: the night porter in our hostel turned out to be a high court judge. We met people from every background and religion and marvelled at the international flavour and theme of love and giving that emanated from everyone in this holy place.

The rooms were built around an open courtyard. Our bedroom was a bit of a shock – a far cry from the luxury we were used to: it had four walls, a window and a door into the bathroom. The only decoration in the room was the picture of a smiling swami. On the bare floor was a dressing table, with no mirror, and two single iron-framed beds with steel springs. The beds had austere paper-thin mattresses, with an overlying sheet and an excuse for a duvet. Clothes were to be hung from a clothesline strung across the room. The en suite bathroom was equally austere, but at least there was a flushing loo and the thrill of a cold shower.

Trying to get comfortable, we pondered this situation. Christianity had always motivated our lives, yet here we were meeting Swami, whom many people considered as some type of deity. Was this a challenge to our Christian faith or should we reject him as an impostor vying against our own Christian religion?

We had always opened our medical practice to all denominations and creeds. Among my patients were bishops and clerics, Coptic priests from Sudan, archbishops of the Greek Orthodox Church, a holy man in Burma, the Muslim mufti of Jerusalem and countless rabbis, as well as untold numbers of leaders of the Hindu, Buddhist and Muslim faiths.

Veronica and I talked through the night about the importance of respect and the right of all to have allegiance to their chosen calling. We agreed that each being must be free to determine their religion and the influence it would have to guide them through life. Amazingly, that night increased not only our own faith but gave us an added tolerance to understand others. We ended our long meditation by reading a quotation from a book about Bhagavan Sri Sathya Sai Baba.

'I have come to light the lamp of love in your hearts, to see that it shines, day by day, with added lustre. I have not come on a mission of publicity for a sect or creed or cause, nor have I come to collect followers for a doctrine. I have no plan to attract disciples or devotees into my fold or any fold. I have come to tell you of this unitary faith, this spiritual principle, this path of love, this virtue of love. This way of love, which leads into the real truth of life?'

With these words still sounding in our ears we fell into a deep sleep, only to be woken at four in the morning by the Muslim call to prayer. We were due in the Ashram for the morning prayers just as dawn was breaking. All the ladies wore brightly coloured saris, so the hall was as pretty as the Chelsea Flower Show.

Hundreds of schoolchildren came in a single file to take their places in the hall and squatting cross-legged on the ground took out their textbooks to continue their studies. The buzz of conversation ceased when Sai Baba entered the Ashram and made across the hall and up the steps to the veranda. He came straight up to me and said: 'Please bring in your wife and guest.'

I stood up in front of the thousands of the assembled congregation and gesticulated to my wife, some hundred yards away, to follow us into Swami's sanctum. Sai Baba invited several other guests to join him. After two minutes, Veronica and Pam came into the room. Seeing me sitting against the left-hand wall, they immediately joined me. Looking rather amused Swami said: 'Come come ladies, you cannot do that here. You are not in London now.'

Once Veronica was seated in the correct place, Baba gave her his full attention: 'Do you believe in me?' Veronica was surprised and did not know how to respond. She looked to me for guidance and I nodded my head, which suggested that we wished to have his friendship.

'Yes, I believe,' said Veronica.

Sai Baba lifted his right arm above his head and produced from thin air a gold pendant bearing his image. Over the next years Veronica always wore this Sai Baba medallion around her neck, along with her enamel Russian Orthodox cross, which so symbolized her Christian commitment in life.

Sai Baba next looked at me and said: 'Come closer to me.'

In my squatting position, I shuffled across the floor towards him. He once again lifted his right arm and produced a large gold ring, with a Peridot stone, which he placed on my finger. This part of the proceedings over, he stood up and ushered Veronica, Pam Austin and myself into yet another and smaller room. Swami sat in the middle of this room, with Veronica on his left and me on his right. Pam Austin sat on the floor in front of us. Baba turning to me said: 'You are a kind man, but you have a conflict, which in the course of time you will resolve and come to understand.'

It was as if he had heard our discussion last night! He then turned his attention to Veronica. Here we were, the two of us, talking to Swami in private audience, while thousands of devotees were waiting in the hall, anxious for his reappearance.

He said to Veronica: 'This is your home, and you are welcome to return here any time you wish.' During the minutes we had been talking together, Swami had been gently tapping my hand. After some minutes, he turned to me and said: 'You can now leave to start operating on my patients.'

'Swami,' I said, 'I will do my best.'

'No,' he replied, 'it will be the best.'

With that we left his presence.

The Sri Sathya Sai Hospital was like a miniature Taj Mahal. In the centre of the complex was a large dome, central to two main wings – one serving renal and the other ophthalmic conditions. Blockages of the urinary tract were a major problem in that part of the world because the levels of calcium in the water were so high. As in the rest of India, the other scourge was the opacification of the lens, a cataract, which could affect patients at any age. Sai Baba had built this specialist hospital with the aim of relieving the suffering of patients with renal or ophthalmic problems. Subsequent to our visit a cardiac unit was developed.

We entered through the central domed area, marvelling at the two-ton Venetian glass chandelier, which had been donated by the president of Italy. As in the rest of the hospital, the floor was paved with marble. We changed and entered the sterile area of the ophthalmic theatre and found ourselves in a perfectly appointed unit. It had closed-circuit television for watching the surgery in progress, and all the latest equipment, including a brand new phaco machine. Our function was to train the ophthalmologists to use this machine. In three days we had to teach the surgeons how to do an operation that normally took at least 50 hours to master.

I demonstrated the first two operations and thereafter acted as assistant to Dr Deepak Khoshla and his surgical team. We operated throughout the first day, only breaking off to attend prayers in the Ashram. As always, Veronica was by my side giving her support and at times advice, having witnessed many such days in other hospitals around the world. The following morning, after prayers, we again went to the hospital and examined the post- and preoperative patients before starting the surgery for the day. The first patient on whom I had operated the previous day had been blind for 20 years, despite being only in his mid-50s. When his eye dressing was removed, he leapt out of his chair and ran around the outpatient department, yelling in Hindi: 'I can see, I can see.' He finally ended up on Veronica's lap and started to hug her and cry, with thanks for his visual salvation. All the other patients had normal results and we continued to teach for the next few days, with Pam Austin teaching her counterparts how to handle the instruments. Inevitably there were some difficulties and complications, but on the whole the week passed without any major incidents.

By the Saturday afternoon our training session had been completed and it was time to say goodbye. With Jit and Haim Aggarwal, we went for final prayer session in the Ashram. I sat as usual in the front row, finding it more and more difficult to sit cross-legged, as the minutes drifted into hours. That evening Sai Baba did not give audiences but spent the time wandering through the hall talking to members of the congregation. We were in the Ashram from 4.30 pm until 7 pm and finally had to take our leave during the final prayers.

We left the city as dusk was falling and started the long drive back to Bangalore. Daylight driving is difficult enough in the narrow roads of India, but in the dark it's a nightmare. All the oncoming lorries drive in the middle of the road, often with one or no headlights, and will swerve to avoid a collision only at the last possible moment. Our journey was made even more uncomfortable by the fact that our driver, Ismile, decided to stop for his dinner in a village with a large unmade road, on which all the inhabitants with their animals seemed to be wandering. There were no street lights and the only illumination came from the surrounding stores and stalls. Ismile walked off into the night leaving us three Westerners alone in the car and, while the natives were in no way threatening, we did feel a long way from home. After some half an hour, Ismile returned and we continued on our journey.

As we were approaching Bangalore, I began to feel anxious as to whether or not I had really fulfilled my function of training the surgeons at that hospital. Some new techniques and minor improvements had been introduced to phaco procedures in recent years. Howard Gimbel, from Calgary, had developed a method of making a circular tear in the anterior capsule of the lens, which gave the rim of the opening more tensile strength. He also introduced the 'divide and conquer' technique for emulsifying the nucleus of the lens. While formerly we had phaco-emulsified the intact nucleus, making it smaller and smaller as the procedure continued, Howard advocated splitting the nucleus before removing the fragments with the phaco. A rock-hard nucleus was easier to emulsify and remove when split into two or more fragments. I had totally omitted to teach this advanced form of phaco-emulsification to the ophthalmic surgeons in Puttaparthy.

I sat in the car feeling more and more miserable as we approached Bangalore. Veronica and I were due to have two days holiday in the hills, before returning to the UK. As we arrived at Bangalore, at midnight, I turned to Veronica and said: 'Darling, I am terribly sorry, but I will have to return to Puttaparthy to finalize the training.'

With incredible grace she replied: 'Sitting next to you in the car I realized that you had a problem, and of course I will come back with you.' Any disappointment that she may have felt at forsaking our holiday was not shown. Shrini Shrinivasan, the Indian manager of Alcon, said that he would personally act as our chauffeur for the long day's return trip.

On Sunday we had a respite from our teaching duties. In the morning we went to a totally unsatisfactory Anglican service, where the theme of the sermon was 'Beware of false prophets'. We never did find out whether or not the insinuations referred to Sai Baba. That afternoon we took a taxi to the Nandi Hills, some 1000 feet high and filled with ruins of old Muslim fortresses. We had a walk along a cliff, which had a sheer drop down to the plains below.

At 4.30 am on the following morning, Veronica, Shrini and I started on our journey back to Puttaparthy. It was a clear sunny dawn and we saw the Indian countryside at its best, arriving at 8.30 am. By now the ophthalmic surgical team were quite adept at doing the phaco procedure, so I was able to introduce the advanced procedure without too much difficulty.

During the first phaco operation of the morning, under my supervision, Dr Dhipal Khoshla made a neat microincision into the anterior chamber of the eye, following which he tore the anterior capsule, as advocated by Howard Gimbel, and produced a neat circular opening in it. Following this he injected a small amount of fluid between the inner surface of the lens capsular bag and the contained lens contents, thus mobilising the lens nucleus. I sat by his side, full of admiration at the way he had mastered this form of surgery. Next he performed the part of the operation that had necessitated our return to the theatre. Using the tip of the phaco machine, he made a deep groove on the exposed upper surface of the nucleus. Into this groove was put the phaco tip and the end of a spatula, and, with counter pressure between the ends of these two instruments, he started to split the nucleus into two halves. Bingo! He had succeeded in completing this modification to the operation. He then removed each fragment of the split nucleus and finished the operation in the usual way.

By the time we were called to prayers in the afternoon, I knew that we had completed our mission. Before leaving Puttaparthy we went to the Ashram for the evening prayers, knowing that we would have to leave before the end of the service. I once again was ushered to the front row of the veranda and assumed that Swami would bid us farewell before we left his city.

I sat cross-legged, anticipating a fond farewell from Swami and grateful thanks for the work we had done. My wishes were not fulfilled. Feeling slightly chastened, I followed my hosts to our car, which was parked close to the entrance of the Ashram. Veronica and the ladies joined us a little time later, with many of our friends and ophthalmic colleagues.

As I climbed into the car, I said to Veronica: 'I am a little hurt that Swami did not say goodbye to us.'

Veronica looked at me and produced from her handbag a picture of Swami, with his right arm held up in a gesture of farewell, which was signed 'With love, Baba.' She explained to me, that while sitting with the ladies and thousands of other members of the congregation, an elegant Greek lady had come and asked her: 'Are you the doctor's wife?'

'I am a doctor's wife,' Veronica replied.

'No, you are *the* doctor's wife,' she replied, 'and Swami asked me to give you this picture of his farewell to you.'

I came away feeling that Sai Baba was one of the most dynamic and fascinating men I've ever met. Many years later when Veronica was ill, the 'vibuti' dust that Sai Baba gave to those who needed healing became more important to her than the chemotherapy she was receiving. There was a trust between us all that was very tangible but not once did it compromise our faith in Christ.

We felt totally inspired that Sai Baba intended us to do further work for the blind patients of India. Shrini gave us a statue of Ganesh, a symbol of unity and cooperation on a long-term project. It was during that drive that the three of us prepared the concept of the mobile eye phaco operating unit, which would be the first in Asia.

CHAPTER 35
The Eye Institute of Gibraltar

Before the year was out we made one more trip to Russia, this time accompanied by Gerry Nash. We stayed at the Fyodorov Hilton Hotel alongside the Eye Institute in Moscow and were escorted everywhere by Natasha Guomeniouk. Natasha was a pretty young Russian, whose looks were slightly affected by the hair loss she had suffered as a result of exposure to nuclear radiation after the Chernobyl explosion. On our first night in Moscow we attended the Moscovitch Theatre and saw Prokofiev's *Romeo and Juliet*, and on the second we watched the Bolshoi School of Ballet. Our days were taken up meeting Yuri Lagarev, with other members of the eye institute, to organize the ordering of equipment for the Gibraltar clinic. We went with Svyatoslav to St Petersburg for one day to take part in festivities to mark the 10th anniversary of the local Fyodorov Eye Institute. The hospital was full of television companies and journalists, and it was patently obvious that there was no need for this clinic to spend money on advertising.

In the evening we sat next to Yuri Lagarev at a banquet given for the 200 members of his staff. While in St Petersburg with Gerry Nash, Elena and young Slava we visited the breathtakingly beautiful Tsarskoye Selo, otherwise known as Pushkin's Village, and the Sheremetzer Palace. Veronica enjoyed these trips to Russia more than those to any other country, and in St Petersburg she had so much pleasure seeing the officer cadet military establishments, where her father had been trained in the earlier part of the century. On our last night in Slavino there was more than a foot of snow on the ground, with an outside temperature of −30°C. That evening a Korean dinner party had been arranged in the Slavino Fyodorov Hotel to celebrate our partnership, and we had to contend with traditional Russian hospitality. Initially all went well, and before dinner we played billiards while enjoying our aperitifs. Problems arose the moment we had commenced the Korean feast. Slava stood up and said: 'A toast to Veronica!' Everybody rose and downed a glass of vodka in one gulp. With glasses recharged, Slava immediately called for another toast. Each member of the party was individually toasted before the horizon was enlarged and the toasts became more general. I realized that Veronica, Stephen, Gerry Nash and I had reached the limits of our capabilities to toast. Standing up, I thanked our hosts for their hospitality and suggested that we should continue the evening without further ceremonies.

'Oh Eric, you do not love us,' said Irine Fyodorov in an assumed aggrieved voice. My pleas had fallen on deaf ears and our celebrations continued. At some stage in the evening Irine entertained us by singing Russian folk songs with an exquisite voice. I was carried down the stairs of the hotel at the end of the evening, propped up by Stephen and Svyatoslav. None of our British party fared any better than myself, but that evening did further cement a friendship that was already very close.

At this time, along with our ever-increasing involvement with Russia, we were committed to the development of the mobile phaco eye unit for the eye camps of India. Having spent some months developing the groundwork for the development of this unit, Mother Fortune smiled on us.

A week after returning from holiday, a patient came to our practice in Harley Street for a final postoperative check-up. Jafar Askari was a very successful Armenian who lived between Saudi Arabia, New York and France. On this final visit to my consulting rooms after his ophthalmic operation, I heard him talking to my manageress, Joy, who said: 'I am glad you came today, as last week Mr Arnott was away in Germany collecting his new Mercedes SLK.'

'I could easily have supplied him with one of those cars,' he replied.

I pricked up my ears and immediately became interested as to whether or not he could help us in our charity. I gave Jafar an examination and found that his vision was entirely normal. He could now return to his normal jet-executive life. After finishing his consultation I told him: 'We have a dream to produce a mobile phaco eye unit, which would be driven out to the remote villages of India to treat blind patients with cataract.'

Jafar was a no-nonsense businessman and immediately replied: 'I will help your dream and give you a Mercedes Benz truck.'

Up until this time in the spring of 1998, no other funds had been raised, but Tony Spooner agreed to act as treasurer on our, as yet, non-existent charity. Veronica needed someone else to support her as a fundraiser and she asked Lyn Wood, a friend of Tania's, to become involved. Veronica herself spent many hours a day striving to raise the necessary funds. Miranda Cordle, who had grown up with Veronica, and her husband, Anthony, allowed us to piggyback on their charity, the Penny Trust. Not only had Jafar Askari persuaded the directors of Mercedes to donate a lorry, but we were also allowed to use their name and call our charity the Penny Trust Mercedes Benz Mobile Eye Unit, or MBMEU for short.

Immediately after setting up this trust, Veronica and I went to Charleston, West Virginia, for a small international congress organized by David Apple, who was the professor of ocular pathology at the Storm Eye Institute. David Apple held a unique position in American ophthalmology, having been given the responsibility to analyse, in his laboratory, any intraocular lens implant that had to be removed from a patient's eye in any of the states of the US. In this way, David became the world authority on complications associated with cataract extraction and lens implantation. He had written a number of books, including a 1000-page atlas on lens implantation, and was much sought after as an international speaker. Also with us were a few other ophthalmic colleagues, such as Charlie Kelman, and we had all been invited to discuss the current state of cataract surgery.

Following this meeting, Veronica and I flew with David and Ann Apple to Tucson, Arizona, to spend a few days at a health centre, where we invited the Apples to join us in the Gibraltar project, which was to be called the Fyodorov Arnott Apple International Eye Institute of Gibraltar.

With our team now complete, we returned to Gibraltar. Svyatoslav and Irine Fyodorov flew in from Russia, bringing with them Boris Feldman, their hospital designer. We ourselves had come over from the UK with Pieter van der Westhuizen, of Hemax Health Care, who would be in charge of equipping the operating theatres, and Max Elliot, the architect. On the managerial side, Gerry Nash joined Stephen. To complete our group, David and Ann Apple arrived from America. With this group we made our first visit to Europort, which we hoped would house our new hospital. This was a vast, still totally empty complex, built on reclaimed marshland by the side of the docks. The centre block had been designed as a hotel and to either side were two extensive multi-storey wings. The whole building, which had been beautifully architected with pale yellow marble-like walls and large blue-tinted windows, faced south and overlooked the Mediterranean. While we were shown around the western wing, Boris Feldman, the Russian designer, suggested that for reasons of security and privacy, we should be housed on the second rather than, as had been planned, the ground floor. With the Fyodorovs and Apples, we wandered around the vast empty space of this floor, establishing where we would have the outpatient department, administrative offices, inpatient ward, a laboratory and operating suites. As we envisaged having teaching seminars and demonstrations, we also planned for a congress hall and library. Throughout this visit to our proposed clinic, the Mediterranean sun poured in through the windows and outside was the blue shimmering sea.

We met Albert Isola, our Gibraltan solicitor, to discuss the legal complexities of the proposed clinic. With the help of the chief minister, Peter Caruana, planning permission had been granted and contracts signed. It would be many months before we would even start to construct this unit, but we looked forward to having eventually the most unique international eye institute in Europe, if not the world. We finalized our meeting by having a lunchtime party on a sailing schooner, which was skippered around the island. Once again with 'the labours of the week completed,' our diverse group of Russian, American and British comrades had a fine party. I slightly disgraced myself by falling overboard halfway through lunch.

We stayed over in Gibraltar for the weekend to learn about the place that would soon become our second home. Svyatoslav had hurt himself the previous week, falling off his Harley Davidson motorbike, and retired to bed with a thrombosis in his leg. Stephen and Kathy stayed up until 4.30 in the morning, talking with Gerry Nash and Albert Poggio, the director of the Gibraltar office in London.

On Sunday morning we had time to appreciate the real beauty of this ancient city: we visited St Trinity, the holy cathedral of Gibraltar, and the King's Chapel and then wandered along the Queensway Wharf before being taken to explore the rock's labyrinth of tunnels. For the flight back, our large group had now diminished to the two Fyodorovs and the four members of our family. With Svyatoslav's previous connections with Gibraltar, having had the ophthalmic ship anchored offshore for some years, it was expected that he would be the one most fêted during our stay. But at the British Airways counter, our air hostess said: 'Thank you Mr Arnott, you operated on my father at the Charing Cross Hospital last year and saved his sight.' This one simple remark restored the confidence we had been seeking.

With the realization that we would have to spend some time every year in Gibraltar, we reluctantly decided to leave Majorca. We hoped to have a small substitute home in the Sotogrande and travel daily from this to our ophthalmic institute when working in Gibraltar. We had one last summer holiday in our treasured Anchorage flat, inviting in turn all our children and grandchildren to stay with us. Finally the day arrived when Veronica and I sat on the steps of our apartment as we supervised the removal of the last of its contents.

CHAPTER 36
The pink truck

In the autumn of 1998 we made another trip to India with Major Upadhyay, going to Indore at the invitation of the vice chancellor of Indore University, Professor Bharat Chaparwal. We flew out to Mumbai, where two old friends of the major met us at the airport. Dr Janki, a gynaecologist, has her own clinic and treats the majority of her patients for no fee, while Albert Fernandis runs a shipping company. These two exceptional people, one a Hindu and the other a Roman Catholic, were both Swami devotees, and lived together a life of dedicated faith and love to others. On countless occasions at all hours of the night, we would be met at Mumbai airport by their smiling, welcoming faces. On this evening they drove us to the Taj Mahal Hotel.

We spent the next three days in Mumbai, where I was one of the guest lecturers at the Indian international congress. On the Sunday we experienced yet another special service at All Saints Church. It was situated next to the botanical gardens, which was filled with exotic colourful shrubs and palm trees, and lay alongside a large pit, into which a certain sect of the Indians were thrown after death to lay in rest. The mass of vultures floating overhead ensured that the pit never became overfilled. The service in this church, with its mystical surroundings, was so different to the one we had suffered in Bangalore one year previously. The Reverend K Divasirvadham gave a service on racial cooperation. The octagonal-shaped Victorian church, with its full congregation of Indians, seemed such a symbol of the best of our former colonialism.

We were as yet totally ignorant of the purpose of our Indore visit. Professor Indira Bhargava, a patient on whom I had previously performed surgery, and his wife, Gan, met us at Indore airport. After checking into the Taj Residency Hotel, we were driven to a small private ophthalmic hospital run by two brothers, Pradeep and Nadil Sethi. Pradeep was the administrator and his brother Nadil was the ophthalmic consultant, who had an assistant colleague, Dr Hemlata. We were shown around the hospital, which was typical of many other Indian hospitals. The wards, large, airy and clean, averaged 15 beds with just a little side table. There was no other furniture in the wards, apart from the occasional chair, and the walls, although freshly painted, were not decorated. The operating theatres were equally austere and sparse, with only the bare essentials required for surgery.

At the newly built outpatient department, we found all the staff and patients of the hospital congregated in the courtyard. We had arrived for the opening ceremony of the new outpatient department which, unbeknown to us, was to be performed by Veronica. After years of travelling in India, nothing any longer came as a surprise. Veronica accepted this honour and, showing no shyness or embarrassment, made an excellent impromptu speech, wishing success in the future for the unit and benefit to those receiving treatment. She then unveiled a plaque recording the date and the unit named after her.

This very memorable day was only just starting. Indira and Gan Bhargava next drove us to a small village, set in woods, which lay a few miles from Indore. This complex housed the abandoned children from the city and was in the charge of a young Indian paediatrician, Dr Mameswari, and his wife. All the children were well clothed, looked healthy and well fed and exuded enthusiasm and happiness. Our arrival had obviously been expected, as all 30 of them were waiting for us in the middle of the road with their benefactors.

The Mameswaris painted the red symbol of welcome on our foreheads, and garlands of flowers were hung around our necks. The children were bemused: many were sucking their thumbs and all were staring at this strange white couple, as if we'd come from another planet. A little boy, who was obviously the leader, came forward and looked us up and down quizzically. Suddenly realizing that we were friends, he clutched Veronica's hand and held tightly to it for the rest of the proceedings. Following a singsong that was given by the children, we inspected the children's schoolwork for the term, which had been specially laid out on tables around the room.

By now we had been accepted as part of the family, and the children vied as to who could get the closest to Veronica, clutching at her dress, as we made our way along the tables. Each child would give a screech of merriment when we examined his or her work, which was of an excellent standard. Veronica, most impressed by the care the young doctor and his wife had given to his protégés, asked if we could adopt this village as part of our charitable commitment. She said that we would send a teddy bear to each child in the village and open some 30 accounts with the Bank of India and place £1 in each. Who knew in the years ahead how much these accounts would grow from the humble beginnings we had started for them on that day. We left that village, once again impressed with what can be achieved for the deprived by the sacrifice and dedication of others who care.

Later that morning we entered the enormous precincts of Indore University. Each department was fields away from its neighbours and it was very easy to become hopelessly lost in the confines of the complex. Most people used bikes to get around. Our host, Bharat Chhaparwal, an ENT surgeon and the first medic to have been given this academic university post, gave us a tour of the whole university, where English was the preferred language for teaching. Our conversation was quite formal until the subject of Sathya Sai Baba was raised. Immediately we became not casual acquaintances but friends with a mutual bond of interest. It transpired that some two years earlier Bharat had been asked by the government of India to inspect the schools of Puttaparthy. As we had two years ago, he thought that this would be just another routine trip. But he found that the educational standards and quality of teaching was second to none. While in Puttaparthy he attended prayers at the Ashram and met Swami. His few days impressed him greatly and he left with a high regard for Sai Baba.

Dr Upadhyay and I were to be made honorary visiting academic professors of the university, the Devi Ahilya Vishwavidyalaya, Indore – only the second time this honour had been awarded. Some 10 years previously, Indira Bhargava had been similarly awarded for his international work on the development of the triple vaccine, which was now available for all the children of India. We were being recognized for our work in advancing the development of ophthalmic surgery in India. In my thanks for the honour that had been bestowed on us, I included a small address on 'concepts of cataract'. I could see Veronica looking up at me with tears in her eyes. It meant so much to both of us that, having tried to help others in some little way, so much was now being bestowed on us.

We returned to the Leika Hotel in Mumbai, planning to set out the next morning to Ahmedabad for an ophthalmic congress organized by Dr Abhay Vasavada. Abhay is an outstanding international surgeon who, with ease, could phaco even the densest Indian cataract. But at the Leika, we were so entranced by the 'Arabian Nights' décor and Indian sense of tradition and peace, we decided to stay for an extra day, as I wasn't due to speak until later in the congress. It was so rare and wonderful to have a full day on our own, with no appointments or planned functions. We lay in bed together for some time before having a late room-service breakfast and did not leave our bedroom till four o'clock in the afternoon. We made full use of the hotel writing paper and wrote thank-you letters to all our new-found friends, who had made the previous week so memorable. This was one of those rare times, when we could enjoy just being together, far away from the outside world, with almost nobody knowing where we were. There was also plenty of time to reflect on how we would raise the considerable finances needed to complete our unit.

At midday on New Year's Eve, in 1998, Veronica and I were disturbed at Trottsford by the sound of a heavy diesel-engined vehicle coming down our drive. Our new Mercedes Benz 'Atego' truck had arrived. This model had only been on the market for a few weeks and the two members of the Mercedes staff, Keith Fairly and Steve David, presented it to us with obvious pride. Although valued at £60,000 it was in a rather skeletal state, having essentially only a cab, chassis engine, gearbox and back axle. Tony Spooner, the treasurer of our Penny Trust MBMEU, was with us for the occasion, as was Jeff Jeffery, our neighbour, and we all had great fun driving it around our small farm. It was stored, in its bare state, in our farmyard for some months, while Veronica strove to raise more finances for its continued construction.

Veronica and Stephen drafted a letter to our many thousands of patients, asking for donations to our trust. Once again we had a magnificent response and enough funds were raised for the Mercedes truck to be moved to Rohills in Andover for the construction of the body of the eye unit.

One of the letters that we circulated had a dramatic response. Robin Tavistock, the Duke of Bedford, had suffered some years earlier from a ruptured artery in the brain while walking on his estate, Woburn Abbey. The farm manager rushed Robin to hospital and undoubtedly helped to save his life. The subsequent care and love given by Robin's wife, Henrietta, after he had received resuscitation in hospital, added considerably towards his recovery. Robin came to consult me about the ophthalmic results of his stroke. One eye was deviating outwards and had severely restricted vision. Over the months, with ophthalmic surgery and remedial treatment, Robin's appearance returned to normal and his vision improved.

Despite the fact that my treatment had required normal not remarkable skills, the Bedfords were very grateful for my small contribution towards his recovery. It is well documented in the press that Robin's rather abrasive middle-aged attitude to life dramatically changed after his brush with death. I only inherited him as a patient after his accident, but his response to our circular letter was typical of his generous personality. He handed his letter to the manager of the Woburn Safari Park, Chris Webster, with the comment 'Look after them.'

On an early spring day Veronica, Tony Spooner and I drove to Woburn Abbey and on to the safari park to meet Chris Webster. We had a meeting with him and his secretary, before embarking on a tour of the safari park. We drove around the wood with the monkeys dropping onto the bonnet of his Land Rover, past the lakes with the hippos wallowing in the mud, the pastures with the deer and llamas and scrubland in which was the one Bengal tiger. We ended up in the enclosure in which were the three treasured Asian calf elephants, Raja, the bull, and Chandrika and Damini. The Asian elephant is an endangered species, and Robin had done a deal with the Indian government to bring these animals to Woburn Safari Park to procreate and increase the species, with a view to sending their progeny back to India. These elephants were amazing – we saw Raja busily painting an impressionist painting, with the paintbrush held firmly in his trunk and a box of oil colours by his side. No doubt they will markedly influence Indian art in the future! Chris Webster gave us Raja's first oil-colour impressionist painting, which, who knows, may one day be worth thousands of pounds. It looked like a Picasso, with criss-crossing lines and swirls of all the colours of the rainbow.

Chris had a personal interest in ophthalmology, having retired from the Brigade of Guards with an eye problem. He told us: 'Every year we have one day in which a chosen charity can have the use of the safari park. I'm prepared to offer you full use of the park and conference centre, with all monies going to your project.' We were speechless, as the most we had expected was one hour's proceeds. Veronica and I had visions of having to organize one big party, and we realized that there was a great deal of preparation to be done in a very limited time. To match Chris's very generous gesture, we agreed that half the profits of the day would go towards the rebuilding of the elephant house.

Veronica and her supporters in the Penny Trust decided to invite, with sponsorship, the children of the Sunshine Homes from all around the country. We also sponsored the children of our local Montessori school in Kingsley. Dr Khalid Hameed, chief executive of the Cromwell Hospital, London, offered to host a lunch, and Mike Gallagher, the marketing manager, offered us his services. We invited friends, patients and staff and organized an auction for the event.

We attended a press conference in the safari park, at which we joined the Duke of Bedford, Count and Countess Pejascevish, who had been great supporters of this function, and Chris Webster, with his staff, Cheryl Williams and Lucy. For the first time we saw the mobile eye unit in its finery, with the body attached. It was parked in the middle of a field, well away from the other activities of the safari park, where it was less likely to be vandalized. Artist Moray Tabac had designed the external decor and it looked truly magnificent. It was painted a delicate shade of pink, with white side stripes, within which was the flag of India. There was also Swami's motto 'Love all, Serve all, and Help all' engraved discreetly in the rear corner on each side of the truck. A plaque on the door of the cab gave recognition to the generosity of Mercedes Benz.

As yet, it was just a hollow shell, totally lacking all the internal fittings required for a top-quality ophthalmic operating theatre. Another £150,000 had to be raised to equip the unit with compressors, sterile air-conditioning, theatre beds, microscopes, phaco machines, surgical instruments, cupboards and shelves.

We all had a big laugh at being photographed with the elephants outside our 'Pink Truck'. Veronica symbolically handed over the keys of the mobile phaco eye unit to Robin, with Raja, Chandrika and Damini placed on either side of them.

The day for this charity event was Saturday 3 July 1999. Veronica and I had spent the previous night at the Bell Hotel, Woburn, with Mike Gallagher, his wife Susan and daughter Helen. Also staying with us were David and Ann Apple, our partners in the Gibraltar Eye Institute project. Our entire family joined us for this exceptional day: Stephen and Kathy with Oliver, Lara and Isabella; and Tania with Nick and Timmy, Natasha and Telisa. Robert, still being a bachelor, came alone.

The safari park had taken on the appearance of a carnival. Arriving in their gaily coloured Sunshine Home minibuses, 2500 children were revelling in the joys of the park with its lake and paddleboats. We'd invited all the blind Asians in the country with their helpers. 'Miss Rachel', the teacher of our local Montessori school, was shepherding her pupils and many of our friends also mingled with the throng. One of my patients, Mr Sharma, who owned the largest Indian catering company in the country, with restaurants all around Britain, had generously prepared a picnic box lunch for the thousands of Sunshine Home children, which we had hoped would be eaten in the open areas of the park. We had also booked a van to bring meals for the 300 blind Asians and their helpers.

Unfortunately, many of the children, preferring burger and chips to an Indian picnic, went to the safari park restaurant. The van for the blind Asians was involved in an accident on the way, so the canteen was very much overstretched, and I did my best to placate my hungry guests before returning to the outer complex for the opening ceremony.

I missed the Duke of Bedford's address, welcoming the Deputy High Commissioner of India, Mr Patel, Khalid Hameed and all the other thousands of visitors to Woburn Abbey. My absence was not noticed, as Veronica had already spoken on behalf of our Penny Trust MBMEU. In the presence of some 130 guests at lunch in the conference centre, Alan Downer held an auction that included, among other items, one day's trout fishing at West Wycombe Park, which was donated by Sir Edward Dashwood. The spirit of the day was well exemplified by the action of Brian Robinson, chairman of Rohills, the company that had hand-built the body for our unit. During lunch, he stood up and said he would donate £500 if his offer could be matched. It was, and we saved £1000 on the cost of the body of our unit.

We had planned to offer tea to our guests in the restaurant of the conference centre but instead watched with huge pleasure as the still-hungry blind Asians ate every last bit of food in the complex.

When all our guests had left, Veronica and I met Michael Gallagher, the marketing manager of the Cromwell Hospital, which had sponsored our guest's lunch, with his staff Julie Rampton, Joan Crowley and Madeleine Delaney, in the conference centre. They had all helped enormously to organize that perfect day. While discussing the events of the day, we were joined by Robin Tavistock, who had driven over from the abbey on his trike. The generosity and hospitality of the Bedfords, Websters, Dr Hameed and Mr Sharma had contributed to making this a very special occasion, which those thousands of children who were with us would never forget.

During the next few months, the unit was fitted with its internal equipment. Pieter Van Der Westhuizen, of Hemax, was in charge of this part of the construction and took it on as his own charitable contribution. I had worked in one of his operating theatres and knew that he was a top expert in his field. His expertise was stretched to the limit by having to design a theatre that was not only half the size of a conventional one but would be used by two surgeons at once.

Little by little the interior of the mobile eye unit took shape. A box appeared on the roof of the body and another under it for the 'cooler' and laminar airflow systems. Brackets fixed to the wall would hold the operating microscopes in place. Our dream mobile eye phaco unit was at last becoming a reality.

CHAPTER 37
More than 50 years on

The year of 1999 was a turning point: at the age of 70, it was time to hand over the practice in Harley Street to Richard and Fiona Packard. As well as the original associates, Major SK Upadhyay, Dr M Islamullah, John Grindle and Lyn Jenkins, four other surgeons had joined our group. Ken Nischal had been headhunted as a paediatric ophthalmic consultant from the children's hospital in Toronto, Canada, to Great Ormond Street Hospital and was a very welcome addition to Arnott Eye Associates. David O'Brart is a consultant glaucoma and refractive surgeon at St Thomas' Hospital. Dominick McHugh specializes in conditions affecting the retina of the eye, and Naresh Joshi is an oculo-plastic surgeon. Naresh had previously been my senior registrar at Charing Cross Hospital and joined our team with a colourful background, his father having been the ophthalmic surgeon to the Sultan of Brunei. A leaving party was arranged for us, at which we were presented with six millennium champagne goblets.

Veronica, Stephen and I made our final farewells to our very loyal ladies – Joy Andrews, Hazel Saunders, Valerie Horsford and Clare Ruocco – after everyone else had left the office. We said goodbye 'for the last time' – only to return a few minutes later, as Veronica had left her scarf behind. We found all four girls in floods of tears. We were acutely aware of what we were leaving behind us and were sad at saying farewell to a staff with whom, over the course of many years, we had shared such a close relationship.

While still being committed to our charity work and the proposed FAA Eye Institute in Gibraltar, Veronica and I now had the opportunities to spend our time together, relaxing without the responsibilities of a large practice. We had more time for the simple pleasures of life, including boating on the south coast with relatives such as Tony and Nickie Laurence or friends like our vicar Peter Bradford.

We spent one week on the Isle of Wight staying at the Crossways Hotel, East Cowes, attending a course by Paul Wise on the fashioning of Windsor fan-back chairs. Veronica and I would bicycle the two miles to Paul's house to work in his rather cold garden shed. Every day we built a little more of our wooden chairs. The legs and backstays had to be cut and turned on a lathe. The backrest needed to be fashioned and bent. The seat was hacked out with an axe and finely curved to the imprint of the sitter's buttocks. On the final day we put the chairs together and sandpapered off the remaining rough edges. We finally had two perfect reproduction chairs, but no doubt Paul Wise had rectified our manufacturing faults every day, after we had left for the evening. Veronica and I had really enjoyed this week, competing against each other and turning our hands to such an unaccustomed craft.

That year, Veronica and I had time to take a holiday in the Caribbean, totally away from ophthalmology. We flew to Barbados and checked into a small hotel called Cobblers Cove, where we had a chalet on the edge of the woodland in the constant company of monkeys and birds. This was a real 'honeymoon retreat', and we were able to enjoy a few days totally on our own, although we joined our fellow guests for meals. We met Judy Dench and her husband Michael Williams, who she was so soon to lose from cancer; but during this holiday they seemed to have not a care in the world and, like us, spent hours frolicking in the calm warm sea.

We explored the island on bicycles, and on the Sunday we rode to the local church for the 8 am service. Thinking that, in this far outpost of the empire, the service would be informal and the church almost empty, we both wore T-shirts, shorts and tennis shoes. We were mortified to see the local women all beautifully dressed in multi-coloured silk dresses and the men wearing dark suits, with ties and bowler hats. Entering the packed church to join this elegant congregation, Veronica and I were overcome with embarrassment. We need not have worried, as the ushers seemed not to notice our inappropriate apparel, or the fact that we were the only two Europeans present. Our hosts, in their devotions, could not have more warmly welcomed us into their house of worship. After an uplifting service we bicycled back to Cobblers Cove, grateful to realize that the real standards of love and Christian thinking were still the norm in this part of the world.

The second part of our Caribbean holiday was in another extreme. We flew to Antigua, as guests of John and Anthea Kendall, on their classic 80-foot yacht 'Zenna', which was anchored in English Harbour, for the Antigua Classic Yacht Races.

With the other crew, Andrew and Caroline Platter – two young Australians who were skipper and cook – and Eoin and Joe Ashton-Johnson, we met in the famous tower that overlooks the bay and saw our ship dwarfed by the huge classic yachts of the world, which were some 120 feet long. The first three days of sailing were very disappointing, as the normally strong seasonal wind was absent, and for much of the time the yachts lay becalmed in a placid sea.

The fourth day's racing was totally different, with a fresh easterly wind of 22 knots. The race of 32 miles was to be run over a four-mile course running from north to south, which had to be traversed four times. In the run up to the start, all the yachts congregated in Antigua Bay and barely avoided collision as their captains jockeyed for the best starting position. Being the timekeeper, I had to yell to John Kendall the countdown – first in minutes and finally in seconds. Such is John's seamanship skill that when the gun was fired we were upwind to all the other yachts and only two meters from the starting line, which we raced across well ahead of all our pursuers. Looking astern of 'Zenna' we witnessed the spectacle of the finest collection of classic yachts in the world, with sails fully filled with the wind coming on the port beam, listing heavily to starboard, as they ploughed through the foamy sea.

Despite having a crew that included amateurs such as Veronica and me and competing against some of the best professional sailors in the world, we came in, after the handicap had been taken into consideration, second overall in the race. We beat the yacht that came into third place by 45 minutes.

The following day we sailed back to Royal Antigua Bay for the start of our home journey.

Later that year we celebrated the 50th anniversary of lens implantation. Sir Harold Ridley was still alive but, being well into his 90s, was naturally very frail. The American Society of Cataract and Refractive Surgery invited Harold and his wife Elisabeth to be the honoured guests at the annual meeting in Seattle, Washington. We were to be their chaperones. It must have been quite a strain for this very elderly couple to travel halfway around the world to be fêted by a society with 10,000 members. Minor problems did occur on several occasions. Before take off, Elisabeth Ridley thought she had mislaid her passport. The flight was delayed for several minutes before it was found in the recesses of her handbag. From then on, Veronica took charge of all their documents.

At the congress, one whole afternoon was taken up with a presentation of Harold's life, produced by David King of the Carlin Company, which included a film of one of his first implant operations. Harold and Elisabeth had not been away from their little thatched cottage in Wiltshire for some years, and Veronica and I had to watch over them continuously in this bustling city. At night we would see that they were safely locked in their bedroom, so they did not wander out of the hotel.

We left them in the custody of a colleague for only one afternoon while we went to the meeting to give my presentation. On returning to the hotel we found that they had been lost for several hours! The whole building was searched to no avail. The reception for them that evening was a disaster, as the guests of honour were missing. Eventually the Ridleys were found in a hotel on the other side of the city, having been left unescorted at its entrance by the driver of their limousine. Despite these few blips, their presence was a great success, and all attending appreciated meeting one of the great pioneers of our profession. Veronica and I particularly enjoyed one day when we went in a minibus with the Ridleys and Peter and Diana Choyce to the Snoqualmie Falls. We only lacked John Pearce, who had drowned some two years previously, to make the quorum of early British implant inventors.

In November of that year, 1999, Veronica and I returned to the USA for another very special meeting of the ASCRS to acknowledge the pioneer work of the innovators of modern cataract surgery. Having just spent a week with Svyatoslav and Irine Fyodorov, we boarded a plane for Florida and spent a few days with Charlie and Ann Kelman in Boca Rota before going on to the meeting in Los Angeles.

The Kelmans' house in Boca Rota was, by all accounts, rather special. As 631 Ocean View, it backed onto the Atlantic Ocean and in the front was a patio that led onto a large inland waterway. The house was spacious and filled with Charlie's musical recordings and sporting gadgets. As in all of Charlie's houses, there was a Steinway piano in the hall, which he frequently played to entertain his guests. One of the garages had been converted to accommodate a virtual-reality golf course.

Earlier that year Charlie Kelman had collapsed in the operating theatre during the middle of a surgical list. He was rushed to hospital, where it was diagnosed that he was suffering from a collapsed lung, with cancer of the lung and a secondary in the brain. Over the following months he had laser-knife therapy to the lesion in the brain and extensive chemotherapy for the primary in the lung. When we arrived, however, Charlie was on the golf course with his 10-year-old son Evan, and Ann was romping around the hall with the younger twins, Seth and Jason. We had a very relaxed evening and dinner together, without any evidence of Charlie's health problem.

The next morning, we found Ching, the ever-faithful helper to the family, preparing an American breakfast , as the twins were playing in their pen. A little later Charlie and Ann joined us and we had a very happy hour all together before Charlie drove us to collect our nephew, Alex Arnott, who was a student in the local university. Charlie was an Anglophile and always drove a British car, at this time a white convertible Rolls Royce Corniche. Charlie, Veronica and I made a spectacular entry into the university in this car with the roof down, which was rather dampened when, on parking, Charlie heavily reversed into another car. Alex spent most of the day with us, before we had to leave to go to Los Angeles.

For the flight to Los Angeles, Charlie hired a twin-jet Hawker 1000 and spent the trip deeply absorbed in a book about natural golf. The journey took one hour more than normal, as the pilots had to fly at reduced speed to conserve fuel because of a limit to the amount that could be carried due to the runway at Boca Rota being short and having weight limitations. A friend, Peter La Haye, the founder of Iolab (one of the original American lens implant companies), perished the following year in a Learjet, which crashed after it had run out of fuel.

On arriving in Los Angeles, Charlie went to see his elder son David, one of his three children from his earlier marriage to Joan, who, although only in his early 30s, had a colostomy and was suffering from diabetes. Veronica and I drove to the Century Plaza Hotel, which had for many years been used for the earlier annual meetings of the American Society of Cataract and Refractive Surgery. Over the previous 10 years, the society had spread its wings, with meetings in New Orleans, San Diego, San Francisco, Seattle, Boston and elsewhere.

We had a whole spare morning, so we escaped to the West Lake Golf Course. We had been so amused the previous day by Charlie's enthusiasm for natural golf that we decided to give it a go ourselves. We had a two-hour lesson with the golf coach, Joe Buttita, and ended up buying two sets of clubs. We later had many hours trying to master the golf swing, which was more akin to playing a cricket stroke with a straight bat.

It was rather nostalgic returning after a gap of a decade to this venue. So much had happened over the intervening years. Manus Kraff, one of the pioneer phaco surgeons with a large practice in Chicago, had recruited David and Ann Karcher, business executives, to manage the ASCRS, which had become one of the major political influences in American and world ophthalmology. Over the years, the membership had grown from hundreds to some 10,000. The annual meetings, with demonstrations of live surgery, teaching courses and didactic presentations, progressively advanced the frontiers of ophthalmology.

At this very special meeting were all those who had created the inventions to make ophthalmic surgery what it was at this present time. The elderly statesmen of the profession reminisced and shared their ideas with the next generation of innovators. That evening we attended the official reception for the meeting of the ASCRS. So many of our great ophthalmic friends were there, but Svyatoslav Fyodorov, John Pearce, Bill Vallerton, Bill Harris and John Sheets were sadly missed.

Present were Charlie Kelman and Bob Sinskey (with his wife Loraine) – the two American surgeons who had been so pivotal to our relationship with American ophthalmology over the previous 35 years. Along with them were numerous colleagues and friends, each of whom brought memories of fruitful and happy occasions. The following are a few who have done much to further their profession: Herve Byron (with his wife Bryn), who as well as being a pioneer phaco surgeon, has written countless articles on the medico-legal aspects of ophthalmology; Herb Gould, the epitome of an American gentleman, who enjoyed his hunting as much as ophthalmology; Henry Clayman, by origin a London cockney, who had emigrated to America and became a leading surgeon in Miami (he once assisted me at surgery during one of my teaching courses in Charing Cross Hospital; the patient chosen for surgery had developed a severe preoperative complication that, with the help of Henry, we resolved); Bob Drews, one-time president of the ASCRS, who had been instrumental in promoting John Pearce's one-piece posterior-lens implant in America and had invited me to be his guest lecturer during his presidency; Jared Emery, from Odessa, Texas, who with me had developed the diamond keratome knife that became the norm in cataract surgery; and Gerald Faulkner, who had entertained us so well when we lectured in Hawaii.

Also there were: Norman Jaffe, from Miami, probably the foremost lens-implant pioneer in America, with whom we had indirectly battled over lens patent rights – despite our past differences we admired him as a surgeon and for the very large contribution he and his son had made to ophthalmology; Malcolm McCannel, from Minnesota, who had introduced a stitch to secure a wayward lens implant – he would light up any party with his wit and fund of jokes; Jack Dodick, with his wife Lyn, who developed an alternative form of phaco cataract treatment using laser as the form of energy; Jack Holliday, who had been instrumental in developing techniques for measuring the required strength of a lens implant; and Herbert Kaufman, from New Orleans, one of America's pioneer surgeons in refractive corneal surgery. In the early 1980s, Herbert had been a guest surgeon at an international eye congress that Emanuel Rosen, Bill Haining and Veronica and I had organized in Venice. We had been rather too ambitious, having the meeting in a hotel on the Lido and the surgery in a hospital in Venice, to which we were to be taken by boat. In his enthusiasm to see that preparations for his surgery were in order, Herve took the boat alone to Venice at 8 am. The other surgeons were thus isolated at the Lido, with no other boat available and the surgical list was delayed some two hours. Herbert did a masterful restorative procedure on the eye of an Indian boy who had been flown in from Bombay. Finally, present was Bill Maloney, who had relentlessly taught Howard Gimbel's modifications in phaco at congresses all around the world. He continued to be a top-line surgeon despite grappling with arthritis.

Many other great pioneers and friends of ours were at this meeting: Paul Fechner, Miles Galin, Howard Gimbel, Spencer Thornton, Howard Fine, Bruce Wallace, Henry Hirschman, John Hunkeler, Gerry Freeman, Paul Ernst, Stephen Brint, Guy Knolle and Bob Asher – to name but a few. All of these surgeons made a great contribution with their example and teaching, helping the conversion of thousands of their colleagues to adopt similar methods of surgery.

Europe had its own representatives, including Jean Jacque and Danielle Aron Rosa. Danielle had perfected a YAG laser that could non-invasively open the posterior capsule of a lens that had lost its transparency weeks or months after cataract extraction and lens implantation. For some time we did not have this instrument in the UK, and many of my patients went to Paris for this treatment. I was rather sorry when we eventually bought our own YAG laser and there was no longer an excuse to send our patients for a holiday in France! Other surgeons included Richard Packard, Michael Roper-Hall, Emanuel Rosen, Helen Seward and Arthur Steele from Britain, Jan Worst from Holland, Bo Phillipson from Sweden, Philippe Sourdille, Patrice De Large and Philippe Crozaphon from France, Ulrich Dardenne, Jorg Draeger and Karl Jacobi from Germany and Lucio Buratto and Fabio Dossi from Italy. All of these Europeans were foremost anterior-segment surgeons in their own country.

Also at this meeting were the younger generation of surgeons who were making their own mark in our profession.

Steve Obstaum and Doug Koch are two innovative surgeons who combined surgical ability with political expedience. Both have been presidents of major ophthalmic societies and have been able to support the contributions of their colleagues. Soon after this meeting, Doug Koch became president of the International Intraocular Implant Club, which was founded by Harold Ridley and Peter Choyce and was host to my final contribution to ophthalmic meetings.

Sam Masket for many years promoted my style of totally encircling loop lens for complicated cases. He studied under Miles Galin and introduced many improvements, including 'scleral pocket incision' into the eye, stitching techniques and the management of astigmatism in cataract surgery. He is currently professor at the Jules Stein Eye Institute.

Howard Fine, as previously mentioned, is probably the foremost 'second-generation pioneer surgeon', along with Howard Gimbel, Bill Maloney and a few others. His clinical and research output is prodigious. As well as his own inventions in instrumentation, he is well known for analysing any new product that comes onto the market. His motivation for progress cannot be overestimated.

Roger Steinert, collaborating with Steve Trokel and Carmen Puliafito, worked from 1982 on the development of lasers. Carmen and Roger Steinert founded a laser research laboratory at Massachusetts Ear, Eye and Throat Infirmary to study the excimer laser. Their counterpart in the UK was Professor John Marshal. These researchers have produced an explosive development of refractive surgery, which can correct the optical errors of patients suffering from long or short sight.

Dick Lindstrom and his wife Jackie had been partners in our Laser Vision Centre in Harley Street.

Marguerite McDonald has probably done more to promote refractive surgery than any other ophthalmologist, with 353 abstracts, 66 books and 165 peer-reviewed articles. She headed the research team that performed the world's first excimer laser treatment to eliminate or reduce the need for glasses and contact lenses. Marguerite is on the editorial board of several publications and at a young age was the first female president of the ASCRS.

Stephen Lane, clinical professor of ophthalmology at the University of Minnesota, Minneapolis, past president of the ASCRS and member of ORBIS International, was a foremost pioneer in excimer refractive surgery.

Priscilla Arnold has had a very busy career in ophthalmology, combining her clinical life with contributions to numerous committees and boards and was the second lady to become president of the ASCRS. Without the participation of members such as Priscilla, our societies would come to a grinding halt.

It was this august group that Veronica and I joined, on that evening, in the ballroom of the Century Plaza Hotel.

The following day, the meeting started with papers that were more senti-mental than scientific. Bob Sinskey was in the chair for the opening session, entitled: 'The Way We Were'.

Historical videos were shown, which included a scene when a very young Veronica rescued Svyatoslav Fyodorov's artificial leg from the beach in Malibu when he did his ocean swim with me.

The second session, chaired by Norman Jaffe, was more scientific. Skip Bechert discussed the development of PMMA lens implants. I followed with my paper, jointly written with Richard Packard, on the first foldable lens.

On the second day of the meeting, Manus Kraff chaired another session entitled 'Do you remember?' This was an excellent meeting with brilliant anecdotes about the past. The meeting was closed with a lunch, at which Charlie Kelman gave the last address. With his usual sense of humour it was called 'Looking back can give you a stiff neck.' James Carter was at this meeting and later became very active in promoting Charlie Kelman's lenses.

In Britain, several events were still to be held later in the year to mark the 50th anniversary of the lens-implant operation. Rayner, the company that had made Harold Ridley's original lenses, organized, with the support of Ann and David Apple, a banquet at the Science Museum in Exhibition Road, London. Full television news coverage was arranged for this event. As an introduction to the Sky TV news bulletin, I was asked to be filmed examining a patient who had had cataract extraction and lens implantation. Accordingly, I invited an old friend Antonia Gibbs, on whom I had operated, to join me in a consulting room at the Cromwell Hospital. The directors of Rayner, Donnie Munro and Ian Collins, were also in attendance, as was Antonia's husband Michael. We had quite a laugh doing this mock-up examination, but Antonia was a real star and looked very good on television. Michael and Antonia were asked to join the banquet, as were some other guests I particularly asked for, including Svyatoslav and Irine Fyodorov, with their business partner Mark Klabin.

John Howard Worsley, the artist, brought with him a painting of the plane flown by Mouse Cleaver, whose operations had been so instrumental in ophthalmic progress, entitled 'One Ran up the Clock'. Although Mouse Cleaver was no longer with us, his sister-in-law Jennie Adams and husband Peter represented him.

Some 150 diners were invited, including many of the current leaders in ophthalmology, as well as representatives from the royal society, Houses of Parliament and other interested parties. Thomas Stuttaford wrote a full-page article for *The Times* the next day. The main organizer of this function, David Apple, was recovering from an operation, but his wife, Ann, had flown from America to be present.

The banquet was held, rather appropriately, in the part of the Science Museum that housed the historic airplanes. Ann Apple and Lord Hunt made the opening speeches, and John Howard Worsley, the artist, presented me with a painting of the Hurricane plane flown by Mouse Cleaver. I gave my speech standing inches below the Vickers Vimy IV plane in which Alcock and Brown had made their epic first flight across the Atlantic. Peter Choyce made a moving address about Harold Ridley, who then replied, looking very bemused at the magnitude of the evening.

Having been much fêted and honoured by the world, Veronica and I thought it would be appropriate to organize a more personal evening for the

Ridleys. We made a booking in a small Riverside Inn, near to their home, and asked Harold and Elisabeth to draw up their own guest list for the occasion. They included in this, the theatre sister of St Thomas' Hospital and the surgical assistant present at the first operation. The medical interns of St Thomas' and Moorfields, who had worked with Harold in the pioneering period, were also invited. Their sons Nick and David joined them, with their wives Loretta and Elspeth. Spencer Thornton came as the official representative for American ophthalmology. In total, 41 guests sat huddled together in the cramped confines of the candlelit Swan Inn, with the Ridleys surrounded by colleagues and friends who had never deserted them in the earlier years of dissension.

Two days after this dinner, we ourselves were honoured at a party given in Claridge's Hotel, London. The occasion was the Millennium Dinner for the Medical Committee of the Cromwell Hospital, which was hosted by Khalid and Gazelle Hameed, with Michael Portillo, the local MP, and the guest of honour. One of my colleagues, Derek Packham, and I were to be made emeritus surgeons of the hospital. Knowing we would have to compete with a seasoned after-dinner speech by Michael Portillo, Veronica and I took considerable time compiling my own. We were able to pass on several jokes that we had picked up on our recent travels to America, as well as introducing an element of formality. In my opening remarks, I said:

'We must all be grateful to have the company of Michael Portillo, who has broken away from his busy schedule to be with us tonight. In my own family there was one notable MP, my Great Grandfather, Sir John Arnott, who had a seat in Kinsale, County Cork, during the 1860s. He entered parliament to introduce the Irish Poor Law Relief Bill, which, with the support of some fellow members, became law. This act enabled the city unions of Ireland to release slum children from the poor houses to the farmlands. They restocked a countryside, which had been decimated of its youth by the recent potato famine, typhus, and mass emigration to America. Many of these children went on to run the farms of the homes into which they had been adopted. A terrible situation had been relieved and the Irish land was slowly able to revert to normality.'

To our complete surprise, all 200 guests present at the dinner gave a standing ovation, as a tribute to our ancestor.

For some months, our younger son, Robert, had been taking out an Australian girl, Kate Ward, and they invited us to join them in Australia to welcome in the new millennium. Two days after Christmas we flew to Sydney, where we were met at the airport by a radiant couple, who announced that they had just become engaged. Despite the 24-hour flight, Veronica and I stayed up well into the night celebrating with Bob and Kate.

We had previously met Kate's mother Georgina on several occasions on her visits to England, and we felt so blessed that we had such a great extended family. After a long journey, we passed through Cootamundra, a town noted as the birthplace of the cricketer Sir Donald Bradman, and drove on a few more miles to their place in Gilgal.

The Ward family had left their previous home some 150 years previously, as it became severely flooded every year. Their new ranch, Gilgal, was named after the biblical promised land, which lies beyond the waters. The head of the family, Stephen Ward, a promising prospective member of parliament, had been involved in a fatal air crash a few years earlier, and Georgina was now running the 12,000 acre farm, with the help of David Alexander – the farm manager.

The house seemed to emphasize the vast spaces of this country. It is a large, very elegant 'colonial style', single-storeyed dwelling, with almost every room having French windows opening onto lawns and pastures that gently slope down to a valley filled with Cypriot trees. These woodlands teem with white cockatoos, which fill the air with the sound of their constant squawking. The surrounding land, lush green after the spring rains, takes on the dusky brown hue of a desert after the frequent summer droughts. Some half a mile from the house is a hill topped by a large rock, which had been split in two, many decades previously, by a bolt of lightning.

It was on 'Split Rock' that Bob had proposed to Kate during a violent rainstorm. The two lovers, soaked to the skin, were so wrapped up in themselves that they were unaware of the surrounding vista, which, as far as the eye could see, is Ward property. Cattle and sheep graze the land. The Merino sheep had recently been introduced and, although only useful for their wool, were proving a success.

Arriving at the busiest time of the year, Veronica and I spent hours, sitting on fences, watching the stock-taking and branding of the cattle and the shearing of the sheep. We were truly welcomed into the family. We met Kate's sister Sophie, husband Lev and son Sam. Before returning to Britain we spent several days at a family reunion in a villa overlooking the sands of Bondi Beach.

Bob and Kate had a relatively short engagement, with the wedding, to be held at Gilgal, arranged for 29 April. We booked flights to Australia for all of our immediate family, with a stay in a resort in Queensland for the week before the wedding. On the weekend of the wedding we all arrived in a minibus at Cootamundra, where most of the guests were staying. We could have been in a small town in the Home Counties of England, as every pub resonated to English accents. Bob and Kate's British friends were most supportive, and 27 flew out for the occasion, including Bob's boss in Pereire Tod, Steve Bradley, and his brother Jules.

The Wards were very generous with their wedding list and allowed us to invite our best American friends and ophthalmic colleagues, Charlie and Ann Kelman and Bob and Loraine Sinskey and my cousin Guy Arnott. 'Bobbles' spent his last evening as a bachelor dining in a restaurant in Cootamundra with his immediate family, our four American friends – one of whom, Charlie, was his godfather – and my cousin Guy.

The weather was perfect for the day of the wedding, which was just as well, as the ceremony was to be conducted in an open-sided hay shed situated on the crest of a hill one-mile from the house. Only one month earlier a kangaroo had been disturbed in its interior. This unlikely setting was transformed, with coconut matting on the floor, silk draped across the ceiling and magnificent floral displays. The effect was impressive and dramatic, as the setting sun changed the light every few minutes in this temporary church, which from then on became known as the 'cathedral'.

The service was conducted by Gill, the local priest, who was the spitting image of Dawn French in *The Vicar of Dibley*. As she raised her hands over the heads of the couple to give the blessing, the family Australian cattle dog, Maggie, decided to add her own congratulations. Walking up the aisle, she headed towards the altar, before turning to sit between the priest and the wedding couple. Gazing at Kate, Maggie outstretched a paw towards her and then moving sideways made the same gesture to Bob. With these salutations completed, she slowly retraced her steps and left the church. During this unrehearsed interlude, the congregation remained silent, but after the blessing was finally given, the guests erupted with laughter. Gill quickly quipped: 'Now you can appreciate why dog is God spelled backwards.'

One year after our day at Woburn Abbey, we held another major fundraising event. Our chaplain friend from Majorca, Mike Brotherton, had introduced us to one of his naval friends, Liam Byrd, who offered to let us use HMS President to host a celebration of the mobile eye unit before it was shipped to India.

Once again, Veronica had a massive amount of organizing to do, with the ever-faithful support of Lyn Wood and Tony Spooner. Dr Khalid Hameed and Mike Gallagher of the Cromwell Hospital sponsored the wine and salmon, while Mr Sharma, my patient, agreed to present a traditional Indian dinner laid out on silver salvers.

Our committee meetings were held in the cramped space of the ward room on Her Majesty's frigate *HMS Grafton*, where Liam Byrd was serving. How different this charity evening was going to be from the space of Woburn. HMS President was a building supported by piles sunk into the bed of the River Thames adjacent to Tower Bridge. A shipping company had formerly owned it before it was bought by Sir Donald Gosling, of National Car Parking (NCP) fame, who donated it to the Royal Navy.

On 3 July 2000, our pink mobile phaco unit, now fully equipped, was parked directly in front of the entrance to the ship. Inside the building, we found ourselves in a hallway lined with dark oak panels, in the middle of which was an ancient helm. The large hall had a balcony running down one side of it, decorated with naval flags. In one corner were windows that exposed a panoramic view of the River Thames. On the opposite side was a stage, with doors leading to the other function rooms of the 'ship'. Half of the hall had tables laid for the expected guests of the evening, while the other half was bare like a parade ring.

Veronica had booked a suite in the Tower Bridge Hotel, so that we could entertain the naval personnel of HMS President and other friends and our immediate family of Arnotts, Whishaws and our new Australian relatives, Georgina and Kate. Veronica, as usual looking rapturous, was nervously going over the lines of the speech she was due to give later that night. Her theme was to compare the growth of her charity to the biblical mustard seed. As she left to check all was ready in the hall, we could hear her muttering: 'A mustard seed is the smallest of all seeds, which grows into the biggest of all plants...'

By the time we made our second entrance to the naval base, a transformation had occurred. At the entrance to the hall was a six-foot high ice statue of a dolphin, which was just beginning to show the heat of the evening. Female sea cadets stood holding trays laden with drinks. The hall soon became packed with our friends, many of whom had never before been in a naval base. They wandered around the rooms, admiring the historic artefacts. We had no seating plan, and, as always, our guests tended to sit with their own personal friends. Our chief guests, Dr Khalid Hameed and the Deputy Indian High Commissioner Mr H Pavel and his wife, sat at a table with the commodore of the base and Jafar Askari, who had so generously donated the Mercedes truck.

Most of the staff from our various hospitals and the Arnott Eye Centre was there to support us. Both Mike Brotherton and Liam Byrd, who had sanctioned this event, seemed to enjoy sharing the facilities of the navy with all our friends. Between courses at dinner, the Cadet Bands of the Royal Navy played naval themes, marching up and down the 'parade ground' alongside our tables. Angela Thomas, draped in a Union Jack Flag, sang *Rule Britannia* and *Amazing Grace*. She subsequently sat at our table and invited us to her Cornish inn, the Halzephron, at Gunwalloe in Mounts Bay, where she would organize a small charity event for us.

The country chairman of Sotheby's South, Tim Wonnacott, conducted an auction, at which a football signed by George Best went for £1000 and a large teddy bear was bought by one of Bob's friends. Jafar Askari bid for frescoes of Nelson Mandela and his wife, which had been designed by Nils Burwitz. Both socially and financially, the event was a great success, with more than £25,000 being raised for the Penny Trust MBMEU. As thanks to the Royal Navy, Veronica and I presented a silver engraved trophy as a perpetual challenge cup to be awarded to the best athletic naval cadet of the year.

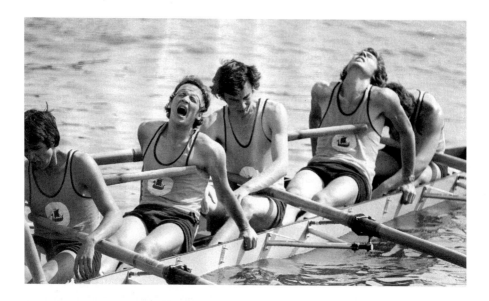

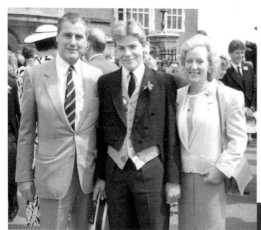

Top: The exhausted Shiplake College first eight after being beaten by Eton College in the semi-final of the Princess Elizabeth Cup. Nick Whishaw (left) and Stephen Arnott (second left) as in the Observer newspaper - Henley Regatta, 1979

Above: Eric, Robert and Veronica Arnott at Bill Yard for Harrow School speech day -1986

Right: Tania Arnott (far left) dancing with the Royal Festival Ballet (later the English National Ballet) in their production of La Sylphide - 1985

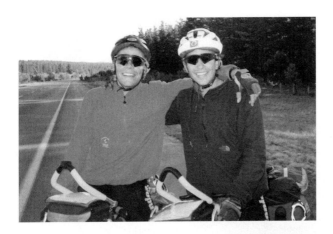

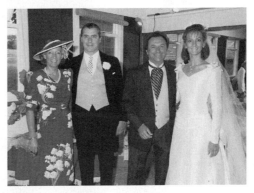

Above: Robert Arnott and Steve Norton on Operation Eyeball, an around-the-world bicycle trip, entering Sydney, Australia - 1994

Right: Veronica and me with Charlie and the bride, Tania Arnott, before her marriage to Nick Whishaw - Trottsford, 1986

Below: Kathy Thompson with Stephen and Veronica Arnott skiing in Davos, Switzerland - 1988

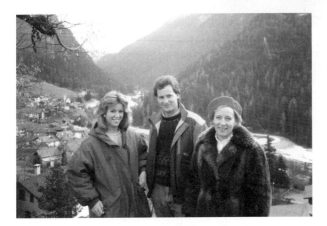

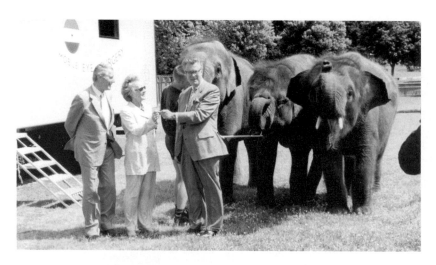

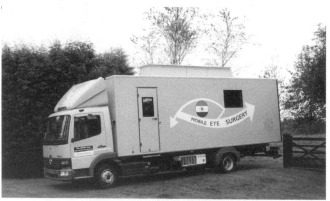

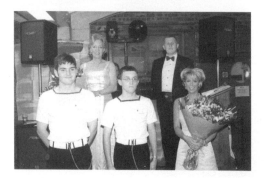

Top: The first major fundraising event for the Mercedes Benz Mobile Eye Unit. Veronica and I symbolically hand over the keys of the unit to Robin Tavistock, the Duke of Bedford, watched by the elephants Raja, Chandrika and Damini, at Woburn Safari Park - July 1999

Centre: The 'Veronica' Mercedes Benz Mobile Phaco Unit leaving Trottsford at the start of the journey to India - September 2000

Bottom: The last major fundraising event for the MMBEU. Veronica Arnott and Lyn Wood, with Lieutenant Liam Byrd and sea cadets on HMS President, London - July 2000

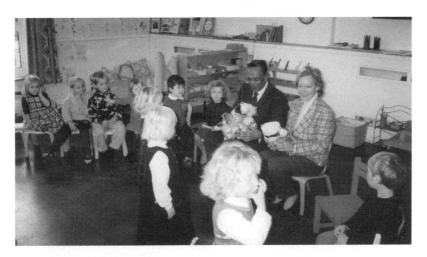

Top: Veronica collecting teddy bears from local schoolchildren to give to Professor Indira Bhargava for our adopted village in India at Kingsley School, Hampshire - November 1999

Centre: The last tug of war in aid of the Penny Trust MBMEU, Halzephron Inn, Gunwalloe - July 2000

Bottom: Family photograph taken at the wedding of Robert Arnott to Kate Ward. (From left to right) Isabella, Stephen, Veronica and Oliver Arnott. Robert and Kate. Lara Arnott. Nick, Timothy, Telisa, Tania and Natasha Whishaw, me and Kathy Arnott in Cootamundra, Australia - April 2000

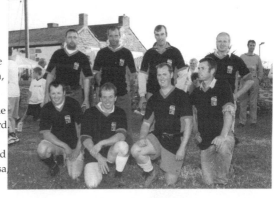

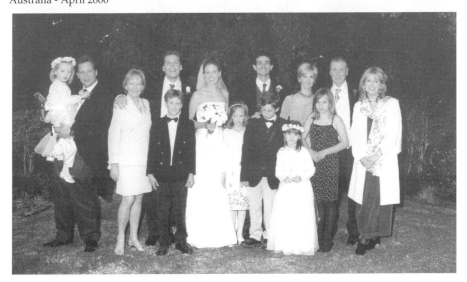

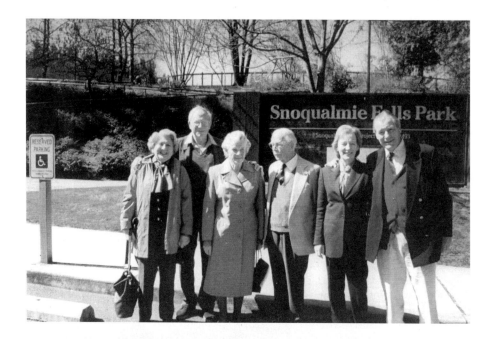

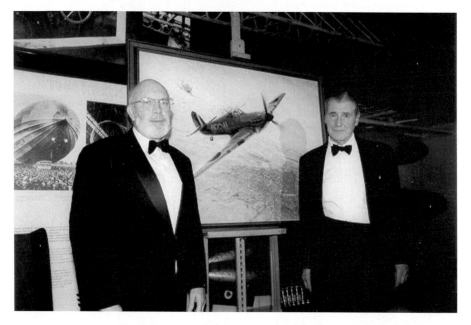

Top: Harold Ridley, the inventor of the lens implant, with Diana and Peter Choyce, and his wife Elisabeth with Veronica and me, last of the early British implant pioneers - Washington, US, 1999

Bottom: John Howard Worsley, the artist, presenting the painting of 'One flew up the clock', which depicted an incident in the Battle of Britain that prompted the beginning of intraocular lens implants. The occasion was the banquet for Sir Harold Ridley to celebrate the 50th anniversary of this invention at the Science Museum, London - November 1999

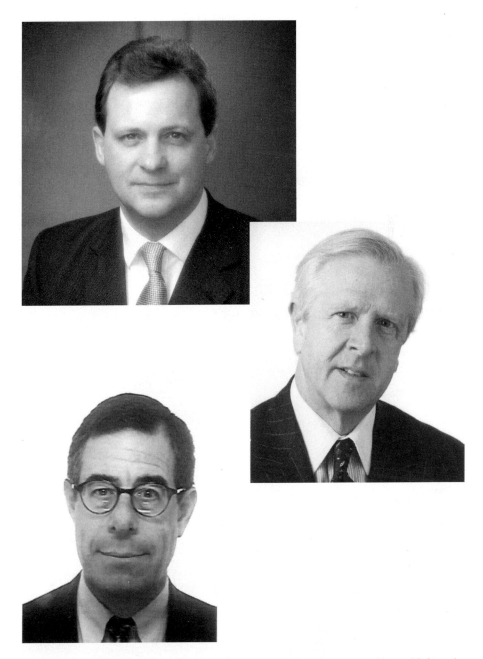

Top: Stephen Arnott, who partnered with me for 15 years and was instrumental in establishing the Arnott Eye Centre and the development of our lens implant designs

Centre: Our good friend and American attorney Bradley G Geist, who successfully defended, with Stephen, our patent rights, against stiff resistance from major multinational pharmaceutical companies

Bottom: Mr Richard Packard, FRCS, who took over Arnott Eye Associates and is a leading international phaco and lens implant surgeon

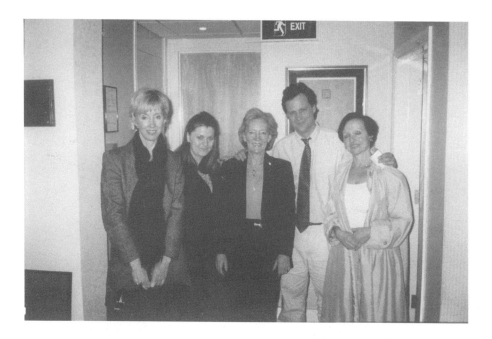

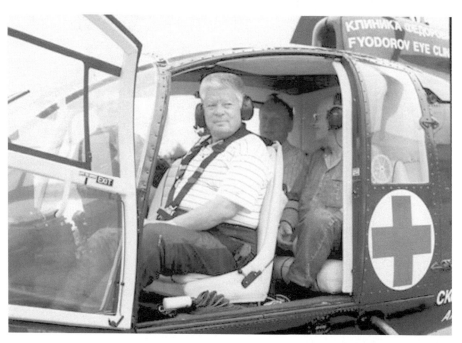

Top: We say farewell to our staff (from left to right) Joy Andrews, Clare Ruocco, Veronica and Stephen Arnott, Hazel Saunders at 22a Harley Street, London, 1999

Bottom: Svyatoslav's final flight (courtesy of Leo Boris) - Russia, June 2000

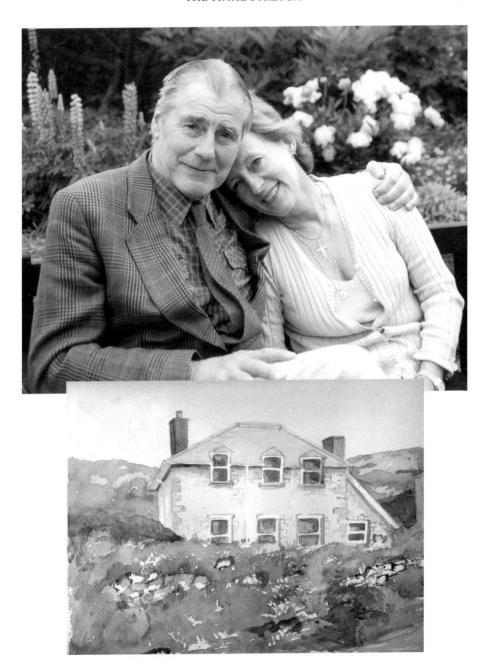

Top: Veronica and me on my 70th birthday - Trottsford, June 1999

Bottom: Watercolour, by Susie Cattley, of the cottage overlooking the Atlantic Ocean in Mounts Bay, which we bought for our retirement and where the hopes for our future became the dreams of the past - Tripolitania, Porthleven, Cornwall, July 2001

Part Nine. Journey's end

CHAPTER 38
Thanksgiving to Svyatoslav, and Veronica's fight

On a Saturday morning, in the first week of June 2000, Svyatoslav Fyodorov made a routine visit to one of his ophthalmic clinics, some 200 kilometres from Moscow. Before climbing into his helicopter for the return trip home, he gave an interview to the local TV news. Standing on the steps of his hospital, he discussed its future, as well as dwelling on the general political situation in Russia. The helicopter was being flown by a pilot, with Svyatoslav and an engineer sitting in the rear. As they approached the suburbs of Moscow, the rear rotor blade fell off and the helicopter violently swayed from side to side as it started to descend. In an effort to lose ballast, the entire luggage was thrown overboard, including a cake that Svyatoslav was bringing back to Irine for their wedding anniversary that weekend. Having almost made the safety of a field, the helicopter clipped a tree, causing it to turn turtle and crash heavily into the ground by the side of a road. Irine Fyodorov heard about the tragedy on the one o'clock Russian television news.

The following morning, after church, we received an unexpected telephone call from Harold Ridley, who had always hated using the phone. In a frail voice, filled with emotion, he told us the news. George Milford-Haven also rang us up, distressed that the helicopter he had indirectly supplied should have been involved in this accident. He told us that this must have been its first flight of the year after winter storage in a hangar. Veronica and I had been with Slava for the last flight from Moscow to Slavino the previous year. Svyatoslav's next flight would be his last.

Veronica and I were mortified on hearing the news and immediately contacted Irine, who did not want us to attend the funeral but asked us to come to the service on the fortieth day, which is when, according to the Russian Orthodox Church, the soul ascends to heaven. We had lost a great Russian friend, who had embodied all the sentiments and feelings of Veronica's ancestors. He typified his people, with his rather square angulated face topped by closely cropped hair, which over the years had changed from black to grey. Like Veronica's own father, he had a strong dominating character and a very warm, affectionate and gentle personality. They had both been true patriots and shared the loss of what their country had once been. Veronica saw in Svyatoslav the same ideals and values of honesty, love and dependability that had been instilled during their upbringing in a turbulent country. In truth, Veronica saw in Svyatoslav a younger image of her own Russian father, Arvid. Bonded in this relationship was the total devotion of Irine to Svyatoslav and Veronica to myself.

At Slavino, we found Irine sitting on the balcony with only the husband of her housekeeper and her own daughter, Elena, for company. She was in an abject state of grief and despondency. We sat silently with her, while the darkness of the night encompassed us, until summoned for dinner.

The following morning we had a hair-raising drive to the crash site. Irine had misjudged the time, and we left the dacha much too late for a ceremony that had been planned. In our chauffeur-driven Mercedes, we hurtled along the Russian roads weaving around traffic, going from one side of the road to the other. Travelling at more than 100 miles an hour, we came out of a corner to find a stationary line of cars ahead of us. I sat mesmerized in the front passenger seat, as we prepared ourselves for a pile-up. At the last moment, a gap appeared in the oncoming cars, and we swerved to safety on the other side of the road. Veronica had been sitting over the rear axle of the car, wedged in her seat between Irine and Elena. At the end of the journey she was visibly distressed and complaining of severe stomach pain.

The press and a large crowd had arrived to witness Irine Fyodorov lay the foundation stone for the construction of a chapel to be built on the exact site of the helicopter crash. We made a more leisurely return to the dacha for mass in the Church of the Nativity of Our Lady in Slavino. Following this service, there was a reception in the congress centre of the complex, the windows of which were wide open for the easier release of Svyatoslav's soul to a better abode.

Irine was seated among many dozens of guests, which included the elite of Russian society. Alexander Solzhenitsyn, the writer of many novels including *Cancer Ward*, and one of the first Sputnik cosmonauts were there, along with numerous politicians, scientists, surgeons and theatrical personalities.

Veronica and I were sitting to the left of Irine, with her daughter Elena and grandson, Slava. The director of Moscow Television gave the first address, with a long incantation in Russian extolling the virtues of Svyatoslav and wishing him well on his trip to paradise. For some minutes after this speech, we all quietly sat in our chairs, appreciating the importance of the open windows. The spell was broken when Irine, in a loud voice said: 'Eric, as you and Veronica are our overseas guests, would you please say something about my husband.' We were taken by surprise, as we had not expected that a foreigner would be asked to speak in this almost totally Russian gathering. I rose from my chair and, via a Russian interpreter, recalled many of the happy and memorable times Veronica and I had shared with this 'giant' of a man and his wife.

We left Russia with sadness, having lost not only one of our greatest friends but, of subsidiary importance, our place in the participation of everyday Russian life. We also realized that this was the end of our hopes for the Gibraltar Eye Institute. Only three days before the helicopter crash, Svyatoslav had telephoned, saying: 'V-e-r-o-n-i-c-a, we are only a matter of two weeks away from the final contract of our Fyodorov-Arnott Apple unit.'

We accepted Angela Thompson's invitation to stay with her in Cornwall. In mid-July, two of our grand-children, Oliver Arnott and Timothy Whishaw, joined us for this short holiday in Cornwall, which was very special for us. Leaving our home, Trottsford, in the early morning, we had a picnic lunch beside a country lane in Wiltshire before staying the night with Veronica's aunt, Hester Cattley, and her cousin Susie and friend, Di Stockwell. Veronica had always enjoyed the company of these relatives and their part of the country. That evening we took Oliver and Timmy to Wonwell Estuary and sat by the ebbing channel of the river, while they explored the smoked fish kiln, salmon pool and creeks that we had discovered so many years before.

Angela Thomas had organized the 'tug-of-war championship' at her Halzephron Inn. The local team, who had last supported this event some 20 years earlier, was fully mustered for the occasion, as were many others from the neighbourhood. The contest took place in a field behind the inn, and hundreds of the locals from Gunwalloe and the neighbouring villages turned up for the spectacle.

Royal Naval Air Station Culdrose, the local naval helicopter base, was most supportive, and the commodore joined us for the evening, as did Reverend Mike Brotherton, the naval chaplain. Their base produced a helicopter that hovered over the event with the flag of St George suspended under its fuselage. Drinks for the evening were 'on the house', and, as a result of this, few funds were actually raised for our charity. Nevertheless, the event was a great success, and everyone hoped that this would help to revive this ancient Cornish sport.

We enjoyed this area and the company of the locals so much that we thought it might be an idea to invest in a small property in Porthleven for our retirement. On Sunday morning, before going to the naval base at Culdrose for Mike Brotherton's service, we stood on the quayside of Porthleven, taking in the beauty of this little port. At the entrance to the harbour was a neo-Gothic building with a clock tower that resembled a church but was in fact the library. Extending from this famous landmark and lining the hill was a terraced row of Victorian houses all painted in different colours. Higher up the hill was an old convent with a large cross on its turreted front wall. Directly opposite us was the Harbour Inn, unchanged from the days when this port had a thriving shipbuilding industry. In the harbour were a number of Cornish fishing boats, carrying out a trade that had not, as yet, totally vanished in this remote part of the country. The four of us looked at these surroundings, wondering where we might fit in with this community.

Later that summer, Veronica and I had planned to take a cruise in the Baltic with Tom and Cline Kilner. Tom had been at school with me, and Cline had shared a flat with Veronica in their premarital days. Veronica was so looking forward to this cruise, which would include visiting cities associated with the lives of her grandparents. In Riga, we hoped to visit the Russian embassy, which had once been their family home.

Veronica had, for some months, been suffering from a distended abdomen, and we decided to seek medical advice before taking this holiday. We consulted a physician in the Cromwell Hospital, a long-standing colleague, who found that Veronica's liver was very enlarged and her liver function tests were grossly abnormal. Because of our frequent trips to Russia, he wondered if Veronica had picked up Legionnaires' disease, but, as a precaution before starting antibiotic therapy, he wished her to have a liver scan.

Veronica and I were still treating her condition with some nonchalance and, on the day of the liver scan, I took one of our grandchildren for a sailing lesson in Bosham while Veronica drove to the Cromwell Hospital. Stephen held her hand during the scan. During the next few minutes, our world changed forever. Veronica rang me at Trottsford saying: 'All is not well. In the middle of the scan, the radiologist rushed from the room to contact my physician. There is a big problem.' We returned the following week to reconsult our physician, who said there were tumours involving both lobes of the liver and a biopsy was required. Thus started the constant trek, to and fro, from hospital to hospital.

The liver biopsy was carried out at the Lister Hospital. I felt helpless at taking Veronica to have tests performed, and seeing her worried and suffering without being able to do anything to help. We could however share the mental anguish, which is the inevitable accompaniment to this situation. A few days later we got the phone call confirming that Veronica had cancer in both lobes of her liver. Dazed and bewildered, I looked at my beautiful wife, who looked so well, and could not believe that this was happening to us. Was this all a bad dream, from which we would soon awake? After some minutes of feeling numb, I realized we had to be progressive and fight back with everything at our disposal. From now on despondency must go, and we would only have hope for what may lie ahead.

The rest of that Saturday was spent making calls all around the world, to Scandinavia, Russia and hospitals around the UK. All this international exploring ended up with us booking a PET scan at our own hospital, the Cromwell, which would determine the site of the primary tumour and if it had spread to any other part of the body. This scan confirmed involvement of the liver, but no sign of any primary lesion or other secondary.

Feeling a little heartened by this result we made an appointment to see Professor Cunningham, a renowned oncologist, at the Sutton branch of the Royal Marsden Hospital. Over the months this would become almost a second home. Despite the 'doom and gloom' surrounding the patients, the staff of the hospital, with their informal and cheerful attitude, did much to allay the fears of their patients.

David Cunningham confirmed the diagnosis of secondaries of the liver, probably from the local biliary system, but wished to defer treatment until after the approaching August bank holiday weekend.

'Can we go away for the weekend?' I asked.

'I do not advise you to travel far, but a weekend in Brighton would do you no harm. Where are you planning to go?' asked the Professor.

'To India,' replied Veronica.

This Veronica, Tania and I did. With no expense spared, we took three first-class tickets to Mumbai and from thence travelled on to Puttaparthy to see Sai Baba. Our whole life was radically changing. The former top international ophthalmic surgeon, coming with his proud wife to teach in the hospital, was now returning to humbly seek help. During one of Sai Baba's walks around the Ashram, he went up to Veronica and placed his hand on her liver. Veronica felt immediate relief and from then on the liver played little part in the ever-changing scenario of our future. On our return, our physicians were amazed at the improvement they could see.

During that autumn we enjoyed an 'Indian summer' and were able to carry on an almost normal life. In early September, I was scheduled to give the Medal Lecture at the Annual International Intraocular Implant Club meeting, to be held in Belgium, by the invitation of the President, Dr Douglas Koch. Veronica and I flew to Brussels where, on leaving the airport, we were mugged at the taxi stand and relieved of my travel bag, which contained our passports, travel documents and cash. Worst of all, my diary for 2000, which I have written every night since 1949, was also taken.

Veronica and I had a golden weekend in Brussels. For many months, Veronica had helped me prepare this paper, with the assistance of David King of the Carlin Company, a film producer, working with ASCRS. David Rowswell, who was supplying the lens implants for my cataract surgery, was partially sponsoring my paper. Before the meeting we watched as all our older colleagues and their younger counterparts walked across the lobby into the congress hall.

That evening I gave the most important lecture of my life to the dozens of foremost international ophthalmologists who had followed the lead of the original pioneers and were now the mainstay of world cataract and lens-implant surgery. The evening started with the IIIC society dinner, throughout which, on Veronica's orders, I did not touch a single alcoholic drink.

The theme of my PowerPoint presentation was 'A Tale of Three Cities', in which I elaborated on the debt we owed to Harold Ridley in London, Charlie Kelman in New York and Svyatoslav Fyodorov in Moscow. Going down memory lane, the 'Hurricane' plane with the PMMA plastic canopy was shown, along with the original phaco unit, which looked like a large tea trolley. Finally, the site of Svyatoslav's helicopter crash appeared on the screen. This address was given to the world's foremost ophthalmic surgeons, who had been instrumental in fusing these three fragments of ophthalmic history into the surgery of the moment.

As I spoke, I was moved by the looks of concentration etched on the faces of the audience and the rapt glow of love and pride on Veronica's face. At the end of my address there was a moment of silence before Gerry Freeman stood up and clapped. We ended our ophthalmic career with a standing ovation from the senior members of our vocation.

A few days after this meeting in Brussels, on 14 September 2000, we held a farewell service at Trottsford Farm, before the departure of our unit to India. At this time, there was a fuel strike in the country, and, with a few exceptions, only our local friends made the event. These exceptions were John Grindle and the Major – both of whom had been extremely supportive ophthalmic colleagues over the years. Our local choir attended in clerical gowns, and the Reverend Peter Bradford conducted a communion and farewell service. Our mobile eye unit was placed some 10 yards in front of a marquee put up for our guests.

After communion, Peter Bradford blessed the unit. Christians, Hindus, Muslims and Jews alike all partook of the bread and wine. The major draped a garland of flowers over the altar cross, at the rear entrance of the truck, as a symbol of religious unity. Our mobile eye unit was finally driven across the lawn and out through the gates of our home to the accompaniment of the hymn *Thou whose almighty word...let there be light*. There was not a single dry eye in the congregation. As a thank you for all their hard work, Veronica gave Tony Spooner and Lyn Wood a Waterford cut-glass eagle.

This felt like our final commitment to ophthalmology, and we now had time to centre on our family. Despite Veronica's illness, we enjoyed one of the most perfect periods of our life. For some weeks we were allowed a respite, when she seemed to be in almost perfect health. We enjoyed trips to Cornwall, where we found our 'dream' cottage, overlooking the cliffs in Porthleven. We employed David and Phil Winn as builders, and Veronica enjoyed ringing David up on a weekly basis, planning the reconstruction of this house, which became almost a hobby. Working together on our little home helped us to dispel any fears for the future.

Veronica was determined to carry on as normal. She continued to do Pilates classes with our daughter, Tania, and we had a modest social life. We attended the wedding of Veronica's goddaughter, Cheska Wood, and the reception in Pavilion Road. We sat on two chairs while the guests milled around us, with the occasional one bending down to talk to us. On another occasion we went to the Oyster Bar at Selfridges, where we were entertained by the jokes of Jack Berger, one of my patients, who happened to be lunching there with his wife, Su-Su.

Problems started towards the end of the year, when it was advised that Veronica should have a colonoscopy. This rather unpleasant examination caused her excruciating pain and had a very deleterious effect. In November of 2000, David Cunningham decided to put Veronica on chemotherapy, at a time when there were signs of jaundice. Unknown to us, Stephen had researched Veronica's condition and had advised Tania and Robert that their mother's symptoms gave a prognosis of only a few months. Thus, to coincide with our 40th wedding anniversary, they treated us to a week at Hartwell House Hotel near Aylesbury, where King Louis XVIII had held court while in exile. Veronica and I were given the Royal Suite, and we spent the next few days exclusively in the company of our children, enjoying a very pleasant holiday together – not knowing that this was meant to be a farewell party. On one day we visited Veronica's old school, the Arts Educational School in Tring, where we sat watching a class being given by her old teacher, Eve Pettinger. Eve afterwards showed us around the premises, which had hardly changed since Veronica's time in the school.

On Christmas Eve, the Reverend Peter Bradford came to Trottsford and gave a communion service for our children and grandchildren. Veronica wanted to give very personal thanks to her loving and supportive family: to Stephen she gave a bronze violinist, to Tania a necklace and to Bob a silver carriage alarm clock. Veronica presented me with a Napoleon-hat handmade mahogany clock for the mantelpiece in Tripolitania, our Cornish house overlooking Mounts Bay. Throughout this serious ceremony, which so expressed the sincere inner feelings of Veronica, there was the banter of laughter and fun in a family that had always been so totally united.

By the start of the year 2001, the storm clouds were beginning to accumulate over us. Veronica was starting to have signs of breathing problems, which were exacerbated by the failure of our Aga cooker at Trottsford, which was emitting toxic fumes. We had to abandon our farmhouse for many weeks and spent this time in our little maisonette in Chancellor's Wharf, London. Here we spent our 'sunset', living day by day.

As over the previous years, we would start the day with prayers and readings from the *Bible* and Sai Baba, lying on our bed overlooking the beauty of the River Thames. While having our early morning tea, we would discuss the happenings of our family and friends before embarking on our duties of the day. These were now seriously curtailed, with my retirement and Veronica's incapacity. We had much time to be together, unencumbered by other distractions, and it was possible to be united in the fulfilment of our partnership of over 40 years. On one occasion, Veronica said to me: 'No matter how close we can be together, I cannot merge into your body. We are two separate individuals and no matter what we wish, we cannot be one.' In that one thought, Veronica had expressed the vulnerability of our position.

There were times when sunshine seeped through a gap in the clouds. We went to the Chelsea Flower Show and debated building a conservatory at Trottsford. Walking through the tents, we admired a stall full of agapanthus, Veronica's favourite flower. We ambled through the rose gardens and stopped to admire the roses on the Harkness stand. One year later, this company would be displaying the Veronica Arnott – a bush rose with clumps of pale yellow, highly scented flowers, which was named in her memory. Having done more walking than on any other day over the previous months, Veronica was feeling rather tired as we made our way towards the exit. We passed a tent that was a champagne bar, and as there was an empty table by the entrance we could not resist taking it. A pretty waitress brought us a half bottle of Moët & Chandon, and we relaxed enjoying our drink while watching the crowds go by.

On going to the snack bar for a sandwich, I saw a long queue stretching into the distance. Realizing that we had gatecrashed further increased the pleasure of our champagne.

For my birthday in June 2000, Veronica, Stephen and I went to Budock Vean – a country-house hotel overlooking the Helford Estuary. Veronica coped well with the long journey down to Cornwall and was well enough to enjoy the birthday party in our bedroom. Veronica gave me a pool table, which we would place in the summerhouse in Tripolitania. The following day we drove over to our new home, which was almost finished. David Winn and his builders were there, which gave us an excuse for a house-warming party. Stephen had spent all of the previous night by himself in Tripolitania, hurriedly hanging pictures and arranging the furniture. We were all but ready to move into our retirement retreat, where, having recently bought a new paint box, Veronica could paint the local landscapes, while I hoped to do some writing.

Veronica's breathing became progressively more laboured, and in early July she had to be admitted as an emergency to Mount Alvernia Hospital in Guildford. As Stephen and I drove her from Trottsford, we little realized it would be for the last time. I stayed the night on a camp bed next to her. All was well until, at midnight, the patient in the next room fell out of bed with a crash, which must have woken up the whole ward. From then onwards it was a downhill struggle. As Veronica was feeling breathless and rather panicky, I sat by her bedside for hours holding her hands. We didn't speak, but our eyes and hands said everything about the absolute love and devotion we had always given to each other.

At six o'clock in the morning, the night sister came into the bedroom and gently tried to help Veronica sit up, but she immediately collapsed. Efforts were made to revive her, but to no avail. I sat in the hallway of the ward, waiting for Stephen, Tania and Robert, knowing that I had reached rock bottom. We later went into Veronica's bedroom and gently removed her Russian Cross, Sai Baba's emblem and her engagement ring.

Some months earlier, while Veronica and I had been watching a television play in bed, she had said: 'If I don't make it, I would like the same service as my brother Charles in St George's Hanover Square, conducted by Mike Brotherton, Jim Hawthorn and Peter Bradford.'

'Don't be silly,' I had retorted. 'I never want you to talk like that again.'

Veronica's wishes were carried out, and the church was filled to capacity. Charlie Kelman's wife, Ann, and Bradley Geist flew over from America and sat with us during the service. Miranda Cordle, who had been so helpful throughout Veronica's illness by reading the *Bible* to her, although herself dying, sat with us in a wheelchair.

As those who have suffered a similar loss will know it is impossible to even start to express one's feelings, which are maybe best kept to oneself. I know however, with the strongest conviction possible, that Veronica's presence is always near at hand. In the weeks that followed the 3rd of July, I found in the books that Veronica had read multiple passages with ink markings in the margin, expressing so visibly her thinking. Emphasized were the needs for faith to be backed up by deeds and tribulation to be met with perseverance. Veronica was very aware of the temporary nature of the body, loaned for life to act as an expression and outward manifestation of the soul, which is everlasting.

This account of the life that Veronica and I enjoyed together is being completed, as I sit at my desk, in our house overlooking the sea in Mounts Bay on the southwest tip of England. Up the coast is Land's End and to the south the Lizard. Behind me lies the whole land mass of our country, and this could act as an analogy of our lives. The hills and mountains represent the high and happy times and the valleys the low points. Each city, town and village equates to all the incidents that occurred – some of great importance, some trivial. The inhabitants are all the people who were associated with us during our journey. Many hopefully were helped, and if any were wronged, it was inadvertent.

In front of me is the Atlantic Ocean, stretching thousands of miles into the distance. Every day it changes. A grey sky may merge into an equally murky sea. The Atlantic may be tumultuous, with angry waves pounding into the cliff a few yards in front of this house, throwing up spray that looks like rain on our window panes. There may be a flat calm, with the horizon separating the darker blue of the sea from the lighter azure of the sky above. At all times, the sea and sky reflect the majestic mystery of the creation and are symbolic of eternity. Somewhere out there beyond our gaze, there must be 'a new beginning in sight'.

POSTSCRIPT

After 3 July 2001, the day that I lost Veronica, the next three years were spent recording from my diaries of the previous decades the wonderful partnership I had enjoyed with my wife and the exceptional circumstances in which I associated with the inventors and pioneers of modern ophthalmic surgery.

The Royal Horticultural Society named a new variety of rose the Veronica Arnott, which, produced by Harkness Roses, was previewed at the Chelsea Flower Show in May 2002. The Diocese of Winchester Cathedral allowed the commissioning of a stained-glass window for her family in St Mary's Church, East Worldham.

The first eye camp in India, using the Penny Trust Mercedes Benz Mobile Eye Unit, was held in the Province of Madhya Pradesh in July 2003. At the inaugural ceremony held in the Hall of Indore University, the chief minister, Mr Digvijay Singh, named the unit 'Veronica', and it was then driven some 300 km to Aron, a small village in the heart of Bengal Tiger Country.

In the UK during this time we lost Sir Harold Ridley. The memorial service was in the chapel of his beloved St Thomas', within which hospital he had perfected so many of his achievements. His most ardent follower, Peter Choyce, also died. Charlie Kelman has also left us. His wife Ann arranged a celebration of his life in St James Theatre on Broadway. I spoke on this occasion about his major contribution to ophthalmology. Posthumously, Charlie has been awarded the Albert Lasker Medical Research Award, one of the biggest honours the US can give. Robert Sinskey, still very active, has been honoured by entering the ASCRS hall of fame.

Personal changes have occurred. Our older son Stephen has set up a company with his old school friend, Sam Jones, providing business solutions for the insurance sector. Our daughter Tania, with her family, has moved into Trottsford Farm, the scene of so many of our memorable times. Robert is now a city broker, and, with his wife Kate, they have introduced two more members to our family, Oscar and Elke.

Nearly two and a half years after I lost Veronica, I was travelling to India again; feeling rather lost without her company, although I did have the companionship of the Major. Having travelled to Madhya Pradesh, there was a ceremony in which the Maharajah blessed the unit and called it the Veronica Arnott Unit. This was a nostalgic moment for me being in the same theatre that I had received my degree some years before. I so remember the abiding presence of Veronica on that day with tears in her eyes, full of emotion. Following this ceremony, our cortege made its way into the hinterland in the Maharajah's personal helicopter. At one point, the Maharajah, full of excitement, gesticulated and pointed out where he had shot his first tiger. In our party were Bharat Chhaparwal, the vice chancellor, whose department was looking after the unit, and the Major. When we reached our destination, the helicopter circled over the Maharajah's palace and in the foreground could be seen our pink unit snuggling below the heights of the fortress.

After the ceremony, one had a sense of total unreality, stepping from the outside into the air-conditioned Veronica Arnott Unit, which was state of the art. Inside the unit were two Indian surgeons and their assistants performing phaco surgery. The walls of the theatre were just like those of any London teaching hospital and had in fact been copied from the Wellington Hospital.

At the presentation, we received a plaque commemorating the occasion, which Nils Burwitz has shown in the illustration on page 299.

So life carries on. After fulfilment and happiness, inevitably there come times of sorrow, which are followed by, yet again, a new start.

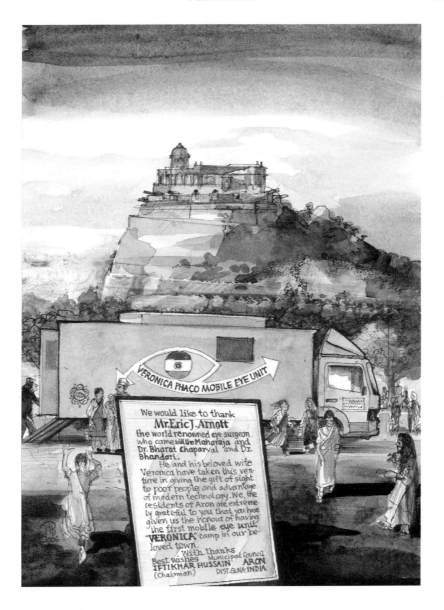

Index